Non-Hodgkin's Lymphomas

Edited by

P. Solal-Céligny
Hôpital St-Louis, Paris, France

F. Reyes
Hôpital H.-Mondor, Créteil, France

N. Brousse
Hôpital Necker, Paris, France

C. Gisselbrecht
Hôpital St-Louis, Paris, France

B. Coiffier
Centre hospitalier Lyon-Sud, Pierre-Bénite, France

With contributions by

C. BAYLE, S. BELAÏCH, A. BOSLY, N. CERF-BENSUSSAN, J.-M. COSSET, C. DARNE,
J.M. DIVINE, J.-P. FARCET, G. FLANDRIN, A. FOURMESTRAUX-RUSKONE, A. GALIAN,
G. GANEM, Ph. GAULARD, J.-L. LEBAIL-DARNE, A. JARRY, J. LECLERC, C. PATTE,
M. PEUCHMAUR, J.-C. RAMBAUD, J.-Y. SCOAZEC, M. SIGAL-NAHUM, M. SYMANN

MANSON PUBLISHING Ltd
London

ÉDITIONS FRISON-ROCHE
Paris

This book is published with the help of the French Ministry of Culture and Communication

Published by Manson Publishing Ltd in association with Editions Frison-Roche, 18 rue Dauphine, 75006 Paris, France

© Editions Frison-Roche, Paris, 1993, ISBN 2-87671-068-4

A CIP catalogue record for this book is available from the British Library.

For full details of all Manson Publishing's titles, please write to: Manson Publishing Ltd, 73 Corringham Road, London NW11 7DL, UK.

ISBN 2-874545-07-3

CONTENTS

Part 4. EXTRA-NODAL NON-HODGKIN'S LYMPHOMAS
Edited by P. Solal-Céligny, N. Brousse

Part 5. TREATMENT OF NON-HODGKIN'S LYMPHOMAS
Edited by C. Gisselbrecht, B. Coiffier

Acknowledgements

The authors gratefully acknowledge the helpful and patient secretarial assistance provided by S. Larnier and V. Ribondin and permission by Laboratoires Roger Bellon to reproduce figures from the first edition of *Lymphomes malins non hodgkiniens* (1986).

LIST OF CONTRIBUTORS

C. BAYLE, M.D.
Service de cytologie, Institut G. Roussy, Villejuif, France.
Prof. S. BELAÏCH
Service de dermatologie, Hôpital Bichat, Paris, France.
A. BOSLY, M.D.
Département d'hématologie, Centre Universitaire Mont-Godinne, Yvoir, Belgium.
Prof. N. BROUSSE
Service d'anatomie et de cytologie pathologiques, Hôpital Necker-Enfants Malades, Paris, France.
Prof. B. COIFFIER
Service d'hématologie, Centre Hospitalier Lyon-Sud, Pierre-Bénite, France.
Prof. J.M. COSSET
Département de radiothérapie, Institut Curie, Paris, France.
C. DARNE
M. DIVINE, M.D.
Service d'hématologie clinique, Hôpital H. Mondor, Créteil, France.
J.-P. FARCET, M.D.
Service d'hématologie clinique, Hôpital H. Mondor, Créteil, France.
Prof. G. FLANDRIN
Laboratoire central d'hématologie, Hôpital Necker-Enfants Malades, Paris, France.
A. FOURMESTRAUX-RUSKONE, M.D.
Service de médecine interne, Hôtel-Dieu, Paris, France.
Prof. A. GALIAN
Service d'anatomie pathologique, Hôpital Lariboisière, Paris, France.
G. GANEM, M.D.
Centre d'onco-radiothérapie et d'hématologie V. Hugo, Le Mans, France.
P. GAULARD, M.D.
Service d'anatomie pathologique, Hôpital H. Mondor, Créteil, France.
Prof. C. GISSELBRECHT
Département d'hématologie, Hôpital Saint-Louis, Paris, France.
A. JARRY, Ph.D.
INSERM U 239, Faculté X. Bichat, Paris, France.
J.-L. LEBAIL DARNE
J. LECLERC, M.D.
Service d'imagerie médicale, Institut G. Roussy, Villejuif, France.
C. PATTE, M.D.
Service de pédiatrie, Institut G. Roussy, Villejuif, France.
M. PEUCHMAUR, M.D.
Service d'anatomie pathologique, Hôpital Necker-Enfants Malades, Paris, France.
Prof. J.-C. RAMBAUD
Service de gastro-entérologie, Hôpital Saint-Lazare, Paris, France.
Prof. F. REYES
Service d'hématologie clinique, Hôpital H. Mondor, Créteil, France.
J.-Y. SCOAZEC, M.D.
Laboratoire de biologie cellulaire, Faculté X. Bichat, Paris, France.
M. SIGAL-NAHUM, M.D.
Service de dermatologie, Centre Hospitalier d'Argenteuil, France.
P. SOLAL-CÉLIGNY, M.D.
Département d'hématologie, Hôpital Saint-Louis, Paris, France.
Prof. M. SYMANN
Clinique Saint-Luc, Bruxelles, Belgium.

Foreword

Human lymphomas have become a topic of great interest in recent years, both because of a dramatic increase in our understanding of the different lymphoid cell types which give rise to these tumours, and also because modern modes of treatment, involving surgery, radiotherapy and chemotherapy and, more recently, marrow transplantation, have improved the overall prognosis to a greater extent than in many other malignant diseases. Lymphomas also provide a very fruitful source of insight into the role of oncogenes in cell physiology. For example, the bcl-2 gene product, which appears to play a previously undetected role as an inhibitor of apoptosis (*programmed cell death*) in the lymphoid system, was identified as a direct consequence of studying the 14;18 translocation in follicular lymphoma.

Continued improvement in the clinical management of non-Hodgkin's lymphomas is dependent on a close collaboration between pathologists and basic scientists on the one hand and oncologists on the other, but unfortunately the two groups have not always joined forces in the most effective manner. There is a tendency among pathologists to be distracted by the elusive goal of a perfect classification scheme for lymphomas and for clinicians to respond to the pathologist's complex and contradictory systems by paying too little attention to some of the clinically relevant insights which have emerged from more scientifically directed analysis of lymphoid tissue biopsies.

The joint international effort which culminated in the *Working Formulation* aimed at resolving the problem of divergence between pathology and clinical medicine and generating a new common language which could be used by both groups to describe cases of lymphoma, and which would give due attention to prognostic indicators. This exercise was successful in that many pathologists and clinicians now use the Working Formulation in their routine practice. However, the inherent divergence of interest between pathologists and clinicians in the field of lymphomas remains and a continued effort is needed to sustain the spirit of the Working Formulation project. The present book is written very much with a sense of this importance of making clinico-pathological correlations. The authors include both clinicians and pathologists, and their partnership as authors of this book reflects their professional collaboration and the views which they have developed as a result of discussing clinical problems together.

One important feature of the book, which is found in relatively few publications on lymphomas, is the emphasis on non-Hodgkin's lymphomas in tissues other than the lymph node (for example in the central nervous system, in the spleen and in bone). This section of the book also covers lymphomas involving the gut, a type of lymphoma which in recent years has been of considerable interest both to pathologists and clinicians, and which promises to provide valuable new insight in the future into the physiology of the gut-associated lymphoid system.

In conclusion, this book provides a highly coherent clinico-pathologically based view of lymphomas which offers new insights into this group of diseases for medical practitioners at all stages of development from the immature ("pre-B cell") resident stage to the fully committed (and possibly over-committed!) *"chef de service"*. As they say : *Read! Enjoy!*

D. MASON

Preface

P. SOLAL-CÉLIGNY, N. BROUSSE

No generally accepted definition - both sufficiently general and meaningfully specific - of non-Hodgkin's lymphomas (NHL) can at present be proposed. They can be described as malignant lymphoid proliferations, which is a simple and practical definition. But the denomination of malignant and lymphoid only partially characterizes NHL.

First, a diagnosis of malignancy is applied to clonal proliferations (i.e. arising from a single cell) with a progressive clinical course. In almost all cases, immunocytological and molecular studies have confirmed the monoclonality of NHL. But the clinical course varies considerably from case to case. In some cases, the course is very indolent and spontaneous remissions although very exceptional in other neoplastic diseases - have been reported in numerous cases of NHL.

Immunohistochemical and molecular studies have confirmed the lymphoid origin of almost all histological types of NHL; in particular, so-called histiocytic lymphomas in the Rappaport classification are in fact of lymphoid origin.

Nevertheless, this definition appears too general. First, it includes lymphocytic leukaemias - either acute or chronic - which are not usually considered as NHL and which will not be detailed herein.

The nosology of NHL is also ill-defined and changing with time. In particular, modifications from immunological and molecular studies show that disorders of unknown nosology are in fact lymphoid monoclonal proliferations which must be considered as NHL. The same is true of granulomatous disorders (lymphomatoid granulomatosis, lethal midline granuloma) and digestive or skin diseases (pseudolymphomas, lymphomatoid papulosis). The boundaries of the entire NHL group are ill-defined since a number of clinical forms of NHL display all the characteristics of other disorders *(fig. 1)*, and the choice of diagnosis is often arbitrary. Distinguishing between them is sometimes a controversial topic but often has little bearing on therapeutic choices.

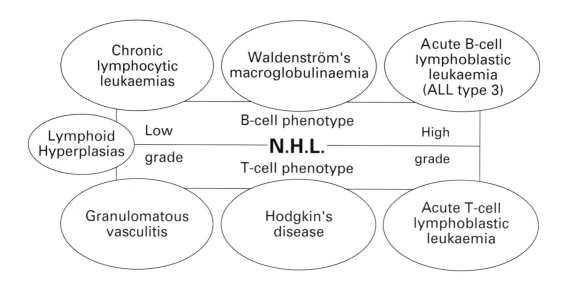

Fig. 1: Schematic diagram showing overlapping between non-Hodgkin's lymphomas and other disorders

1.

LYMPHOMAGENESIS

edited by

F. REYES

Lymphocyte Differentiation

F. REYES

Lymphocytes are haemopoietic cells that express polymorphic, clonotypically distributed antigen-specific receptors. Two main molecular types of receptor exist: the membrane immunoglobulin (mIg) of B lymphocytes and the T-cell receptor (TCR) of T the chains that constitute such antigen-receptors result in their expression at the membrane of the cell. This chapter focuses on several characteristics of lymphocyte differentiation that are relevant to the understanding and investigation of immunoproliferative disorders.

Studies of lymphocyte differentiation have been greatly facilitated by the availability of monoclonal antibodies (mAbs) and the development of molecular genetic techniques. These tools have defined, better than the morphological and cytochemical approaches, the various steps of the differentiation and the functional heterogeneity of lymphocytes. Thus several mAbs identify a panel of antigens expressed by T cells, but not by B cells or other haemopoietic lineages: such antigens are T-cell differentiation markers. Other antigens expressed only by B lymphocytes are considered as B-cell markers. Within T and B lineages, some antigens will be expressed only at early differentiation steps and disappear later when cells mature: such antigens serve as maturation markers. Activation markers are those determinants which appear during the cell cycle in relation to the proliferation process. Complementary DNA probes are now available that serve to identify the genes encoding the TCR and Ig chains and their rearrangements which take place at the earlier steps of T or B differentiation. Thus TCR or Ig gene rearrangements are considered as differentiation markers. In addition they also represent clonality markers since, within each clone, a unique rearrangement of V, D and J genes results in a unique antigen-specific receptor.

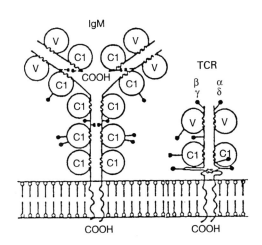

Fig. 1: Schematic view of the antigen-specific receptors expressed by lymphocytes. Because of their structural analogy (see text), the membrane IgM of B lymphocytes and the TCR-αβ and -γδ of T lymphocytes are considered members of the "Ig superfamily" (as also are CD4, CD8 and MHC molecules not shown here). Adapted from (32).

lymphocytes (*fig. 1*). A state of immunocompetence is reached by B or T lymphocytes when the synthesis and assembly of

Phenotype

Monoclonal antibodies recognize epitopes of molecules present in the cytoplasm and the membrane of the cell. A given molecule, usually a glycoprotein, may express several epitopes recognized by the corresponding mAbs. Conversely, several mAbs will define a molecule through the cluster of antigens (epitopes) which it contains. This forms the basis for the cluster of differentiation (CD) nomenclature *(see Table 1, p. 74)*. The identification of molecules expressed at the surface or within the cell by means of immunostaining methods such as immunofluorescence allows phenotypic determination.

Phenotypic markers of T-cell differentiation

CD3

CD3 is a multi-chain complex of five non-polymorphic polypeptides. These invariant CD3 molecules are non-covalently bound to the TCR heterodimeric structures (1) *(detailed below)* and the CD3-TCR complex is expressed on the membrane of T cells.

CD3 and TCR assemble in the endoplasmic reticulum and the complex is processed in the Golgi apparatus before it is transported to the cell membrane.

Anti-CD3 mAbs co-modulate the TCR. During thymic ontogeny, CD3 becomes detectable in the cytoplasm of thymocytes when the TCR β-chain gene has rearranged and RNA transcripts are present *(fig. 2)*. CD3 is expressed by most "double-positive" (CD4+/CD8+) thymocytes *(see below)* and its expression persists in the more mature T cells. Thus CD3 is a "pan-T" differentiation marker. *In vitro,* anti-CD3 mAbs can activate T cells and induce their proliferation; it is generally accepted that CD3 plays an important role in transmembrane signalling (1,2). Thus, antigen binding to TCR induces through the CD3 complex a cascade of

events resulting in T-lymphocyte activation. Finally, CD3 molecules can be revealed by immunofluorescence or related techniques either at the surface of maturing T cells or in the cytoplasm (especially the perinuclear zone) of thymocytes.

T-cell receptor (TCR)

TCR molecules are clonotypically distributed among T cells. They recognize and bind processed antigens. The TCR expressed by the vast majority of mature thymic and peripheral T-cells is a 90 kD disulphide-linked aß heterodimer, which recognizes antigens in the context of self-MHC molecules (3); each α and β chain is encoded by rearranging V and C genes *(fig. 1)*. More recently, two novel rearranging TCR genes have been identified, encoding a $\gamma\delta$ heterodimer expressed by a minor population for both thymic and peripheral T cells (4,5). The expression of TCR $\alpha\delta$ and $\gamma\delta$ is mutually exclusive. The biological role of the TCR-$\gamma\delta$ is currently the subject of investigations aimed at defining the size of its repertoire and the nature of both the antigens and MHC restriction elements that it recognizes (6). There is, however, evidence that most, if not all, TCR-$\gamma\delta$ cells have the potential for NK-like, non-MHC-restricted cytotoxicity. One unresolved question is whether during thymus development cells rearranging the $\gamma\delta$ genes will later give rise to $\alpha\beta$ by further rearrangements or whether productive rearrangements of both $\gamma\delta$ and $\alpha\beta$ genes occur in separate lineages (7,8). In

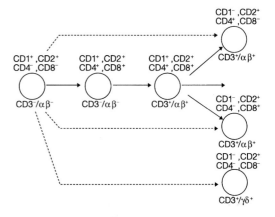

Fig. 2: Model of human thymic differentiation. Adapted from (33)

humans, a mean of 4% of CD3+ cells express the TCR-γδ in fetal and post-natal thymus, peripheral blood and lymphoid organs (9). TCR-γδ cells have been generally referred to as "double negative" (CD4-,CD8-) although a sizeable portion may express low levels of CD8, especially in peripheral lymphoid tissues. In contrast, virtually all TCR-γδ cells express the CD2, CD7 and CD5 pan-T antigens, as do the TCR-αβ cells.

In mice, TCR-γδ cells also account for the vast majority of dendritic epidermal lymphocytes (10) as well as intraepithelial gut lymphocytes (11). In chickens, TCR-γδ cells are similarly located preferentially in the intestinal epithelium whereas the TCR-αβ counterpart is located primarily in the lamina propria (12). This has led some researchers to propose that TCR-γδ cells constitute a class of T cells involved in surveillance of epithelial surfaces (13). The generality of these findings, is however, challenged by recent data in humans showing that TCR-γδ cells do not exhibit an obvious tropism for epithelial microenvironments in gut- and skin-associated lymphoid systems (9). In contrast, in exact homology to the chicken, human TCR-γδ cells seem to reside preferentially in anatomically distinct regions of the organized lymphoid tissues, such as the sinuses of the splenic red pulp (9,12).

Several mAbs have been developed that serve to identify TCR-αβ and TCR-γδ cells, i.e. that recognize epitopes encoded by the corresponding V or C rearranging genes. The WT31 mAb (14) detects a C-encoded epitope of the TCR-αβ heterodimer expressed at the surface of live cells; conversely βF1 (15) recognizes the cytoplasmic β chain both in its free form and in the mature αβ heterodimer and thus can be used for the staining of frozen tissue sections and cytospin preparations. The anti-TCRδ1 mAb which recognizes a C-encoded epitope of the δ chain, identifies all γδ expressing cells and thus represents operationally a pan-TCR-γδ marker (5). Anti-δTCS1 is an example of mAb reacting with a variable epitope (Vδ1) of the δ chain, thus identifying only a subpopulation of normal γδ cells. Another example is the anti-TiγA mAb which identifies a predominant subset

of γδ cells expressing a Vγ9-encoded γ chain. These mAbs can be used on live cell suspensions, cytospin preparations and frozen tissue sections.

Other accessory molecules

A series of mAb-defined cell surface antigens have been identified that function in concert with the CD3-TCR complex to modulate the immune response. These accessory molecules include CD2, CD4, CD8 (and also LFA-1 not described here). They are non-polymorphic molecules that not only increase the avidity with which T cells interact with antigen-presenting cells but are also able to transduce intracellular signals that synergize with those generated by the CD3-TCR complex (*fig. 3*).

CD2, a 45 kD transmembrane glycoprotein is the sheep red blood cell receptor responsible for E rosettes. Monoclonal antibodies have been developed that inhibit E rosette formation by interacting with CD2 epitopes. CD2 is thus expressed on all thymocytes and peripheral T cells, being a "pan-T antigen", as is the CD3 molecule. CD2 is not expressed on circulating B lymphocytes. *In vitro* pairs of anti-CD2 mAbs are able to activate T cells (16). The ligand for CD2 is the broadly distributed glycoprotein LFA-3 (17).

CD4 is a 45 kD transmembrane glycoprotein expressed on helper T lymphocytes.

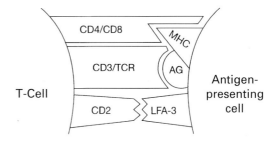

Fig. 3: Structures in the interactions between T-cells and antigen-presenting cells. These structures comprise the CD3-associated TCR (αβ, γδ), the CD2, CD4, CD8 accessory molecules (as well as LFA-1 not shown here) and their corresponding ligands.

CD4 interacts with the class II MHC products expressed by antigen-presenting cells (16).

CD8 is a 32 kD transmembrane glycoprotein, expressed on suppressor/cytotoxic T lymphocytes. CD8 interacts with class I MHC products. Expression of CD4 and CD8 occurs early in thymic ontogeny (*fig.2*). Thus thymocytes can be subdivided into several populations based on the expression of CD4 and CD8: CD4-/CD8- (double negative) cells; CD4+/CD8+ (double positive) cells; CD4-/CD8+ and CD4+/CD8- mature cells. CD4 and CD8 are not pan-T markers but rather serve to delineate functional subsets of mature T cells.

Other pan-T antigens

In addition to CD3 and CD2, CD7 and CD5 antigens are also considered as pan-T markers and commonly studied in the phenotypic identification of T lymphoma cells. CD5, however, also delineates a subset of B cells (*see below*). CD7 is the earliest expressed marker since it is found on the pro-thymocytes present in fetal liver before their entry into the thymus (18), i.e. prior to the onset of TCR gene rearrangements.

Phenotypic markers of B-cell differentiation

B cells synthesize immunoglobulins (Ig). Ig molecules were first used used as a marker for the identification of B cells. The cellular distribution of Ig differs according to the maturational development of B cells (membrane or cytoplasmic Ig). Other mAb-defined molecules can be used as B-cell differentiation markers. Activated B cells express new determinants such as CD23 (IgE Fc receptor) and CD25 (IL2 receptor), the latter being also expressed by activated T cells. B cell differentiation is usually divided into the pre-B, B lymphocyte and Ig-secreting cell compartments (*fig. 4*).

Cellular Ig

In the pre-B compartment, cells progressively express cytoplasmic μ chain (cμ)

without detectable light chain, as revealed by immunofluorescence (19). Thus the phenotype of the most mature pre-B cells is nIg-, cμ+.

The B lymphocyte compartment comprises peripheral and circulating resting (G0) cells that are able to bind antigen by means of their specific antigen-receptor, i.e. membrane Ig (mIg), the latter being easily identified by immunostaining cell suspensions (20). Such B lymphocytes express mIgM, with mIgG+ and mIgA+ cells being few, as revealed by relevant anti-μ, anti-γ and anti-α antibodies. The Kappa/Lambda (κ/λ) ratio for mIg is 2/3. It should be noted that, in addition, most IgM+ lymphocytes co-express membrane IgD, and that mIgM and mIgD share the same κ or λ light chain isotype. Thus the major phenotype of peripheral resting B cells is mIgM, mIgD, κ+. The co-expression of the two heavy chain μ and δ isotypes characterizes a maturational event located between the mIgM+, IgD- lymphocyte (also termed "virgin" lymphocyte) and the Ig-secreting cells.

The compartment of Ig-secreting cells encompasses cells maturing into plasma cells. The mIg are progressively lost and cIg accumulate in the cytoplasm. These cIg+ cells are easily identified in smears and tissue sections. Secretory Ig is present within the endoplasmic reticulum and the Golgi complex as shown by immunoelectron microscopy (21). Since plasma cells are the progeny of B lymphocytes, the antigen specificity of secretory Ig is identical to that of lymphocyte mIg within a given clone. The mIg and cIg share the same light-chain monotypy.

In contrast, the major phenotype is cIgG and cIgA, with IgM and IgD positive plasma cells being few. This results from the isotype switching involving the heavy chain of Ig molecules (μ → γ, μ → α).

Other pan-B antigens

Some glycoproteins, expressed by cells throughout the various compartments of B-cell differentiation, can be identified by mAbs and thus be used as pan-B markers

(22). CD19 is a 95 kD molecule expressed in early pre-B cells, prior to CD10 (*see below*) and cμ. CD19, however, is lost by the most mature plasma cells. CD20 is a 35 kD molecule whose expression parallels that of CD19, although it is not detectable in the earliest pre-B cells. The 140 kD CD21 molecule is virtually absent from pre-B cells and expressed mostly by B lymphocytes. CD21 contains the EBV receptor.

CD10, the antigen previously described as CALLA ("Common Acute Lymphoblastic Leukaemia Antigen"), is expressed by pre-B cells but also by more mature cells such as follicular centre cells. In addition, CD10 also appears to be expressed by certain leukaemic T cells, polymorphonuclears and non-haemopoietic cells. CD5, previously considered as a pan-T differentiation marker, is also expressed by a subpopulation of normal B lymphocytes, as well as by B cells involved in some auto-immune diseases and chronic lymphocytic leukaemia.

Finally the use of mAbs has greatly facilitated the phenotypic identification of malignant cells, such as early pre-B cells with no detectable cytoplasmic μ chain, and non-Hodgkin's lymphoma cells. In addition, the detection of a κ/λ monotypy, as revealed by monospecific anti-Ig antibodies, is generally considered to be strongly suggestive of monoclonality. This has been further confirmed by recent genomic studies (*see below*).

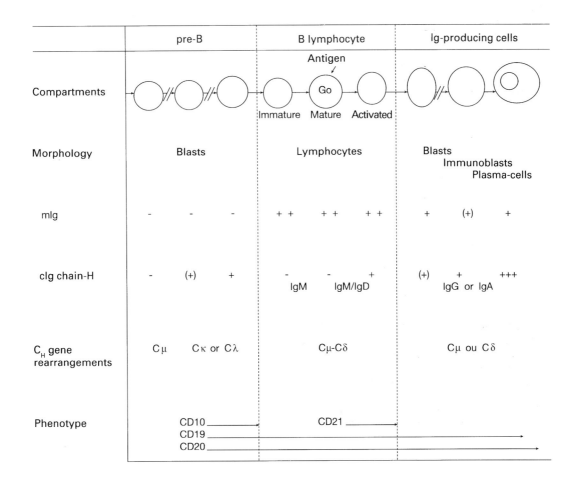

Fig. 4: Schematic view of B-cell differentiation.

Phenotypic markers of activated lymphocytes

Upon interaction with antigen, lymphocytes become activated, which means they leave the G0 phase and progress to G1. This entry into the cell cycle is paralleled by the expression of mAb-defined determinants (23) such as the CD25 molecule of activated T cells which is part of the IL2-receptor. Later on, the S phase of DNA synthesis is paralleled by the expression of other determinants such as MHC class II antigens on activated T cells. Similarly, activated B lymphocytes also express CD25, as well as the CD2 "pan-T" antigen (24) and the CD23 molecule (25).

their antigen-specific receptors. TCR as well as Ig molecules are made up of constant (C) and variable (V) regions. The latter contain the antigen-combining sites and are specific for a given clone and its progeny. Thus TCR and Ig molecules are encoded by genes composed of several V and C subsegments. These V and C gene subsegments are physically separated in their germ-line state. During T- or B-cell differentiation, a process of DNA recombination results in the close apposition of specific V and C gene subsegments to form an active TCR or Ig gene, giving rise to functional RNA transcripts. Such rearrangements create, at the DNA level, markers unique to each individual cell. Thus the detection of uniform rearrangements allows the recognition of a clonal expression and its involvement in T- or B-cell differentiation.

Genotype

The diversity of the repertoire of T and B lymphocytes is explained by the structure of

Ig genes

Ig molecules are composed of two identical heavy (H) and two identical light (L) chains.

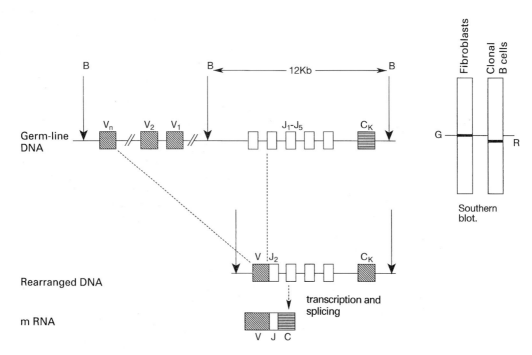

Fig. 5: Organization of kappa gene located on chromosome 2. Vertical arrows indicate restriction sites of the BamHI endonuclease (B). Patterns obtained by Southern blotting using a Ck probe are shown on the right. G, germ-line band; R, rearranged band. Adapted from (34).

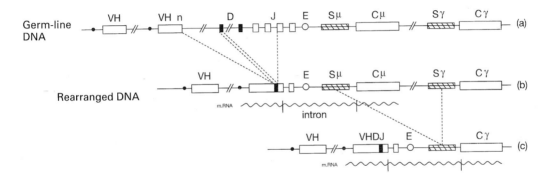

Fig. 6: Organization of the heavy-chain locus on chromosome 14. (a) Germ-line configuration (b) VDJ-C rearrangement resulting in RNA transcription (c) CDJ-C rearrangement leading to the isotype switching of Ig-secreting cells. Enhancer (E) sequence is active in both rearrangements. Adapted from (30).

Thus an Ig molecule has two identical antigen-binding sites resulting from the quaternary structures of VL and VH regions.

Each C region of molecules is encoded by a C gene, each V region being encoded by gene subsegments which are separated in their germ-line state. Thus the V region of a κ or γ light chain (VL) is encoded by a V gene and a J ("junction") gene: the synthesis of a light chain results from the junction of a V and J gene with deletion of interspaced DNA sequences (*fig. 5*). V-J junctions are regulated by an enzyme, termed recombinase, which recognizes "heptamer-nonamer" signals located 3' of V genes and 5' of J genes. The V region of heavy chains (V_H) is encoded by V, J and D ("diversity") gene subsegments (*fig. 6*). Thus the synthesis of a heavy chain results from two sequential rearrangements: $D-J_H$ followed by V_H-DJ_H (26,27). Later on during B-cell differentiation, a further rearrangement will take place, resulting in an isotype switching of the heavy chain (*fig. 6*). Thus the deletion of DNA between switch sequences (S) located 5' of the C_H genes will allow the V_HDJ_H ensemble to be expressed with another C_H gene. Figure 6 illustrates the gene rearrangements leading to the switch from IgM to IgG synthesis within a B cell.

κ, γ and H chain loci are located on chromosomes 2p12, 22q11 and 14q32, respectively. The heavy-chain locus contains about $80V_H$, 50 D, 9 J_H and 11 C_H genes. The κ light-chain locus contains 40-80 Vκ, 55 Dκ and 1 Cκ genes. The γ locus contains 50 Vγ and 6 Jγ and 6 Cγ genes (28).

Ig genes rearrange sequentially during B-cell differentiation. Pre-B cells first rearrange the heavy-chain locus, resulting in the synthesis of cytoplasmic μ chains. This is followed by the rearrangement of the κ locus resulting in the synthesis of a κ light chain which upon assembly with μ chain will allow the expression of membrane IgM (mIgMκ). As a rule, Ig gene rearrangements involve one or both alleles; however, only one rearrangement will be productive, giving rise to full-length mature RNA transcripts. Thus, the κ rearrangement may involve one allele, or, if non-productive, the second allele. If both κ alleles are non-productively rearranged, then the λ locus will rearrange (29). The rearrangement thus implies the deletion of the Cκ gene which results from the rearrangement of a sequence termed "kappa-deleting element", located 3' of Cκ. Membrane Igs (mIg) differ from secretory Igs in their transmembrane portion encoded by exons located 3' of C_H gene subsegments. Differential splicing of primary RNA transcripts determines the expression of either mIg or cIg. Similarly, the coexpression of IgM and IgD in B lymphocytes results from primary transcripts containing both Cμ and Cδ sequences.

TCR genes

As described above, TCR-$\alpha\beta$ and TCR-$\gamma\delta$ are anchored in the cell membrane by their hydrophobic region and are linked to the CD3 polypeptide complex. TCR $\alpha\beta$ is expressed by CD3+, CD4+/CD8- and

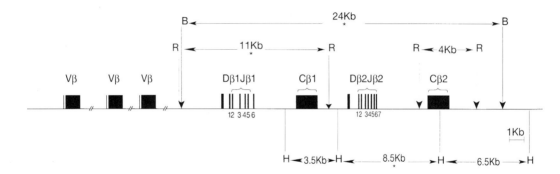

Fig. 7: Organization of the TCR-β chain locus on chromosome 7. Vertical arrows indicate restriction sites of BamHI (B), EcoRI (R) and HindIII (H). Sizes of the corresponding germ-line bands obtained with a Cβ probe hybridizing to both Cβ1 and Cβ2 are shown. Adapted from (30).

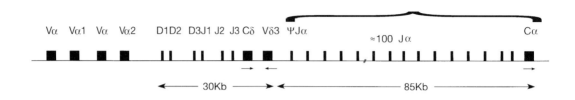

Fig. 8: Organization of the TCR-α and TCR-β chain loci on chromosome 14. The δ locus is located within the α locus and thus is deleted when a Vα-Jα rearrangement occurs. Adapted from (30).

CD3+, CD4-/CD8+ lymphocytes as a disulphide-linked heterodimer. TCR γδ is expressed by CD3+, CD4-/CD8- lymphocytes as a heterodimer, with γ and δ chains being disulphide-linked or not. Like Ig molecules, each α, β, and δ chain of the TCR consists of C and V regions. The C region is encoded by a C gene and the V region is encoded by rearranging V and J (α and γ chains) or V, D and J (β and δ chains) gene subsegments.

Such VJ or VDJ junctions are regulated by recombinase, as in the case of Ig genes (27). The organization of TCR genes has been recently reviewed (30).

The β locus, on chromosome 7q35, contains about 60 Vβ, and a duplicated Cβ gene in homologous two Cβ1 and Cβ2 subsegments with corresponding 5' J and D subsegments (*fig. 7*). The α locus, on chromosome 14q11 contains about 50 Vα, 100 Jα genes and one Cα gene. The Jα subsegments are dispersed over an 80 kb region, resulting in the unusually large size of the α locus (*fig. 8*). The γ locus on chromosome 7q15 contains 14 Vγ, 5 Jγ and 2 Cγ subsegments (*fig. 9*). Cγ1 and Cγ2 (unlike Cβ1 and Cβ2) differ structurally since Cγ1 contains 3 exons, one of which has a cysteine site, whereas Cγ2 comprises 4 or 5 exons with a non-cysteine site. This results in polymorphism in the size of the chains encoded by Cγ2. Due to the absence of cysteine, γ2 chains are non-covalently bound to the δ chain of TCR-γδ. The δ locus is situated within the α locus, 5' of Jα subsegments (*fig. 8*). It contains 3 D, 3 J genes and one Cδ gene. Vδ genes are few (6 have been identified to date), some being located among Vα, and one (Vδ3) being 3' of Cδ.

It is generally accepted that TCR genes rearrange sequentially during thymic ontogeny, although it is in dispute whether productive γδ and αβ rearrangements occur within the

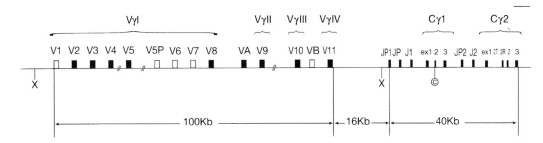

Fig. 9: Organization of the TCR-γ locus on chromosome 7. The 14 Vγ genes are categorized into 4 subgroups. The Vγl subgroup contains 9 V genes, 4 being pseudogenes (open box). Structural differences of Cγ1 and Cγ2 are shown; Cγ1 contains 3 exons whereas Cγ2 contains 4 to 5 exons as a result of a duplication or triplication of exon 2. Exon 2 of Cγ1 has a cysteine residue. Adapted from (30).

same or separate lineages. γ and δ genes rearrange first, followed by β and later by α genes. Productive rearrangements of the γ and δ loci give rise to TCR-γδ cells.

Non-productive γ and δ rearrangements are believed to be followed by VDJ junctions within the β and the α loci, leading to TCR-αβ cells (31). Rearrangement of the α locus results in the deletion of the δ gene (fig. 8). Thus only γ gene rearrangements are detectable in all T cells, whether γδ or αβ.

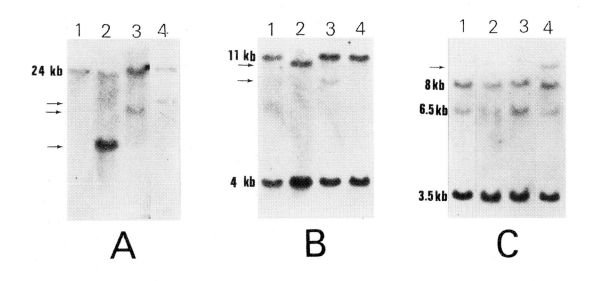

Fig. 10: DNA rearrangements of the β-TCR gene using the Cβ probe after digestion with BamHI (A), EcoRI (B) and HindIII (C). Sizes of the germ-line bands are shown at the top, and arrows indicate the rearranged fragments. Lanes 1, germ-line control; lanes 2 and 3, two T-cell lymphoma samples showing the rearrangement of one allele of the Cβ1 segment; lane 4, another sample showing the rearrangement of one allele of the Cβ2 segment.

References

1. CLEVERS H, ALARCON B, WILEMAN T, TERHORST C
   The T-cell receptor/CD3 complex: a dynamic protein ensemble.
   Ann Rev Immunol, 1968; 6: 629-662.

2. SUSSMAN JJ, BONIFACINO JS, LIPPINCOTT J et al.
   Failure to synthezise the T-cell CD3-ξ chain; structure and function of a partial T-cell receptor complex.
   Cell, 1988; 52: 85-93.

3. MARRACK P, KAPPLER J
   The antigen-specific major histocompatibility complex restricted receptor on T cells.
   Adv Immunol, 1986; 38: 1-17.

4. BRENNER MB, STROMINGER JL, KRANGER MS
   The δT-cell receptor.
   Adv Immunol, 1988; 43: 133-149.

5. TRIEBEL F, HERCEND T
   Subpopulations of human peripheral Tγδ lymphocytes.
   Immun Today, 1989; 10: 186-188.

6. BLUESTONE JA, MATIS LA
   TCR δ cells: minor redundant T-cell subset or specialized immune system component?
   J Immunol, 1989; 142: 1985-1988.

7. ALLISON PJ, LANIER LL
   T-cell receptor γ gene: rearrangement and cell lineages.
   Immun Today, 1987; 8: 293-296.

8. WINOTO A, BALTIMORE C
   Separate lineages of T cells expressing the αβ and γδ receptors.
   Nature, 1989; 338: 430-432.

9. GROH V, PORCELLI S, FABBI M et al.
   Human lymphocytes bearing T-cell receptors αβ are phenotypically diverse and evenly distributed throughout the lymphoid system.
   J Exp Med, 1989; 169: 1277-1294.

10. STINGL G, KONING F, YAMADA H et al.
    Thy-1+ dendritic epidermal cells express T3 antigen and the T-cell receptor chain.
    Proc Natl Sci USA, 1987; 84: 4586-4590.

11. GOODMAN T, LEFRANCOIS L
    Expression of the γδ T-cell receptor on intestinal CD8+ intraepithelial lymphocytes.
    Nature, 1988; 333: 855-858.

12. BUCY RP, CHEN CH, CIHAK J, LOSCH U, COOPER MD
    Avian T-cells expressing γδ receptors localize in the splenic sinusoids and the intestinal epithelium.
    J Immunol, 1988; 141: 2200-2205.

13. JANEWAY CA
    Frontiers of the immune systems.
    Nature, 1988; 338: 804-806.

14. SPITS H, BORST J, TAX W, CAPEL PJA, TERHORST C, DE VRIES JE
    Characteristics of a monoclonal antibody (WT31) that recognizes a common epitope on the human T-cell receptor for antigen.
    J Immunol, 1985; 135: 1922-1928.

15. BRENNER MB, McLEAN J, SCHEFT H, WARNKE RA, JONES N, STROMINGER JL
    Characterisation and expression of the human αβ T-cell receptor using a framework monoclonal antibody.
    J Immunol, 1987; 138: 1502-1509.

16. BIERER BE, SLECKMAN BP, RATNOFSKY SE, BURAKOFF SJ
    The biologic roles of CD2, CD4 and CD8 in T-cell activation.
    Ann Rev Immunol, 1989; 7: 579-599.

17. SELVARAJ P, PLUNKETT PL, DUSTIN M, SANDERS ME, SHAW S, SPRINGER TA
    The T lymphocyte glycoprotein CD2 binds the cell surface ligand LFA-3.
    Nature, 1987; 326: 400-2.

18. HAYNES BF, MARTIN ME, KAY HH, KURTZBERG J
    Early events in human T-cell ontogeny.
    J Exp Med, 1988; 168: 1061-1080.

19. COOPER MD
    Pre-B cells: normal and abnormal development.
    J Clin Immunol, 1981; 81: 1-12.

20. PREUD'HOMME JL, SELIGMANN M
    Surface immunoglobulins on human lymphoid cells.
    Prog Clin Immunol, 1974; 2: 121-129.

21. GOURDIN MF, FARCET JP, REYES F
    The ultrastructural localization of immunoglobulins in human cells of immunoproliferative diseases.
    Blood, 1982; 59: 1132-1139.

22. ZOLA H
    The surface antigens of human B lymphocytes.
    Immunol Today, 1987; 8: 308-311.

23. COTNER T, WILLIAMS JM, CHRISTENSON L, SHAPIRO HM, STROM TB, STROMINGER J
    Simultaneous flux cytometric analysis of human T-cell activation antigen expression and DNA content.
    J Exp Med, 1983; 157: 461-468.

24. WALDMANN TA
    The structure, function and expression of Interleukin-2 receptors on normal and malignant lymphocytes.
    Science, 1986; 727: 232-235.

25. GORDON J, GUY GR
    The molecules controlling B lymphocytes.
    Immunol Today, 1987; 8: 339-342.

26. ALT FW, BLACKWELL TK, DE PINHL RA, RETH MG, YANCOPOULOS GD

   Regulation of genome rearrangement events during lymphocyte development.
   Immunol Rev, 1986; 89: 5-30.

27. YANCOPOULOS GD, BLACKWELL TK, SUH H, HOOD L, ALT FN

   Introduced T-cell receptor variable region gene segments recombine in pre-B cells: evidence that B and T cells use a common recombinase.
   Cell, 1986; 44: 251-259.

28. DARIAVACH P, LEFRANC G, LEFRANC MP

   Human immunoglobulin Cλ6 encodes the Kern+Oz- chain. Cλ4 and Cλ5 are pseudogenes.
   Proc Natl Acad Sci USA, 1987; 84: 9074-9078.

29. KORSMEYER SJ, HIETER PA, RAVETCH JV, POPLACK DG, WALDMANN TA, LEDER P

   Developmental hierarchy of immunoglobulin gene rearrangement in human leukemic pre-B cells.
   Proc Natl Acad Sci USA, 1981; 78: 7096-7100.

30. LEFRANC MP

   Organization of the human T-cell receptor genes
   Eur. Cytoline Net. 1990; 1: 121-130.

31. TIEBEL F, LEFRANC MP, HERCEND T

   Further evidence for a sequentially ordered activation of T-cell rearranging gamma genes during T-lymphocyte differentiation.
   Eur J Immunol, 1988; 18: 789-794.

32. WILLIAMS AF, BARCLAY AN

   The immunoglobulin superfamily-domains for cell surface recognition.
   Ann Rev Immunol, 1988; 6: 381-405.

33. ALLISON JP

   Structure, function and serology of the T-cell antigen receptor complex.
   Ann Rev Immunol, 1987; 5: 503-540.

34. WALDMANN TA, KORSMEYER SJ, BAKHSHI A, ARNOLD A, KIRSCH IR

   Molecular genetic analysis of human lymphoid neoplasms.
   Ann Int Med, 1985; 102: 497-510.

Adult T-cell leukaemia/lymphoma: a model of retrovirus-induced lymphomagenesis

M. DIVINE, J.-P. FARCET

Introduction

Adult T-cell leukaemia-lymphoma (ATL) was first described in 1977 in Japan as a new form of T-cell malignancy (1). At the same time, a retrovirus, termed HTLV-1, was isolated from patients with cutaneous T-cell lymphoma (2). The same virus was subsequently isolated from Japanese patients with ATL (3-5). An aetiological association of HTLV-1 with ATL was clearly established by extensive seroepidemiology which showed the same geographical distribution of HTLV-1 and ATL and HTLV-1 infection in all patients with ATL. The demonstration of the monoclonal integration of the provirus in ATL cells provided direct evidence for the involvement of HTLV-1 in leukaemogenesis (6).

Epidemiology

The development of serological assays for HTLV-1 infection has provided epidemiological information about HTLV-1 distribution and transmission (7-9).

HTLV-1 infection is prevalent in certain geographical areas and sporadically observed in immigrants from these endemic regions, including Southern Japan, the South-Eastern United States and the Caribbean basin (10).

Isolated clusters of infection have also been identified in Italy, New Guinea, the Arctic and Taiwan. Preliminary data also suggest a high prevalence of infection in some areas of Africa, but extensive seroepidemiological data are not yet available.

The highest rates of seropositivity are found in South-West Japan, where up to 30% of the population has been shown to have antibodies to the virus. However, even in highly endemic regions, the prevalence of infec-tion depends on several factors. The rates vary markedly from one area to another. The prevalence of seropositivity increases with age, reaching a plateau in the 50-yr age group; this pattern may result from the increased exposure to virus as age increases or alternatively from the late reactivation of early, latently infected T cells. A slight female predominance in the HTLV-1 seropositive rate is observed. Striking intrafamilial clusterings of seropositive carriers is also reported (11).

The transmission of HTLV-1 infection is not fully characterized because incubation time from exposure to onset of disease may last several decades. The Japanese descriptive surveys suggest that HTLV-1, like HIV-1, is transmitted, although poorly, by the same routes: from mother to child, either across the placenta or by breast-feeding (12), by sexual contact, and by blood transfusion (13). Transmission seems to require the transfer of living infected cells from virus carriers to recipients. In the United States the epidemiological survey of HTLV-1 infection is limited to selected high-risk populations and blood donors, and is hampered by the frequent occurrence of cross-reactive HTLV-2 infection, particularly among drug abusers (14).

Clinical features

A spectrum of clinical patterns has been associated with HTLV-1 infection, ranging from the asymptomatic carrier state to the aggressive prototypic ATL (15). After a long period of latency, only a small proportion of the infected population will develop lymphoma. It has been suggested that the natural course of ATL progresses sequentially from the HTLV-1 carrier state through intermediate states to acute ATL, indicating a process of multistage leukaemogenesis. These different steps of HTLV-1 infection may be recognized at the clinical, haematological and molecular levels.

The first and most frequent condition is the *healthy carrier* state. Healthy carriers are asymptomatic and have a normal white blood cell (WBC) count without atypical lymphocytes; HTLV-1 proviral DNA is not detectable by Southern blot analysis of peripheral blood lymphocytes using HTLV-1 probes. However, as recently reported in some asymptomatic carriers, low levels of HTLV-1 viral transcripts can be detected by more sensitive techniques, such as the polymerase chain reaction (PCR) (16). *Smouldering* ATL is a non-aggressive form presenting as a chronic skin disease (17,18). Patients have normal WBC counts with a few abnormal cells (0.5-5%), and display a monoclonal pattern of HTLV-1 genome integration. It remains uncertain whether this condition always precedes the appearance of overt ATL.

A transitional form between the healthy carrier state and smouldering ATL has been recently recognized by some authors (19). This intermediate state has been defined by Southern blot analysis as a condition in which HTLV-1 proviral DNA is integrated in a polyclonal fashion in peripheral blood lymphocytes.

The *chronic form* is an insidious disease characterized by lymphadenopathy, minimal skin infiltration, and no visceral involvement. Atypical lymphocytes include at least 10% of the circulating nucleated cells. Over time, chronic ATL may progress to the acute form.

The *prototypic acute* form concerns less than 1% of HTLV-1 infected individuals (1,20-22). Typical features usually include hepatosplenomegaly, lymphadenopathy that spares the mediastinum, frequent skin lesions, and an elevated WBC count. Bone-marrow involvement is often slight, irrespective of the degree of lymphocytosis. The latter is composed of pleomorphic malignant cells ranging from small to large cells, with pronounced nuclear convolutions. ATL usually has an aggressive course with rapid dissemination, visceral involvement with pulmonary, leptomeningeal and/or liver infiltration, increased bone resorption leading to lytic lesions and hypercalcaemia, and frequent life-threatening infections by opportunistic agents such as *Pneumocystis carinii, Cryptococcus neoformans* and *Cytomegalovirus*. Response to intensive combination chemotherapy is often short, and median survival usually does not exceed one year. Thus ATL is regarded as a high-grade non-Hodgkin's lymphoma.

Almost all patients and carriers have serum antibodies directed against HTLV-1 structural proteins. Molecular studies usually show excellent correlation with the results of serological surveys: indeed, leukaemic cells of ATL patients, regardless of the stage of disease (smouldering, chronic, acute), contain the viral genome and are found to be monoclonal with respect to the integration site of proviral genome (23). However, some differences between serological and molecular data have occasionaly been described. Seronegative healthy infected subjects from highly endemic areas (11,24) and seronegative patients with typical ATL have been reported (25,26). In these cases, novel approaches, such as the highly sensitive PCR procedure, are well-suited for detecting HTLV-1 DNA sequences (27).

Virological aspects of HTLV-1 infection

HTLV-1 is an RNA-containing C retro-virus. "Type C" refers to the morphology of the virus during budding. The sequence of 9032 bases of the complete HTLV-1 proviral genome was determined in 1983 by Seiki et al. (28). Like other retroviruses, HTLV-1 contains the structural genomic regions gag, pol, env, and two identical long terminal repeat sequences (LTRs) at the ends. The LTRs carry transcriptional control elements, known as promoters and enhancers. However, a unique feature of HTLV-1 is the presence of an unusual sequence, now termed pX, between env and the 3' LTR. This sequence is common to all members of the HTLV family which includes HTLV-1, HTLV-2, STLV-1 and BLV. Unlike classical oncogenes, it has no known homogeneous c-onc sequences in the cellular genome.

The gag gene encodes a 53 kD (p53) precursor polypeptide which is cleaved to the three major components of the virion core, p19, p24 and p15. Expression of the pol gene is detected as reverse transcriptase activity but the pol gene product has not yet been identified in HTLV-1 infected cells. The env gene encodes two glycoproteins, gp46 and gp21, which are products of the cleavage of a precursor protein, gp61. On mature viral particles, gp46 represents the outer component of the viral envelope. gp21 is the transmembrane envelope component which anchors the glycoprotein complex to the viral nucleocapsid.

The pX sequence contains four overlapping open reading frames between the env gene and 3' LTR. Three products, Tax (also designated as p40x, tax1 or tat-I), Rex(p27x), and p21x have been identified. The great majority of Tax and Rex are found in the nucleus; p21x is localized in the cytoplasm. Tax and Rex are essential for viral replication (29). Thus, Tax activates transcription from the promotor in the viral LTR sequences (30); Rex regulates the splicing of genomic RNA, allowing synthesis of the virion structural proteins.

Cell-virus interactions

Phenotypic and genotypic features of ATL cells

ATL cells display a mature T-cell phenotype CD1-, CD2+, CD3+, CD5+ and belong to the CD4+ T-cell subset (31). *In vitro* studies of Pokeweed mitogen-induced immunoglobulin synthesis suggest that the leukaemic cells are CD4+ inducers of suppression (32). A CD8+ phenotype of tumour cells has occasionally been described in the setting of polyclonal CD8 lymphocytosis in patients co-infected with HTLV-1 and HIV-1 (33).

The surface density of the CD3 antigen on ATL cells is lower than on normal T cells. The expression of the antigen recognized by WT31 monoclonal antibody (mAb), a common epitope of the $\alpha\beta$ T-cell receptor (TCR), is also decreased in ATL. The CD3 antigen on ATL cells can be modulated by anti-CD3 mAb, suggesting that CD3-TCR complexes can still be regulated (34). The retroviral genome has been suspected of playing a causative role in the specific down-regulation of CD3 gene transcription.

The configuration of TCR β and γ genes in ATL cells has been extensively analysed by the Southern blot method. TCR β genes are monoclonally rearranged in all neoplastic ATL cells. Rearrangements of TCR γ genes are also detected in the leukaemic cells of most ATL patients. Comparative studies of the patterns of TCR gene rearrangements and of the nucleotide sequences of the variable regions (Vβ) of TCR β genes indicate that ATL cells do not utilize any specific Vβ gene (35).

ATL cells are also known to constitutively express the p55 chain (Tac) of the Interleukin-2 receptor (IL-2R) detected by the anti-CD25 mAb. Fresh ATL cells usually give a weak staining; however, expression of IL-2R antigens is enhanced by 24-hour incubation. IL-2R displays some differences as compared with IL-2R on normal activated T-cells. The Tac antigen on ATL cells is not down-regulated by anti-CD25 mAb; furthermore, the number of IL-2R does not decline with time of culture (36). The biological significance of the expression of

IL-2R on ATL cells is intriguing, since most ATL cells do not respond to exogenous IL-2. As will be detailed in the last section, a model of autocrine growth is proposed at early stages of leukaemogenesis. In support of an autocrine loop, some authors have identified primary ATL tumour cells (37) and ATL cell lines (38) whose proliferation, at least in part, involves the simultaneous display of IL-2R and the production of IL-2.

No HTLV-1 antigens are generally detected in fresh isolated tumour cells from ATL patients, when either protein or mRNA is assessed (39). Absence of viral antigens from ATL cells could explain how infected T-cells elude immunosurveillance mechanisms.

After being cultured for a few days, ATL cells express enhanced amounts of both IL-2R and HTLV-1 transcripts (40), suggesting a close association between IL-2R expression and HTLV-1 expression in ATL cells. Alternatively, *in vivo* expression of viral genes may not be required for the constitutive expression of IL-2R on ATL cells, although it may represent an early event in ATL development. It is also possible that trace levels of viral transcripts, as detected only by PCR, are sufficient to maintain constitutive expression of IL-2R (41).

Experimental data

Several steps of the virus growth cycle are subjected to regulation. First, viral adsorption and transmission are mediated through the interaction of viral glycoproteins and specific binding sites on the target-cell membrane. Second, HTLV-1 proviral genome is integrated randomly into target-cell DNA. Finally, proviral DNA is transcribed through the activation of the LTR sequences.

Cellular binding sites

Assays of syncitium induction (cell fusion), virion binding, and propagation of vesicular stomatitis virus pseudotypes bearing the HTLV-1 envelope glycoprotein allow detection of HTLV-1 receptors on a broad range of human and mammalian cells (42,43). Thus, human B and T lymphocytes, fibroblasts, endothelial cells and many different cells of several species possess cell-surface receptors for HTLV-1. However, a direct positive correlation between HTLV-1 adsorption and integration of HTLV-1 proviral DNA in target cells is most often limited to human lymphoid cells. Thus, not all receptor-positive cells are susceptible to infection, indicating that the cellular receptor restriction is not the major determinant of cell tropism of HTLV-1. Susceptibility of cells to infection can be controlled at later points in the virus growth cycle beyond virus-cell binding. Quantitation of HTLV-1-cell binding by flow cytometry using purified labelled virions shows that T lymphocytes express higher levels of HTLV-1 receptors than do non-T cells. Furthermore, the number of HTLV-1 receptors increases upon *in vitro* mitogenic exposure of the target T-cells.

Retroviral env glycoproteins have major functions in viral infection. gp46 contains the binding domain of the T-cell surface receptor. Likewise, gp21 contains the fusion domain involved in syncitium formation and also in virus penetration.

T-cell activation represents the main early event occurring *in vitro* after viral attachment to the membrane (44). Indeed, binding of viral particles to the target T-cells induces expression of IL-2R and synthesis of IL-2, and triggers polyclonal T-cell expansion. Thus, envelope glycoproteins are not only involved in virus-cell binding but are also potent mitogens. The initial target T-cell activation could define a preleukaemic event, favouring viral integration and viral replication in actively dividing T cells. HTLV-1 receptors might be related to signal-transducing receptors on the T-cell membrane, the CD3-TCR complex or the CD2 molecules, which define the two classical activation pathways (45). However, the identity of HTLV-1 receptors is still unknown.

Cellular infection by HTLV-1

Transfer experiments demonstrate that HTLV-1 can be transmitted *in vitro* to a wide variety of target cells, inducing lymphoid human cells and T-lymphocytes from several other species.

HTLV-1 transfer studies usually consist in co-culturing irradiated HTLV-1-producing cells with recipient cells. Indeed, cell-to-cell transfer assays appear more efficient than cell-free virus infection.

Successful transmission can be monitored by analysis of integrated proviral DNA, reverse transcriptase activity, and/or intracellular HTLV-1 core antigen p19 expression. Furthermore, cytological, phenotypic, and functional changes define the cellular transformation that is specifically exhibited by human T-cells, after *in vitro* HTLV-1-transmission. Transformed T-cells display lobulated nuclei similar to those of ATL cells, express IL-2R, and progressively acquire IL-2-independent growth. Thus, the *in vitro* transformation of T cells morphologically mimics the *in vitro* leukaemic process.

Susceptibility of the lymphoid cells to *in vitro* virus transmission depends on their type, source and activity state (46). CD4+ T-cells are the preferential target cells for virus replication. Under some experimental conditions CD8+ T-cells can also be transformed by the virus. Conversely, large granular lymphocytes with natural killer activity seem to be resistant to HTLV-1 infection. Cord-blood and bone-marrow cells appear to be more sensitive than PBL. Finally, prior activation of target T-cells with mitogen and IL-2 before HTLV-1 transfer enhances the efficiency of HTLV-1-induced transformation.

HTLV-1-infected T-cell lines can be established from long-term cultures of leucocytes from patients with ATL. ATL cell lines share phenotypic features with fresh uncultured leukaemic cells. However, karyotypic and genotypic profiles, such as integration sites of HTLV-1 and configuration of TCR-β genes, differ from those of fresh leukaemic cells (47). These findings indicate that most cell lines do not derive from the primary leukaemic cells, but from T cells infected *in vitro*.

HTLV-1-induced cellular transformation is a slow process *in vitro*, requiring a delay of two to five weeks before the first cytoplasmic p19 core antigen can first be detected. During the early stage of infection, proviral integration sites are polyclonal. Later on, after three to six months of culture, a monoclonal selection is observed, while the cells become IL-2-independent during their growth. These events are observed when either normal helper or cytotoxic clones are used as target cells. After transformation, cells proliferate autonomously, some of them losing their functional properties (48).

Trans-activation of cellular genes

Unlike many other transforming animal retroviruses, HTLV-1 lacks a typical oncogene. Furthermore, it does not insert at any specific site within the host genome (49). Hence, a cis-acting viral promoter cannot account for ATL development. Thus a trans-acting viral function must be involved in the leukaemic process.

The Tax protein seems to play a crucial role in HTLV-1-induced T-cell transformation, by means of trans-activating transcription of a set of cellular genes involved in T-cell growth.

Several studies have analysed the expression of endogenous or transfected genes upon Tax activation. The inductive effects of Tax are usually restricted to certain human T-cell lines (JURKAT, HSB-2) (50). This apparent restriction may reflect a particular state of differentiation of target cells or the cellular distribution of some co-factor required for Tax function. First, endogenous IL-2 and IL-2R genes have been shown to be induced by transfection with Tax-expressing plasmids (50). Second, activation of various cellular genes has been ascribed to Tax, mainly through co-transfection experiments; cellular genes encoding for granulocyte-macrophage colony-stimulating factor and for the nuclear proto-oncogene c-fos have been shown to be induced by Tax (51-54).

The molecular mechanism by which Tax trans-activates its target genes is still unclear. The spectrum of cellular genes regulated by Tax appears to be restricted. Tax does not bind the DNA. It seems rather to function in an indirect manner by modifying the expression of host transcription factors.

On the basis of experimental data, a model of autocrine pathway has been proposed for the development of ATL at early stages (52,54-56). Infection by HTLV-1 of T cells leads to expression of Tax at low levels. Tax induces expression of IL-2R and the production of IL-2, thereby leading to an early phase of uncontrolled autocrine polyclonal T-cell growth. Additional antigen stimulation may be necessary for full activation of the IL-2 gene and completion of the IL-2 autocrine loop.

The ensuing period of oligoclonal T-cell proliferation may facilitate the occurrence of chromosomal events required for completion of T-cell transformation.

A variety of cytogenetic abnormalities has been described in ATL cells, such as deletion of chromosome 6, insertion on 14 and trisomy 7 (57). No relationship to known oncogenes has been recognized. Chromosomal events could provide T-cells with an additional advantage of autono-mous growth and favour the emergence of a monoclonal proliferation.

However, the underlying mechanisms in the final development of ATL *in vivo* still remain to be determined. Identification of the viral receptors and of the primary target molecule of Tax should lead to a better understanding of the virus-target cell interactions.

References

1. UCHIYAMA T, YODOI J, SAGAWA X, TAKOTSUKI K, UCHIMO H
   Adult T-cell leukemia: clinical and hematologic features of 16 cases.
   Blood, 1977; 50: 481-491.

2. POESZ BJ, RUSCETTI FW, GAZDAR AF, BUNN PA, MINNA JD, GALLO RC
   Detection and isolation of type C retrovirus particles from fresh and cultured lymphocytes of a patient with cutaneous T-cell lymphoma.
   Proc Natl Acad Sci USA, 1980; 77: 7415-7419.

3. YOSHIDA M, MIYOSHI I, HINUMA Y
   Isolation and characterization of retrovirus from cell lines of human adult T-cell leukemia and its implication in the disease.
   Proc Natl Acad Sci USA, etc. 1982; 79: 2031-2035.

4. POPOVIC M, REITZ MS, SARNGADHARAN MG, et al.
   The virus of Japanese adult T-cell leukaemia is a member of the human T-cell leukaemia virus group.
   Nature, 1982; 300: 63-66.

5. WATANABE T, SEIKI M, YOSHIDA M
   HTLV type I (US isolate) and ATLV (5 Japanese isolates) are the same species of human retrovirus.
   Virology 1984; 133: 238-241.

6. YOSHIDA M, SEIKI M, YAMAGUSHI K, TAKATSUKI K
   Monoclonal integration of human T-cell leukemia provirus in all primary tumors of adult T-cell leukemia suggests causative role of human T-cell leukemia virus in the disease.
   Proc Natl Acad Sci USA, 1984; 81: 2534-2537.

7. HINUMA Y, KOMADA H, CHOSA T, et al.
   Antibodies to adult T-cell leukemia-virus-associated antigen (ATLA) in sera from patients with ATL and controls in Japan: a nationwide sero-epidemiologic study.
   Int J Cancer, 1982; 29: 631-635.

8. BLATTNER WA, BLAYNEY DW, ROBERT-GUROFF M et al.
   Epidemiology of human T-cell leukemia/lymphoma virus.
   J Inf Dis, 1983; 147: 406-416.

9. RATNER L, POIESZ BJ
   Leukemias associated with human T-cell lymphotropic virus type I in a non-endemic region.
   Medicine, 1988; 67: 401-430.

10. GALLO RC
    The human T-cell leukemia/lymphoma retrovirus (HTLV) family: past, present, and future.
    Cancer Res, 1985; 45 (suppl): 4524s-4533s.

11. SARIN PS, ACKI T, SHIBATA A et al.
    High incidence of human type-C retrovirus (HTLV) in family members of a HTLV-positive Japanese T-cell leukemia patient.
    Proc Natl Acad Sci USA, 1983; 80: 2370-2374.

12. KOMURO A, HAYAMI M, FUJII H, MIYAHARA S, HIRAYAMA M
    Vertical transmission of adult T-cell leukemia virus.
    Lancet, 1983; i: 240.

13. SATO H, OKOCHI K

   Transmission of human T-cell leukemia virus (HTLV-1) by blood transfusion: demonstration of proviral DNA in recipients' blood lymphocytes.

   Int J Cancer, 1986; 37: 395-400.

14. LEE H, SWANSON P, SHORTY VS, ZACK JA, ROSENBLATT JD, CHEN Y

   High rate of HTLV-II infection in seropositive IV drug abusers in New Orleans.

   Science, 1989; 244: 471-475.

15. KUEFLER PR, BUNN PA

   Adult T-cell Leukaemia/Lymphoma.

   Clinics in Haematol, 1986; 15: 695-720.

16. TOMOHIRO K, MASANORI S, KENSEI T et al.

   Detection of mRNA for the tax/rex1 gene of human T-cell leukemia virus type I in fresh peripheral blood mononuclear cells of adult T-cell leukemia patients and viral carriers by using the polymerase chain reaction.

   Proc Natl Acad Sci USA 1989; 86: 5620-5624.

17. YAMAGUCHI K, NISHIMURA H, KOHROGI H, IONO M, MIYAMOTO Y, TAKATSUKI K

   A proposal for smoldering adult T-cell leukemia: a clinicopathologic study of five cases.

   Blood, 1983; 62: 758-766.

18. KAWANO F, YAMAGUCHI K, NISHIMURA H, TSUDA H, TAKATSUKI K

   Variation in the clinical courses of adult T-cell leukemia.

   Cancer, 1985; 55: 851-856.

19. KAZUNARI Y, TETSUYUKI K, KIYONOBU N et al.

   Polyclonal integration of HTLV-I proviral DNA in lymphocytes from HTLV-I seropositive individuals: an intermediate state between the healthy carrier state and smouldering ATL.

   Br J Haematol, 1988; 68: 169-174.

20. CATOVSKY D, ROSE M, GOOLDEN AWG et al.

   Adult T-cell lymphoma-leukaemia in blacks from the West-Indies.

   Lancet, 1982: 639-643.

21. BLAYNEY DW, JAFFE ES, BLATTNER WA et al.

   The human T-cell leukemia/lymphoma virus associated with American adult T-cell leukemia/lymphoma.

   Blood, 1983; 62: 401-405.

22. BUNN PA, SCHECHTER GP, JAFFE E et al.

   Clinical course of retrovirus-associated adult T-cell lymphoma in the United States.

   N Engl J Med, 1983; 309: 257-264.

23. YOSHIDA M, SEIKI M, YAMAGUCHI K, TAKATSUKI K

   Monoclonal integration of human T-cell leukemia provirus in all primary tumors of adult T-cell leukemia suggests causative role of human T-cell leukemia virus in the disease.

   Proc Natl Acad Sci USA, 1984; 81: 2534-2537.

24. BLATTNER WA, NOMURA A, CLARK JW et al.

   Modes of transmission and evidence for viral latency from studies of human T-cell lymphotropic virus type I in Japanese migrant populations in Hawaii.

   Proc Natl Acad Sci USA, 1986; 83: 4895-4898.

25. SHIMOYAMA M, KAGAMI Y, SHIMOTOHNO K et al.

   Adult T-cell leukemia/lymphoma not associated with human T-cell leukemia virus type I.

   Proc Natl Acad Sci USA, 1986; 83: 4524-4528.

26. GIBBS WN, LOFTERS WS, CAMPBELL M et al.

   Non-Hodgkin's lymphoma in Jamaica and its relation to adult T-cell lymphoma.

   Ann Intern Med, 1987; 106: 361-368.

27. KWOK S, EHRLICH G, POIESZ B, KALISH R, SNINSKY JJ

   Enzymatic amplification of HTLV-I viral sequences from peripheral blood mononuclear cells and infected tissues.

   Blood, 1987; 72: 1117-1123.

28. SEIKI M, HATTORI S, HIRAYAMA Y, YOSHIDA M

   Human adult T-cell leukemia virus: Complete nucleotide sequence of the provirus genome integrated in leukemia cell DNA.

   Proc Natl Acad Sci USA, 1983; 80: 3618-3622.

29. VARMUS H

   Regulation of HIV and HTLV gene expression.

   Genes & Development, 1988; 2: 1055-1062.

30. SODROSKI JG, ROSEN CA, HASELTINE WA

   Transacting transcriptional activation of the long terminal repeat of human T-lymphotropic viruses in infected cells.

   Science, 1984; 225: 381-384.

31. HATTORI T, UCHIYAMA T, TOIBANA T, TAKATSUKI K, UCHINO H

   Surface phenotype of Japanese adult T-cell leukemia cells characterized by monoclonal antibodies.

   Blood, 1981; 58: 645-653.

32. MORIMOTO C, MATSUYAMA T, OSHIGE C et al.

   Functional and phenotypic studies of Japanese adult T-cell leukemia cells.

   J Clin Invest, 1985; 75: 836-843.

33. HARPER ME, KAPLAN MH, MARSELLE LM et al.

   Concomitant infection with HTLV-I and HTLV-III in a patient with T8 lymphoproliferative disease.

   N Engl J Med, 1986; 315: 1073-1078.

34. MATSUOKA M, HATTORI T, CHOSA T et al.

   T3 surface molecules on adult T-cell leukemia cells are modulated in vivo.

   Blood, 1986; 67: 1070-1076.

35. MATSUOKA M, HAGIYA M, HATTORI T et al.
Gene rearrangements of T-cell receptor β and γ chains in HTLV-I infected primary neoplastic T cells.
Leukemia, 1988; 2: 84-90.

36. DEPPER JM, LEONARD WJ, KRONKE M, WALDMANN TA, GREENE WC
Augmented T-cell growth factor receptor expression in HTLV-1-infected human leukemic T cells.
J Immunol, 1984; 133: 1691-1696.

37. ARIMA N, DAITOKU Y, OHGAKI S et al.
Autocrine growth of interleukin 2-producing leukemic cells in a patient with adult T-cell leukemia.
Blood, 1986; 68: 779-782.

38. NOWELL PC, FINAN JB, CLARK JW, SARIN PS, GALLO RC
Karyotypic differences between primary cultured and cell lines from tumors with the human T-cell leukemia virus.
J Natl Cancer Inst, 1984; 73: 849-852.

39. FRANCHINI G, WONG-STAAL F, GALLO RC
Human T-cell leukemia virus (HTLV-1) transcripts in fresh and cultured cells of patients with adult T-cell leukemia.
Proc Natl Acad Sci USA, 1984; 81: 6207-6211.

40. UMADOME H, UCHIYAMA T, HORI Y et al.
Close association between interleukin 2-receptor mRNA expression and human T-cell leukemia/lymphoma virus type I viral RNA expression in short-term cultured leukemic cells from adult T-cell leukemia patients.
J Clin Invest, 1988; 81: 52-61.

41. KOZURU M, UIKE N, TAKEICHI N et al.
The possible mode of escape of adult T-cell leukemia cells from antibody-dependent cellular cytotoxity.
Br J Haematol, 1989; 72: 502-506.

42. SINANGIL F, HARADA S, PURTILO DT, VOLSKY DJ
Host cell range of adult T-cell leukemia virus I. Viral infectivity and binding to various cells as detected by flow cytometry.
Int J Cancer, 1985; 36: 191-198.

43. KRICHBAUM-STENGER K, POIESZ BJ, KELLER P et al.
Specific adsorption of HTLV-1 to various target human and animal cells.
Blood, 1987; 70: 1303-1311.

44. GAZZOLO L, DUC DODON M
Direct activation of resting T lymphocytes by human T-lymphotropic virus type I.
Nature, 1987; 326: 714-716.

45. DUC DODON M, BERNARD A, GAZZOLO L
Peripheral T-lymphocyte activation by human T-cell leukemia virus type I interferes with CD2 but not with the CD3/TCR pathway.
J Virol, 1989; 63: 834-842.

46. MACCHI B, POPOVIC M, ALLAVENA P et al.
In vitro *susceptibility of different human T-cell subpopulations and resistance of large granular lymphocytes to HTLV-I infection.*
Int J Cancer, 1987; 40: 1-6.

47. MAEDA M, SHIMIZU A, IKUTA K et al.
Origin of human T-lymphotropic virus I-positive T cell lines in adult T-cell leukemia.
J Exp Med, 1985; 162: 2169-2174.

48. YARCHOAN RH, GUO G, REITZ M, MOLYISH A, MITSUYA H, BRODER S
Alterations in cytotoxic and helper T cell function after infection of T-cell clones with human T-cell leukemia virus type I.
J Clin Invest, 1986; 77: 1466-1470.

49. SEIKI M, INOUE J, TAKEDA T, YOSHIDA M
Direct evidence that p40x of human T-cell leukemia virus type I is a trans-acting transcriptional activator.
EMBO J, 1986; 5: 561-565.

50. INOUE J, SEIKI M, TANIGUCHI T, TSURU S, YOSHIDA M
Induction of interleukin 2-receptor gene expression by p40x encoded by human T-cell leukemia virus type I.
EMBO J, 1986; 5: 2883-2888.

51. CROSS SL, FEINBERG MB, WOLF JB, HOLBROOK NJ, WONG-STAAL F, LEONARD WJ
Regulation of the human interleukin-2 receptor a chain promoter by the transactivator gene of HTLV-1.
Cell, 1987; 49: 47-55.

52. SIEKEVITZ M, FEINBERG MB, HOLBROOK N, WONG-STAAL F, GREENE WC
Activation of interleukin 2 and interleukin-2 receptor (Tac) promoter expression by the trans-activator (tat) gene product of human T-cell leukemia virus type I.
Proc Natl Acad Sci USA, 1987; 84: 5389-5393.

53. WANO Y, FEINBERG M, HOSKING JB, BOGERD H, GREENE WC
Stable expression of the tax gene of type I human T-cell leukemia virus in human T cells activates specific cellular genes involved in growth.
Proc Natl Acad Sci USA, 1988; 85: 9733-9737.

54. NAGATA K, OHTANI K, NAKAMURA M, SUGAMURA K
Activation of endogenous c-fos proto-oncogene expression by human T-cell leukemia virus type I encoded p40x protein in the human T-cell line, Jurkat.
J Virol, 1989; 63: 3220-3226.

55. MARUYAMA M, SHIBUYA H, HARADA H
et al.

Evidence for aberrant activation of the interleukin-2 autocrine loop by HTLV-I-encoded p40x and T3/Ti complex triggering.

Cell, 1987; 48: 343-350.

56. YOSHIDA M, SEIKI M

Recent advances in the molecular biology of HTLV-1: trans-activation of viral and cellular genes.

Ann Rev Immunol, 1987; 5: 541-559.

57. FUKUHARA S, HINUMA Y, GOTCH YI,
UCHINO H

Chromosome aberrations in T lymphocytes carrying adult T-cell leukemia-associated antigens (ATLA) from healthy adults.

Blood, 1983; 61: 205-207.

Burkitt's lymphoma and Epstein-Barr virus-associated lymphoid malignancies : models for lymphomagenesis

F. REYES

Introduction

Epstein-Barr virus (EBV), a ubiquitous virus that infects populations in all parts of the world, has been associated with two human malignancies: Burkitt's lymphoma and nasopharyngeal carcinoma. EBV was first isolated from a Burkitt's lymphoma culture, suggesting that this tumour was virally induced. More recently, several EBV-associated lymphoid malignancies have been described that occur in the context of immune deficiency, including AIDS.

Relationship between EBV and B-cell differentiation

EBV is a herpes group virus that has a dual tropism for epithelial cells of the oropharynx and B lymphocytes (1-3). EBV was first identified within a malignant lymphoid cell line established from a patient with "endemic" (African) Burkitt's lymphoma (BL). EBV is a potent polyclonal mitogen of normal B lymphocytes equipped with an EBV receptor identical to the C3d receptor (4), now termed the CD21 molecule.

Infection by EBV is followed within a few hours by the presence in the cells of nuclear virus-encoded proteins termed EBNA (Epstein-Barr nuclear antigens) and by the entry of infected lymphocytes into the S phase of the cell cycle (2,5). Subsequently a small number of the target cells will sustain active viral replication leading to the production of new infectious viral particles (virions) and cell death (whose occurrence in epithelial cells accounts for the excretion of virus in the saliva of EBV-carriers).

Alternatively, most of the target B cells will sustain a non-lytic, latent infection based on the persistence of multiple copies of the EBV genome as circularly closed episomal DNA (whereas in EBV virions, DNA has a linear configuration). This episomal genome integration is responsible for intense cell proliferation (6). *In vitro*, such latent (non-productive) infection accounts for the immortalization of B lymphocytes into a permanent lymphoblastoid cell line (LCL) composed of polyclonal diploid B cells maturing into Ig-synthesizing cells. Thus EBV provides the signals necessary for the activation and continuous proliferation of B cells in blood and peripheral lymphoid tissues (7).

The linear virion form of EBV DNA has variable numbers of direct tandem repeats at each terminus. Consequently, the terminal restriction endonuclease fragments, as well as the fused terminal fragments in the episomal form, are heterogeneous in size. Consequently, hybridization with terminus-specific probes reveals the viral genome configuration (circular/latent vs linear/replicative). It also permits assessment of tissue clonality in EBV-infected cells. A single band representing identical EBV-joined termini is deleted in the cells of monoclonal proliferations, such as nasopharyngeal carcinoma and BL, whereas polyclonal LCL contain multiple forms of the joined termini (8,9). Molecular studies have also identified several EBV genes, one of which codes for the major protein EBNA1 responsible for the maintenance of the viral DNA episomal state (10). A second gene, coding for EBNA2, is required for the immortalization of B cells, in conjunction with a gene coding for the "latent membrane protein" termed LMP (10-13). Expression of LMP by latently infected B cells is believed to account for their recognition by cytotoxic T cells and thereby for their control *in vivo*. In addition, the EBNA2 gene induces the expression by B cells of the CD23 activation molecule (12), the soluble form of which may act as an autocrine growth factor (15,16). Thus EBV genome simultaneously codes for proteins which are necessary for both the continuous proliferation of B cells and their long-term control by immune cytotoxic T cells. Following *in vivo* primary infection, EBV particles generated through the lytic pathway elicit a humoral immune response accounting for antibodies such as anti-VCA (viral capsid antigen). The non-productive (latent) pathway leads to a self-limited polyclonal B-cell expansion as a result of efficient T-cell control (2,3,17). Primary EBV infection is usually clinically silent; in some cases it may be accompanied by the clinical symptoms of infectious mononucleosis. The disease is characterized by the early proliferation of latently infected B cells followed by an expansion of controlling T cells which, in blood, gives rise to the designation of "mononucleosis" (2,3,6).

Later on, the healthy carrier-state is defined by:
1) continuous production of virus mostly by epithelial cells and infection of adjacent B cells in the oropharynx; and
2) killing of latently infected B cells by cytotoxic T cells.

This steady-state equilibrium is characterized by:
1) the persistence of low titres of anti-VCA and anti-EBNA IgG antibodies; and
2) the relative ease with which LCL can be established from seropositive individuals. As a consequence this equilibrium can be perturbed by impairment of the T-cell control.

Burkitt's lymphoma (BL)

BL is a well-defined entity based on morphological, phenotypic and genotypic features. The initial cytological and histopathological descriptions are still essential: BL comprises a monomorphous proliferation of blastic cells with a basophilic cytoplasm containing clear vacuoles and a regular nucleus (18). Malignant cells have a B-cell phenotype with monotypic surface IgM, usually no IgD and no cytoplasmic Ig (19). Monoclonality has been further confirmed by gene rearrangement studies (20) and more recently by the detection of a homogeneous EBV DNA episomal population upon hybridization with terminus-specific probes (8,9), suggesting that BL is a clonal expansion of a single EBV-infected target cell. BL malignant cells have an abnormal karyotype showing reciprocal translocations of chromosome 8 (band q24) with chromosome 2, 14 or 22. It was subsequently shown that the genes on both loci participating in the translocation were the Ig genes on chromosome 14, 2 or 22 and the *c-myc* gene on chromosome 8 [reviewed in (6,21,22)]. Thus the cytogenetic abnormalities of BL appear similar to those of plasmacytomas of Balb/c and NZB mice in which a reciprocal translocation also involves the *c-myc* and Ig genes.

Relationship between BL and EBV

BL was first described as a tumour occurring at high frequency in children from Central Africa (so-called "endemic" BL). Because of its epidemiological characteristics the tumour was suspected of having a viral a etiology and this led to the isolation of EBV from a BL malignant cell-line (23). The viral hypothesis was further supported by several observations (1):

1) children with endemic BL had high titres of anti-EBV IgG antibodies and conversely high antibody titres in young children from endemic areas predicted the development of BL;

2) EBNA (detected by immunofluorescence) and EBV genome (detected by genetic probes) were detected in cells of virtually all BL cases in Africa; and

3) EBV was isolated in several permanent cell-lines easily grown from BL tissue biopsies.

The viral hypothesis was subsequently strengthened by the following findings:

1) EBV could immortalize normal B lymphocytes *in vitro* (see above);

2) EBV could induce malignant lymphoma when injected into primates (24); and

3) EBNA and EBV genome were detected in malignant lymphoproliferative disorders (detailed below) that were reported to occur in immune deficiencies, either primary, or secondary to immunosuppressive therapy and to HIV infection (3,25-28).

Taken together, these data suggested that EBV exhibited some oncogenic potential and that BL could be a virally induced tumour. However, it appeared that the association between EBV and BL was not simple and that additional cellular changes had to occur in malignant BL cells: these cells displayed a monoclonal pattern of growth and chromosomal translocations in contrast with non-malignant EBV-immortalized LCL. Nevertheless, it became accepted that BL might occur as a final consequence of the reactivation of latent EBV infection by some immune-deficient state.

Relationship between chromosomal translocations and clonal selection

As stated above, BL is defined by specific chromosomal changes [reviewed in (6,21,22)]. The first described and most common translocation involves the long arm of chromosome 14 (band q32) and of chromosome 8 (band q24): t(8;14) (q24;q32) (*fig. 1*). Subsequently, two other variant translocations were described, t(2;8) (p11;q24) and t(8;22) (q24;q11), respectively. In a given BL cell, the reciprocal translocation involves the Ig non-productive allele, leaving the untranslocated allele fully functional, e.g. rearranging Ig VDJ genes and encoding surface IgM molecules. With few exceptions (29), the variety of translocation correlates with the light chain isotype expressed by the BL cell (30). Thus variants t(2;8) and t(8;22) are found in IgM-Kappa and IgM-Lambda cells respectively, with the common t(8;14) being found in either cell.

Chromosomal translocations, first defined by cytogenetic studies, can be further analysed at the molecular level using cDNA probes specific for Ig and *c-myc* gene subsegments. The *c-myc* proto-oncogene is a nuclear phosphoprotein with DNA binding activity whose function, although not fully understood, involves regulation of cell proliferation (31). It was originally defined as the cellular homologue of the gene transduced by avian oncogenic retroviruses. The *c-myc* gene, which is located at band q24 of chromosome 8, consists of one non-coding (1) and two coding (2,3) exons. The *c-myc* locus is implicated in all BL cases although in different ways, according to the type of translocation. In t(8;14), *c-myc* moves from chromosome 8 to chromosome 14. *C-myc* breakpoints are always located 5' (upstream) of exons 2 and 3, thus leaving the coding region undamaged; the breakpoint on chromosome 14 is usually located around the γ switch region. As a result, the *c-myc* gene is fused to an Ig heavy-chain gene, in head-to-head fashion (5'-5') (*fig. 2*). In variants t(2;8) and t(8;22), the *c-myc* gene remains on chromosome 8 and the Ig light chain loci move to chromosome 8. The breakpoint on chromosome 8 is always downstream (3') of exon 3 and that on chromosomes 2 or 22 is 5' of C κ or C λ. Thus *c-myc* is again located 5' of an Ig constant region, now in head-to-tail fashion (5'-3').

It follows that in addition to cytogenetic studies, the translocations/rearrangements of the *c-myc* locus can be identified by molecular genetic methods using probes specific for *c-myc* exons and appropriate restriction enzymes.

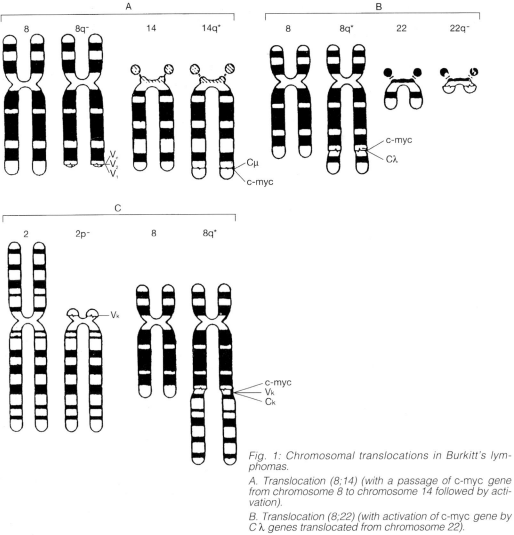

Fig. 1: Chromosomal translocations in Burkitt's lymphomas.

A. Translocation (8;14) (with a passage of c-myc gene from chromosome 8 to chromosome 14 followed by activation).

B. Translocation (8;22) (with activation of c-myc gene by C λ genes translocated from chromosome 22).

C. Translocation (2;8) (with activation of c-myc gene by V κ C κ genes translocated from chromosome 2).

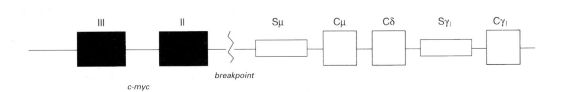

Fig. 2: Chromosomal translocations (8;14) in Burkitt's lymphoma. After deletion of exon 1, the c-myc oncogene is translocated upstream of a switch region of the heavy chain in a head-to-head position (junction between 5' extremities of both chromosomes).

Regardless of the translocation variant, high levels of *c-myc* RNA are found in BL cells. *C-myc* transcripts are derived from the translocated allele whereas the normal allele is transcriptionally silent, suggesting that transcriptional regulation is important in normal cells (31). The mechanisms of *c-myc* deregulation in BL cells remain to be elucidated, although deregulation obviously appears as a consequence of the fusion of *c-myc* with active Ig loci.

It has been generally accepted that the constitutive (non-regulated) expression of myc protein is a critical step in the development of uncontrolled clonal cell proliferation leading to BL. The role of *c-myc* in normal cell growth regulation is beyond the scope of this review. As an example, a rapid increase in myc expression occurs when Go cells of several lineages are sti-mulated to enter the cell cycle by mitogens or growth factors (31). To test the hypothesis that deregulated myc expression predisposes to neoplasia, several strains of transgenic mice have been developed that carry the *c-myc* gene linked to different regula-tors (32). The association between *c-myc* deregulation and BL led to the develop-ment of strains of mice with constitutive expression of *c-myc* restricted to the lymphoid lineage, by using transgenes linking *c-myc* to Ig enhancers, such as *E-myc*. This model proved remarkably potent in inducing monoclonal B cell proliferations. However, several finding imply that deregulated myc expression is not the only critical factor in inducing lymphoma, suggesting that additional oncogenes must collaborate. This model also offered the pos-sibility of studying the pre-lymphoma state in *E-myc* transgenic mice. The most conspicuous change was a poly-clonal expansion of pre-B cells and, to a lesser extent, of mature B cells. Interestingly, pre-lymphomatous *E-myc* B cells in transgenic mice did not prove to grow more easily in culture than their normal counterpart or to exhibit unlimited proliferative capacity (as do BL cells). Thus the *c-myc* gene cannot be considered, *per se*, as an "immortalizing" gene. This again emphasizes the fact that oncogenesis must be a multistep process involving several cooperating factors.

A multistep scenario for the development of BL

Although BL cases have been recognized outside Africa (so-called "sporadic" BL, which, as described below, is not consistent-ly associated with EBV), the EBV-associat-ed African ("endemic") BL first led to the suggestion by Klein (21) that tumours developed in three steps with the following sequence of events:

1) EBV-induced immortalisation of B cells following primary infection;

2) polyclonal expansion of EBV-positive B cells, possibly as a result of malaria co-infection; and

3) occurrence of a chromosomal transloca-tion leading to the development of a malig-nant clone through *c-myc* deregulation.

This model has been very useful in that it stressed the importance of the co-operation of two factors - EBV and *c-myc* -, thus stimu-lating recent molecular research, part of which has been described above. In addition, the EBV-associated lymphoproliferative dis-orders occurring in the context of immune deficiency (see below) were shown to result from progression from an initial polyclonal expansion towards an oligo- or monoclonal process (28). This view was reinforced by the finding that, in some AIDS-related lym-phomas, a step of pre-lymphomatous multi-ple clonal B-cell expansion - presumably induced by EBV reactivation - preceded development of a monoclonal process in which the *c-myc* locus was rearranged, lead-ing to malignant lymphoma (27). Further *in vitro* experiments involving transfer of an activated *c-myc* gene into EBV-immortalized B lymphocytes from AIDS patients showed that co-operation between EBV and *c-myc* was sufficient to induce the malignant trans-formation of B cells, as revealed by growth in semi-solid media, as well as reduced growth factor requirements and tumourigenicity in nude mice (33). This *in vitro* transforming activity of *c-myc* on EBV-infected cells was felt to recapitulate the steps involved in *in vivo* tumourigenesis, giving additional sup-port to the hypothesis that the increased num-ber of proliferative B cells produced by EBV infection might increase the probability of chromosomal translocation leading to a fully malignant phenotype.

Since massive EBV infection in individuals with immune deficiency very likely results from impaired T-cell immunity to the virus (17,34), it is of interest that a defect in the control of EBV-infected B cells by cytotoxic T cells was documented during malaria (35), thereby providing support to step 2 of Klein's hypothesis which postulated that co-infection with malaria favoured the polyclonal increase of EBV-positive B cells.

However, in view of several epidemiological, cytogenetical and molecular arguments that have become available during recent years, an alternative hypothesis must be put forward. It should first be recalled that in 5% of "endemic" BL in Africa, and, most importantly, in 80% of "sporadic" BL cases that occur in low-incidence areas such as Europe and the United States, EBNA and EBV genomes are not detected in malignant cells although they carry specific translocations (6). It is also remarkable that *in vitro* EBV-induced LCL do not display the BL chromosomal changes even if cells are kept proliferating for a long time. Finally, the study of an increasing number of cases with EBV-associated B-cell proliferative disorders developing in patients with immune deficiency has shown that the situation is more complex than initially thought and that BL should not be considered simply a direct consequence of the impairment of immune control of a latent EBV infection.

EBV-associated B-cell lymphoproliferative disorders (BLPD) and HIV-related lymphomas

The importance of immune surveillance has been stressed by the observation that patients with immunodeficiencies were prone to developing uncontrolled proliferations of EBV-positive lymphoid cells, usually classified as diffuse non-Burkitt lymphoma. As an example, such proliferations following primary infection were fatal in children with a genetically determined disorder, named X-linked lymphoproliferative disorder (36). Subsequently, the frequent occurrence of lymphoma in patients receiving immunosuppressive therapy for cardiac or renal allograft was recognized (37). More recently, patients receiving bone marrow transplantation (especially in the context of mismatching and/or T depletion) have been identified as having predisposition to lymphoid malignancy, most often of donor origin (38,39). A similar predisposition was again recently reported in patients with congenital immunodeficiency and is suspected in patients immunocompromised by intensive chemotherapy regimens for acute leukaemia (40).

Moreover, it is now well established that individuals with HIV infection are at increased risk of acquiring malignant lymphoma (27,41-43). HIV DNA sequences are not detectable in lymphoma cells, suggesting that HIV does not play a direct role in lymphomagenesis (27,44). HIV-related lymphomas are aggressive B-cell tumours and they include - besides true BL carrying the specific translocation - a number of cases classified as diffuse large-cell lymphoma. The latter are in many respects similar to those described above and it has become clear that immunodeficiency, whether congenital, iatrogenic, or acquired, predisposes to lymphoid malignancies that represent histologically and phenotypically a spectrum of disease ranging from polymorphous and polyclonal to monomorphous and monoclonal (non-Burkitt-type) proliferations (38,45-47). Collectively these neoplasms have been referred to as BLPD (48). It should be noted that, regardless of histological and phenotypic appearance, they behave in a clinically malignant fashion. Molecular genetic analysis of different biopsy sites in individual patients has shown the multiclonal origin of transplant-associated BLPD and, in some cases, the presence of distinct subclones within individual lesions (39,49), a situation similar to that of malignant lymphoma induced by injection of EBV in primates (50). The observations are consistent with the proposal that BLPD initiate as polyclonal and progress towards a more restricted clonality as shown by analysis of immunoglobulin gene rearrangement and EBV genomic determinants (9,27,49).

Most importantly, the majority of BLPD are associated with EBV (38-40,46,47,49,51), as revealed by the detection of EBNA and multiple copies of EBV genome in proliferating B cells. However, neither chromosomal translocation of the BL type nor rearrangement of *c-myc* were detected in several cases (38,47). Thus EBV probably plays a primary role in the pathogenesis of BLPD developing in immunocompromised hosts.

The same holds true for some AIDS-associated lymphoma although the situation is more heterogeneous. It has been observed that the non-Burkitt type of AIDS-related lymphoma, which we classify here as BLPD, occurs in patients with severe immune deficiency and is rapidly fatal (42). A French co-operative study of a large series of patients has recently confirmed that such non-BL malignancies are usually positive for EBV markers and lack both chromosomal translocation and *c-myc* rearrangement (52, Lenoir G, personal communication). On the other hand, true BL (also termed "small non-cleaved") also account for certains AIDS-related lymphomas. In contrast to BLPD, they occur in HIV-positive patients whose immune function is not yet severely impaired, e.g. without overt immune deficiency. They all display one of the three BL specific translocations and *c-myc* amplification; however, the presence of EBV genome is not consistently demonstrated. Thus some AIDS-related cases of true BL are identical to the EBV-negative "sporadic" BL. This provides evidence that specific BL translocation and *c-myc* amplification also occur in B cells in the absence of overt underlying immune deficiency and reactivation of a latent EBV infection. Such malignant cells can be grown in culture, showing that the possibility of establishment of BL cell lines is not limited to EBV-associated cases (6).

Conclusion

In view of all that has been learned since the pioneer studies of African BL, an alternative model has been proposed by Lenoir (6) in which BL also develops in three steps, although in a different sequence:

1) polyclonal activation of the B-cell system, as a result of persistent stimulation by malaria, or HIV infection;

2) chromosomal translocation resulting in Ig/myc juxtaposition, making some B cells responsive to growth factors in the absence of antigenic stimulus. It is assumed that such cells are not yet immortalized and would presumably die unless a third event occurs;

3) infection by EBV of B cells with constitutive *c-myc* expression, resulting in its autonomous growth. This step could also be reached through other unknown factors in the case of EBV-negative BL.

Chromosomal juxtaposition and EBV infection of a cell remain two critical steps in this model. The hypothesis is consistent with several items of experimental data (see above) showing that myc expression alone is not sufficient for cell proliferation. *C-myc* should be regarded rather as a competence factor making cells responsive to growth signals such as the autocrine circuits established by EBV in B cells (33). Thus EBV would be critical for complementing myc functions. This model is also consis-tent with experimental data suggesting that, upon EBV infection, cells carrying the *c-myc* translocation downregulate expression of EBNA and LMP, as well as LFA-1 adhesion molecules, thus possibly escaping recognition by specific cytotoxic T cells (53,54).

In Lenoir's model, malaria plays a critical role not as a cause of T-cell deficiency but rather as a cause of extensive activation of host B cells. It is indeed remarkable that EBV-associated polyclonal BLPD have not been observed in African populations at risk for endemic BL. On the other hand, the study of pre-malignant lesions in HIV-infected patients should help our future understanding of the development of either BLPD or BL.

References

1. BIRD AG, BRITTON S
   The relationship between Epstein-Barr virus and lymphoma.
   Semin Hematol, 1982; 19: 285-297.

2. EPSTEIN MA, MORGAN AJ
   Clinical consequences of Epstein-Barr virus infection and possible control by an anti-viral vaccine.
   Clin Exp Immunol, 1983; 53: 257-265.

3. PURTILLO DT
   Immune deficiency, Epstein-Barr virus (EBV) and lymphoproliferative disorders.
   New York and London: Plenum Medical Book Company. 1984.

4. FINGEROTH JD, WEISS JJ, TEDDIER TF, STROMINGER JL, BIRO PA, FEARON DT
   Epstein-Barr virus receptor of human B lymphocytes is the C3d receptor CR2.
   Proc Acad. Sci USA, 1984; 81: 4510-4514.

5. WOLF H
   Biology of Epstein-Barr virus.
   New-York and London: Plenum Medical Book Company. 1984.

6. LENOIR GM, BORNKAMM GW
   Burkitt's lymphoma, a human cancer model for the study of the multistep development of cancer: proposal for a new scenario.
   Adv Viral Oncology, 1987; 7: 173-206.

7. FRADE R, CREVON MC, BAREL M et al.
   Enhancement of human B-cell proliferation by an antibody to the C3d receptor, the GP 140 molecule.
   Eur J Immunol, 1985; 73: 15-19.

8. RAAB-TRAUB N, FLYNN K
   The structure of the termini of the Epstein-Barr virus as a marker of clonal cellular proliferation.
   Cell, 1986; 47: 883-889.

9. PATTON DF, WILKOWSKI CW, HANSEN CA et al.
   Epstein-Barr virus-determined clonality in post-transplant lymphoproliferative disease.
   Transplantation, 1990; 49: 1080-1084.

10. YATES J, WARREN N, SUDGEN B
    Stable replication of plasmids derived from Epstein-Barr virus in various mammalian cells.
    Nature, 1985; 313: 812-815.

11. WANG F, GREGORY CD, ROWE M et al.
    An EBV membrane protein expressed in immortalized lymphocytes transforms established rodent cells.
    Cell, 1985; 43: 831-840.

12. WANG F, GREGORY CD, ROWE M et al.
    Epstein-Barr virus nuclear antigen-2 specifically induces expression of the B-cell activation antigen CD23.
    Proc Natl Acad Sci USA, 1987; 84: 3452-3456.

13. YOUNG L, ALFIERI C, HENNESSY K et al.
    Expression of Epstein-Barr virus transformation-associated genes in tissues from patients with EBV lymphoproliferative disease.
    N Engl J Med, 1989; 321: 1080-1085.

14. HAMMERSCHMIDT W, SUGDEN B
    Genetic analysis of immortalizing functions of Epstein-Barr virus in human B lymphocytes.
    Nature, 1989; 340: 393-397.

15. GORDON J, LEY SC, MELAMED MD, ENGLISH LS, HUGUES-JONES NC
    Immortalized B lymphocytes produce B-cell growth factor.
    Nature, 1984; 310: 145-147.

16. KAWATABE T, TAKAMI M, HOSODA M et al.
    Regulation of Fc R2/ CD23 gene expression by cytokines and specific ligands (IgE and anti-Fc R2 monoclonal antibody): Variable regulation depending on cell types.
    J Immunol, 1988; 141: 1376-1382.

17. KONTTINEN YT, BLUESTEIN HG, ZVAIFER NJ
    Regulation of the growth of Epstein-Barr virus-infected B cells.
    J Immunol, 1985; 134: 2287-2291.

18. WRIGHT DH
    Cytology and histochemistry of the Burkitt's lymphoma.
    Br J Cancer, 1963; 17: 50-55.

19. GUGLIELMI P, PREUD'HOMME JL
    Immunoglobulin expression in human lymphoblastoid cell lines with early B-cell features.
    Scand J Immunol, 1981; 13: 303-307.

20. HENNI T, GAULARD PH, DIVINE M et al.
    The respective contribution of the immunophenotypic and immunogenotypic methods for the determination of clonality and lineage.
    Blood, 1988; 72: 1937-1943.

21. KLEIN G
    Specific chromosomal translocations and the genesis of B-cell-derived tumors in mice and men.
    Cell, 1983; 32: 311-315.

22. CROCE CM, TSUJIMITO Y, ERICKSON J, NOWELL P
    Chromosome translocations and B-cell neoplasia.
    Lab Invest, 1984; 51: 258-274.

23. EPSTEIN MA, ACHONG BG, BARR YM
    Virus particles in cultured lymphoblasts from Burkitt's lymphoma.
    Lancet, 1964; 1: 702-703.

24. HENLE W, HENLE G
    Epstein-Barr virus human malignancies.
    Adv. Viral Oncology. G. Klein ed. 1985; 5: 201-238.

25. HANTO DW, FRIZZERA G, GAJL-PECZALSKA KJ

Epstein-Barr virus-induced B-cell lymphoma after renal transplantation.

N Engl J Med, 1982; 306: 913-917.

26. MARTIN JP, SHULMAN HM, SCHUBACH WH et al.

Fatal Epstein-Barr virus-associated proliferation of donor B cells after treatment of acute graft-versus-host disease with a murine anti-T-cell antibody.

Ann Intern Med, 1984; 101: 310-315.

27. PELICCI PG, KNOWLES DM, ARLIN ZA et al.

Multiple monoclonal B-cell expansions and c-myc oncogene rearrangements in acquired immune deficiency syndrome related lympho-proliferative disorders.

J Exp Med, 1986; 164: 2049-2076.

28. SHEARE WT, RITZ J, FINEGOLD MJ et al.

Epstein-Barr virus-associated B-cell proliferations of diverse clonal origins after bone-marrow transplantation in a 12-year-old patient with severe combined immunodeficiency.

N Engl J Med, 1985; 312: 1151 1159.

29. RECHAVI G, BENBASSAT I, BERKOWICZ M et al.

Molecular analysis of Burkitt's leukemia in two hemophilic brothers with AIDS.

Blood, 1987; 70: 1713-1717.

30. LENOIR G, PREUD'HOMME JL, BERNHEIM A et al.

Correlation between immunoglobulin light chain expression and variant translocation in Burkitt's lymphoma.

Nature, 1982; 298: 474-476.

31. CORY S

Activation of cellular oncogenes in haemopoietic cells by chromosome translocation.

Adv Cancer Res, 1986; 47: 189-234.

32. CORY S, ADAM JM

Transgenic mice and oncogenesis.

Ann Rev Immunol, 1988; 6: 25-48.

33. LOMBARDI L, NEWCOMB EW, DALLA-FAVERA R

Pathogenesis of Burkitt lymphoma: expression of an activated c-myc oncogene causes the tumorigenic conversion of EBV-infected human B lymphoblasts.

Cell, 1987; 49: 161-170.

34. BIRX DL, REDFIELD RR, TOSATO G

Defective regulation of Epstein-Barr virus infection in patients with acquired immunodeficiency syndrome (AIDS) or AIDS-related disorders.

N Engl J Med, 1986; 14: 8711-8715.

35. WHITTLE HC, BROWN J, MARSH K et al.

T-cell control of Epstein-Barr virus-infected B cells is lost during P. falciparum malaria.

Nature, 1984; 312: 449-451.

36. PURTILLO DT

Malignant lymphoproliferative diseases induced by Epstein-Barr virus in immune-deficient patients, including X-linked, cytogenetic and familial syndromes.

Cancer Genet Cytogenet, 1981; 4: 251-268.

37. PENN I

Malignant lymphomas in organ transplant recipients.

Transplant Proc, 1981; 13: 736-738.

38. SHAPIRO RS, McCLAIN K, FIZZERA G et al.

Epstein-Barr virus associated B-cell lymphoproliferative disorders following bone-marrow transplantation.

Blood, 1988; 71: 1234-1243.

39. ZUTTER MM, MARTIN PJ, SALE GE et al.

Epstein-Barr virus lymphoproliferative disorders after bone-marrow transplantation.

Blood, 1988; 72: 520-529.

40. JONCAS JH, RUSSO P, BROCHU P et al.

Epstein-Barr virus polymorphic B-cell lymphoma associated with leukemia and with congenital immunodeficiencies.

J Clin Oncol, 1990; 8: 378-384.

41. ZIEGLER JL, BECKSTEAD JA, VOLBERDING PA et al.

Non-Hodgkin's lymphoma in 90 homosexual men.

N Engl J Med, 1984; 311: 565-570.

42. KALTER SP, RIGGS SA, CABANILLAS F et al.

Aggressive non-Hodgkin's lymphomas in immuno-compromised homosexual males.

Blood, 1985; 66: 655-659.

43. KNOWLES DM, CHAMULAK GA, SUBAR M et al.

Lymphoid neoplasia associated with the acquired immunodeficiency syndrome (AIDS).

Ann Intern Med, 1988; 108: 744-753.

44. GROOPMAN JE, SULLIVAN JL, MULDER C et al.

Pathogenesis of B-cell lymphoma in a patient with AIDS.

Blood, 1986; 67: 612-617.

45. FRIZZERA G, HANTO DW, GAJL-PECZULSKA KJ et al.

Polymorphic diffuse B-cell hyperplasias and lymphomas in renal transplant recipients.

Cancer Res, 1981; 41: 4262-4279.

46. KNOWLES DM, INGHIRAMI G, UBRIACO A, DALLA-FAVERA R

Molecular genetic analysis of three AIDS-associated neoplasms of uncertain lineage demonstrates their B-cell derivation and the possible pathogenetic role of the Epstein-Barr virus.

Blood, 1989; 73: 792-799.

47. DONHUIJSEN-ANT R, ABKEN H, BORNKAMM G et al.

    Fatal Hodgkin and non-Hodgkin's lymphoma associated with persistent Epstein-Barr virus in four brothers.

    Ann Int Med, 1988; 109: 946-952.

48. SHAPIRO RS

    Epstein-Barr virus-associated B-cell lymphoproliferative disorders in immunodeficiency: meeting the challenge.

    J Clin Oncol, 1990; 8: 371-373.

49. CLEARY M, NALESNIK MA, SHEARER WT, SKLAR J

    Clonal analysis of transplant-associated lymphoproliferations based on the structure of the genomic termini of the Epstein-Barr virus.

    Blood, 1988; 72: 349-352.

50. CLEARY ML, EPSTEIN MA, FINERTY S et al.

    Individual tumors of multifocal EB virus-induced malignant lymphomas in tamarins arise from different B-cell clones.

    Science, 1985; 228: 722-725.

51. LIST AF, GRECO A, VOGLER LB

    Lymphoproliferative diseases in immunocompromised hosts : the role of Epstein-Barr virus.

    J Clin Oncol, 1987; 5: 1673-1689.

52. RAPHAEL M, GENTILHOMME O, TULLIEZ M, BRYON PA, DIEBOLD J

    Histopathology of the high-grade non-Hodgkin's lymphomas in AIDS.

    Arch Pathol Lab Med, 1990, in press.

53. KLEIN G

    The Ig/myc translocation in Burkitt's lymphoma is a rate-limiting step in tumor development with multiple phenotypic consequences.

    Progress in Immunology, 1989; 7: 464-467.

54. INGHIRAMI G, GRIGNANI F, STERNAS L et al.

    Down-regulation of LFA-1 adhesion receptors by c-myc oncogene in human B-lymphoblastoid cells.

    Science, 1990; 260: 682-685.

t(14;18) translocation and non-Hodgkin's lymphomas

P. SOLAL-CELIGNY

In 1979, Fukuhara et al. identified t(14;18) translocation as a non-random event in NHL and noticed its association with a follicular (nodular) architecture (1). Then, in 1984, Tsujimoto et al. cloned the breakpoint of t(14;18) junction (2). Since these first studies, molecular biology has allowed many important insights into the role of t(14;18) in the development of follicular NHL (3).

Analysis of t(14;18) translocation

The t(14;18) is a reciprocal head-to-tail translocation between the long arms of chromosomes 14 and 18. The breakpoint on chromosome 14 is located on q32, in most cases within or immediately 5' to the joining region (J_H) of the Ig heavy-chain (IgH) gene (4,5) (fig. 1), at the position where the D segments are recombined with the J_H segments during DJ joining to produce an active heavy-chain gene. In t(14;18) cells, D_H segments mediate junction with 18q at the der(18) breakpoint, while Ig joining (J_H) segments fuse with 18q at the der(14) breakpoint (6).

The breakpoint on chromosome 18 is located on q21, on a region called bcl-2 (B cell leukaemia/lymphoma 2). This region has been considered as a proto-oncogene since:

- it is conserved among species (7,8);

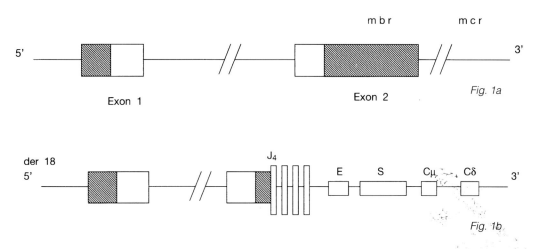

Fig. 1: Schematic view of the bcl-2 oncogene on chromosome 18 (fig.1a) and after translocation on chromosome 14 (fig. 1b). In this case, the breakpoint is located on the mbr region of bcl-2 exon 2 with junction with a J4 gene on chromosome 14.

- it is expressed in normal B cells at certain stages of maturation (mostly at the pre-B cell stage with down-regulation during B-cell differentiation) (7,8) or after stimulation of T and B lymphocytes with mitogens (7); and

- it is increased in its expression in certain tumour cells, i.e. NHL with t(14;18) translocation (9,10).

The bcl-2 gene is composed of 2 exons separated by an intron of more than 50 kb (11) (*fig. 1*). Each exon contains a non-encoding region (on the 5' side on exon 1 and on the 3' side on exon 2) and a region translated into protein. The breakpoints on chromosome 18q21 involved in t(14;18) translocation are located on remarkably limited regions of the gene. Most of them (approximately 60 to 70%) are located on a 500 bp region called the *major breakpoint region* (mbr) in the untranslated part of exon 2 (2,4,10) (*fig. 1*). Twenty to 30% of the breakpoints are located on the *minor cluster region*, up to 20 kb downstream of exon 2 (12) (*fig. 1*). In rarer cases, the breakpoint is located 5' to the bcl-2 gene (13). Whatever the breakpoint location on chromosome 18, the encoding regions of exon 1 and exon 2 of the bcl-2 gene are not disrupted but translocated on chromosome 14.

In cells containing a t(14;18) translocation, the bcl-2 gene is juxtaposed with the IgH gene and this results in deregulated expression of the bcl-2 gene (8,9). The normal bcl-2 gene is repressed but the hybrid IgH-bcl-2 gene is expressed, encoding for an abnormal hybrid mRNA (10,13). In man, bcl-2 transcripts produce 2 proteins, p26 bcl-2α and p22 bcl-2β, by variation of the splicing site (10,11,14,15). Bcl-2β is an integral-membrane protein mostly localized on perinuclear membranes and mitochondria, inserted by its C-terminal hydrophobic domain (14). Haldar et al. have shown that bcl-2α protein has striking identities with several regions of the Ha-Ras or G protein which belongs to the GTP-binding G protein family (16). This result has not been confirmed (17).

Transfection experiments on NIH3T3 cells have confirmed the oncogenic properties of bcl-2 gene (17). The mechanisms by which bcl-2 protein exerts its oncogenic effects are unknown. Unlike other transmembrane oncogenic products (such as v-erb-B protein), bcl-2 protein has no tyrosine-kinase properties. Bcl-2 can cooperate with *c-myc* protein to promote the immortalization of pre-B cells in culture (18,19). In B cells transfected with bcl-2 gene alone, survival was prolonged but cells remained in G_0 phase (18). A fusion gene Ig-bcl-2 transfected in mouse embryonic cells secondarily induces the development of an atypical lymphoid hyperplasia, involving predominantly centrofollicular cells (20). This fusion gene also increases the life span of mature polyclonal B cells (20). Human B cells infected with Epstein-Barr virus and transfected with bcl-2 gene produce unusually high levels of bcl-2 protein and have a growth advantage compared to EBV-infected B cells not transfected with bcl-2 (21).

These biological properties are consistent with the indolent course of follicular lymphomas. Thus bcl-2 may play a role in transduction of mitogenic signals, either transiently during certain normal stages of differentiation, or continuously in t(14;18) B cells, thus favouring a malignant growth. Some preliminary - but very interesting - studies have shown that bcl-2 protein(s) may inhibit *programmed cell death* (apoptosis) of B lymphocytes (23). The transformation of follicular NHL into aggressive NHL is probably related to the occurrence of other gene rearrangements. A c-myc rearrangement concomitant with the transformation of a follicular NHL has been demonstrated in one case (24).

Differentiation of t(14;18) B cells

Several facts strongly suggest that the occurrence of the (14;18) translocation is an early event in B-cell differentiation. More precisely, the t(14;18) is an error during the first step of differentiation, the joining between a Diversity gene (D) and a Joining gene (J) (25). Instead of joining separate segments of the same chromosome *(see the chapter "B-cell differentia-tion")*, a recombinase would join segments on separate chromosomes. This mistake could be explained by structural similarities between chromosome 18q21 regions close to the breakpoints and the heptamer-nonamer sequence bordering each gene segment and used by the recombinase as a recognition signal for DJ joining (25). Such a mechanism of homologous recombination has not been confirmed by other groups (5,6). On the contrary, Cleary and Sklar (5) suggested that translocation may be preceded by deletion of gene segments between D_H and J_H on chromosome 14 and followed by insertion of 1-5 nucleotides at the N-region of the breakpoint by a terminal deoxynucleotidyl transferase.

From the occurrence of t(14;18) at a pre-B-cell differentiation stage, a development scheme for malignant proliferation of mature B cells has been suggested and partially confirmed by experimental data (6,9,25-27). As a t(14;18) precludes the continuation of heavy chain gene rearrangements, either a rearrangement occurs on the other Ig_H allele, or, in the absence of a functional Ig_H rearrangement, there is no production of immunoglobulins (28). As in normal B cells, the heavy chain gene rearrangement is followed by successive kappa and, if not productive, lambda light chain gene rearrangements (27). Furthermore, Ig_H and Ig_L genes are the sites of point mutations (29). These point mutations may express themselves by variations in Ig gene rearrangement patterns. Multiclonality of some lymphomas has been suggested by these variations (30). Nevertheless, all these lymphoma cell populations have the same t(14;18) breakpoint and are subclones derived from a common pre-B progenitor cell in which a single t(14;18) translocation has occurred (31).

Thus, follicular lymphomas are the result of successive transformational events beginning in bone-marrow pre-B cells. However, for reasons that remain unclear, cells carrying the t(14;18) translocation must differentiate further to express their malignant capabilities.

Detection of t(14;18) in lymphoma cells

Besides their interest in terms of follicular NHL pathogenesis, these molecular studies have greatly increased the possibilities of detecting cells carrying a t(14;18) translocation among lymphomatous lesions. Using conventional cytogenetic analysis, a t(14;18) translocation has been found in approximately 70 to 80% of NHL with a follicular architecture (32,33) [67% in a recent review of 262 cases (34)]. Using several DNA probes flanking or within the bcl-2 gene, molecular analysis allows detection of a minority of cells carrying the t(14;18) translocation. The presence of t(14;18) cells is confirmed if there is a co-migration of rearranged chromosome 18 DNA fragments and a rearranged heavy chain gene detected with a J_H probe (4,36-38). Using this technique, a t(14;18) trans-location was found in 69% (38) to 89% (36) of follicular lymphomas. More recently, lower incidences of t(14;18) detection in follicular lymphoma have been reported from Japan [33% (35)] and Europe [51% (34)] using molecular techniques suggesting that chromosome 18 breakpoints may occur outside on the mbr or mcr in a higher percentage of cases (34). The sensitivity of the technique may be increased by the Polymerase Chain Reaction (PCR), using oligonucleotide primers specific for the regions of chromosome 18 [either for the major breakpoint region (39-41) or for the minor cluster region (43)]. Although PCR technique proves to be more complex than initially thought, it could be most useful for the diagnosis of minimal residual disease, especially in bone marrow before autologous transplantation.

Ngan et al. (44) have developed an ususual method for the demonstration of the t(14;18) on frozen tissue sections. Using a rabbit antiserum directed against bcl-2 proteins, and classical immunohistochemical methods, they found a close relationship between the presence of a t(14;18) translocation and staining with these antiserums. Using monoclonal antibodies directed against bcl-2 proteins, Mason et al. could not confirm such a close relationship. They found that lymphoma cells (but not non-malignant lymphoid B cells) could be strained with anti-bcl-2 antibodies in the absence of t(14;18) (45).

The study of t(14;18) translocation has provided substantial insights into the biology of lymphoma cells but several questions remain unanswered. Besides the increase in lymphoid cell lifespan by inhibition of apoptosis, what is the precise role of bcl-2 gene and its products? Which additional events are necessary for the malignant growth of these B cells? Does bcl-2 gene expression play a role in clinically expressed lymphomas or only in the early stages of development?

References

1. FUKUHARA S, ROWLEY JD, VARIAKOJIS D et al.
   Chromosome abnormalities in poorly differentiated lymphocytic lymphoma.
   Cancer Res, 1979; 39: 3119-3128.
2. TSUJIMOTO Y, FINGER LR, YUNIS JJ et al.
   Cloning of the chromosome breakpoint of neoplastic B cells with the t(14;18) chromosome translocation.
   Science, 1984; 226: 1098-1099.
3. ROWLEY JD
   Chromosome studies in the non-Hodgkin's lymphomas: the role of the (14;18) translocation.
   J Clin Oncol, 1988; 6: 919-925.
4. BAKHSI A, JENSEN JP, GOLDMAN P et al.
   Cloning the chromosomal breakpoint of t(14;18) human lymphomas: clustering around JH on chromosome 14 and near a transcriptional unit on chromosome 18.
   Cell, 1985; 41: 899-906.
5. CLEARY ML, SKLAR J
   Nucleotide sequence of a t(14;18) chromosomal breakpoint in follicular lymphoma and demonstration of a breakpoint-cluster region near a transcriptionally active locus on chromosome 18.
   Proc Natl Acad Sci USA, 1985; 82: 7439-7443.
6. BAKHSHI A, WRIGHT JJ, GRANINGER W, et al.
   Mechanism of the t(14;18) translocation: structural analysis of both derivative 14 and 18 reciprocal partners.
   Proc Natl Acad Sci USA, 1987; 84: 2396-2400.

7. REED JC, TSUJIMOTO Y, ALPERS JD, CROCE CM, NOWELL PC
   Regulation of bcl-2 protooncogene expression during normal human lymphocyte proliferation.
   Science, 1987; 236: 1295-1299.
8. GURFINKEL N, UNGER T, GIVOL D, MUSHINSKI JF
   Expression of the bcl-2 gene in mouse B-lymphocytic cell lines is differentiation-stage specific.
   Eur J Immunol, 1987; 17: 567-570.
9. GRANINGER WB, SETO M, BOUTAIN B, GOLDMAN P, KORSMEYER SJ
   Expression of Bcl-2 and Bcl-2 fusion transcripts in normal and neoplastic cells.
   J Clin Invest, 1987; 80: 1512-1515.
10. CLEARY ML, SMITH SD, SKLAR J
    Cloning and structural analysis of cDNAs for bcl-2 and a hybrid bcl-2/immunoglobulin transcript resulting from the t(14;18) translocation.
    Cell, 1986; 47: 19-28.
11. TSUJIMOTO Y, CROCE CM
    Analysis of the structure, transcripts and protein products of bcl-2, the gene involved in human follicular lymphomas.
    Pro Natl Acad Sci USA, 1986; 83: 5214-5218.
12. CLEARY ML, GALILI N, SKLAR J
    Detection of a second t(14;18) breakpoint cluster region in human follicular lymphomas.
    J Exp Med, 1986; 164: 315-320.
13. TSUJIMOTO Y, BACHIR MM, GINOL I et al.
    DNA rearrangement in human follicular lymphoma can involve the 5' or the 3' region of the bcl-2 gene.
    Proc Natl Acad Sci USA, 1987; 84: 1329-1331.
14. CHEN-LEVY Z, NOURSE J, CLEARY ML
    The bcl-2 candidate protooncogene product is a 24 kilodalton integral-membrane protein highly expressed in lymphoid cell lines and lymphomas carrying the t(14;18) translocation.
    Mol Cell Biol, 1989; 9: 701-710.
15. TSUJIMOTO Y, IKEGAKI N, CROCE CM
    Characterization of the protein product of bcl-2, the gene involved in human follicular lymphomas.
    Oncogene, 1987; 2: 3-7.
16. HALDAR S, BEATTY C, TSUJIMOTO Y, CROCE CM
    The bcl-2 gene encodes a novel G protein.
    Nature, 1989; 342: 195-198.
17. MONICA K, CHEN-LEVY Z, CLEARY ML
    Small G proteins are expressed ubiquitously in lymphoid cells and do not correspond to bcl-2.
    Nature, 1990; 346: 189-191.
18. REED JC, CUDDY M, SLABIAK T, CROCE CM, NOWELL PC
    Oncogenic potential of bcl-2 demonstrated by gene transfer.
    Nature, 1988; 336: 259-261.

19. VAUX DL, CORY S, ADAMS JM

Bcl-2 gene promotes haemopoietic cell survival and cooperates with c-myc to immortalize pre-B cells.

Nature, 1988; 335: 440-442.

20. NUNEZ G, SETO M, SEREMETIS S et al.

Growth- and tumor-promoting effects of deregulated Bcl-2 in human B-lymphoblastoid cells.

Proc Natl Acad Sci USA, 1989; 86: 4589-4593.

21. McDONNELL TJ, DEANE N, PLATT FM et al.

Bcl-2-immunoglobulin transgenic mice demonstrate extended B-cell survival and follicular lymphoproliferation.

Cell, 1989; 57: 79-88.

22. TSUJIMOTO Y

Overexpression of the human bcl-2 gene product results in growth enhancement of Epstein-Barr virus immortalized B cells.

Proc Natl Acad Sci USA, 1989; 86: 1958-1962.

23. HOCKENBERY D, NUNEZ G, HILLMAN C, SCHREIBER RD, KORSMEYER SJ

Bcl-2 is an inner mitochondrial membrane protein that blocks programmed cell death.

Nature, 1990; 348: 334-337.

24. LEE JT, INNES DJ Jr, WILLIAMS ME

Sequential bcl-2 and c-myc oncogene rearrangements associated with the clinical transformation of non-Hodgkin's lymphoma.

J Clin Invest, 1989; 84: 1454-1459.

25. TSUJIMOTO Y, GORHAM J, COSSMAN J, JAFFE E, CROCE CM

The t(14;18) chromosome translocations involved in B-cell neoplasms result from mistakes in VDJ joining.

Science, 1985; 229: 1390-1393.

26. RAFFELD M, WRIGHT JJ, LIPFORD E et al.

Clonal evolution of t(14;18) follicular lymphomas demonstrated by immunoglobulin genes and the 18q21 major breakpoint region.

Cancer Res, 1987; 47: 2537-2542.

27. BERTOLI LF, KUBAGAWA H, BORZILLO GV, BURROWS PD, SCHREEDER MT, CARROLL AJ, COOPER MD

Bone marrow origin of a B-cell lymphoma.

Blood, 1988; 72: 94-101.

28. DE JONG D, VOETDIJK BMH, VAN OMMEN GJB, KLUIN-NELEMANS JC, BEVERSTOGK GC, KLUIN PM

Translocation t(14;18) in B-cell lymphomas as a cause for defective immunoglobulin production.

J Exp Med, 1989; 169: 613-624.

29. LEVY S, MENDEL E, KON S, AVNUR Z, LEVY R

Mutational hot spots in Ig V-region genes of human follicular lymphomas.

J Exp Med, 1988; 168, 475-489.

30. SIEGELMAN MH, CLEARY ML, WARNKE R, SKLAR J

Frequent biclonality and Ig gene alterations among B-cell lymphomas that show multiple histologic forms.

J Exp Med, 1985; 161: 850-857.

31. CLEARY ML, GALILI N, TRELA M, LEYY T, SKLAR J

Single cell origin of bigenotypic and biphenotypic B-cell proliferations in human follicular lymphomas.

J Exp Med, 1988; 167: 582-597.

32. LEVINE EG, ARTHUR DC, FRIZZERA G, PETERSON BA, HURD DD, BLOOMFIELD CD

There are differences in cytogenetic abnormalities among histologic subtypes of the non-Hodgkin's lymphomas.

Blood, 1985; 66: 1414-1422.

33. YUNIS JJ, OKEN MM, KAPLAN ME, ENSRUD KM, HOWE RR, THEOLOGIDES A

Distinctive chromosomal abnormalities in histologic subtypes of non-Hodgkin's lymphoma.

N Engl J Med, 1982; 307: 1231-1236.

34. PEZZELA F, RALFKIAER E, GATTER KC, MASON DY

The 14;18 translocation in European cases of follicular lymphoma: comparison of Southern blotting and the polymerase chain reaction.

Brit J Haematol, 1990; 76: 58-64.

35. AMAKAWO R, FUKUHARA S, OHNO H et al.

Involvement of bcl-2 gene in Japanese follicular lymphomas.

Blood, 1989; 73: 787-791.

36. WEISS LM, WARNKE RA, SKLAR J, CLEARY ML

Molecular analysis of the t(14;18) chromosomal translocation in malignant lymphomas.

N Engl J Med, 1987; 317: 1185-1189.

37. LIPFORD E, WRIGHT JJ, URBA W et al.

Refinement of lymphoma cytogenetics by the chromosome 18q21 major breakpoint region.

Blood 1987; 70, 1816-1823.

38. LEE MS, BLICK MB, PATHAK S et al.

The gene located at chromosome 18 band q21 is rearranged in uncultured diffuse lymphomas as well as follicular lymphomas.

Blood, 1987; 70: 90-95.

39. LEE MS, CHANG KS, CABANILLAS F, FREIREICH EJ, TRUJILLO JM, STASS SA

Detection of minimal residual cells carrying t(14;18) by DNA sequence amplification.

Science, 1987; 237: 175-178.

40. CRESCENZI M, SETO M, HERZIG GP, WEISS PD, GRIFFITH RC, KORSMEYER SJ

Thermostable DNA polymerase chain amplification of t(14;18) chromosome breakpoints and detection of minimal residual disease.

Proc Natl Acad Sci USA, 1988; 85: 4869-4873.

41. STETLER-STEVENSON M, RAFFELD M, COHEN P, COSSMAN J

    Detection of occult follicular lymphoma by specific DNA amplification.

    Blood, 1988; 72: 1822-1825.

42. CUNNINGHAM D, HICKISH T, ROSIN RD, SAUVEN P, BARON JH, FARRELL PJ, ISAACSON P

    Polymerase chain reaction for detection of dissemination in gastric lymphoma.

    Lancet, 1989; i: 695-697.

43. NGAN BY, NOURSE J, CLEARY ML

    Detection of chromosomal translocation t(14;18) within the minor cluster region of bcl-2 by polymerase chain reaction and direct genomic sequency of the enzymatically amplified DNA in follicular lymphomas.

    Blood, 1989; 73: 1759-1762.

44. NGAN BY, CHEN-LEVY Z, WEISS LM, WARNKER RA, CLEARY ML

    Expression in non-Hodgkin's lymphoma of the bcl-2 protein associated with the t(14;18) chromosomal translocation.

    N Engl J Med, 1988; 318: 1630-1644.

45. PEZZELA F, TSE AGD, CORDELL JL, PULFORD KAF, GATTER KC, MASON DY

    Expression of the bcl-2 oncogene protein is not specific for the 14;18 chromosomal translocation.

    Am J Pathol, 1990; 137: 225-232.

2.

METHODS

edited by

F. REYES

Histological and immunohistochemical methods

P. GAULARD, M. PEUCHMAUR, N. BROUSSE

Pathology

Histological methods

Superficial lymph nodes may be aspirated or surgically removed. Lymph node biopsy must be carried out on the whole lymph node. Smears are done by touching with slices of fresh lymph node, before putting it into the fixative. Cytological analysis requires May-Grunwald-Giemsa staining. Smears can also be air dried and then stored at -20°C or -80°C for cytological immunophenotyping. A portion of the lymph node is immediately snap-frozen in liquid nitrogen for immunohistological and/or immunogenomic study. The other part of the lymph node must be rapidly fixed. Haematoxylin-eosin, May-Grünwald-Giemsa and reticulin fibre stainings (Gordon-Sweet method) are mandatory for optimal histological study.

Pathological aspects

The involvement of a lymph node by a non-Hodgkin's lymphoma is easy to recognize when the following criteria are fulfilled: disappearance of the normal architecture, obstruction of the sinuses, homogenization of the parenchyma, infiltration of the capsule and spreading into the perinodal fat tissue. But this characteristic pattern is far from being constant. The involvement may be focal, forming clusters of neoplastic cells, as in lymphoblastic NHL. It may be partial, sparing lymph node areas, as in T-cell lymphomas where the neoplastic proliferation is located first in the T-cell – dependent paracortical zone, without involvement of the B-cell – dependent zones such as follicles.

The morphological classification of NHL relies on two main criteria: the architecture of the pro-

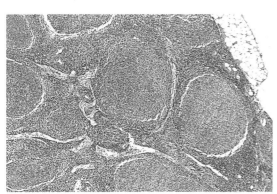

Fig. 1a: Follicular lymphoma.

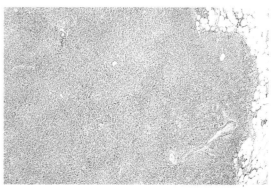

Fig. 1b: Diffuse lymphoma.

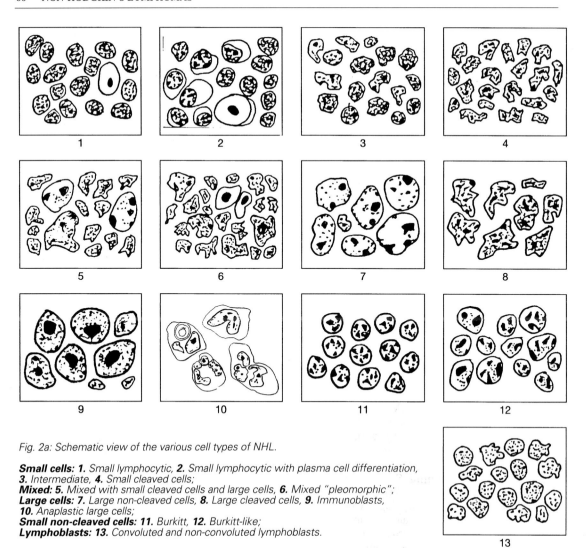

Fig. 2a: Schematic view of the various cell types of NHL.

Small cells: 1. *Small lymphocytic,* **2.** *Small lymphocytic with plasma cell differentiation,*
3. *Intermediate,* **4.** *Small cleaved cells;*
Mixed: 5. *Mixed with small cleaved cells and large cells,* **6.** *Mixed "pleomorphic";*
Large cells: 7. *Large non-cleaved cells,* **8.** *Large cleaved cells,* **9.** *Immunoblasts,*
10. *Anaplastic large cells;*
Small non-cleaved cells: 11. *Burkitt,* **12.** *Burkitt-like;*
Lymphoblasts: 13. *Convoluted and non-convoluted lymphoblasts.*

liferation and the characteristics of the neoplastic cells. Two types of architecture are described: follicular or diffuse *(fig. 1)*. In follicular NHL, the proliferation is organised in nodules separated by interfollicular areas containing numerous reactive cells. In the diffuse type, the proliferation forms a sheet with scattered reactive cells. These two types may coexist in the same lymph node and the pattern is described as follicular and diffuse. They may also be found concomitantly in different lymph nodes in the same patient. The architecture of the proliferation is in most cases easy to recognize and concordance is high among pathologists. If the nodular architecture does not appear clear, reticulin staining may be useful to ascertain the nodularity. Since the prognosis of most follicular NHL is better than that of diffuse NHL and they require different treatments, the follicular architecture must be dearly determined.

Cytological analysis *(fig. 2)* of lymphoid proliferation must be examined at high magnification, and, if necessary, with oil immersion. First, the cell size must be estimated since there are morphological and clinical differences between "large"-cell and "small"-cell proliferations. The best way to analyze the cell size is to compare the size of the nuclei of neoplastic cells with that of normal lymphocytes and/or of macrophages. The diameter of the nucleus of large cells is greater than or equal to 2 times that of normal lymphocytes (or greater than the nucleus of macrophages). A more precise cell classification relies on

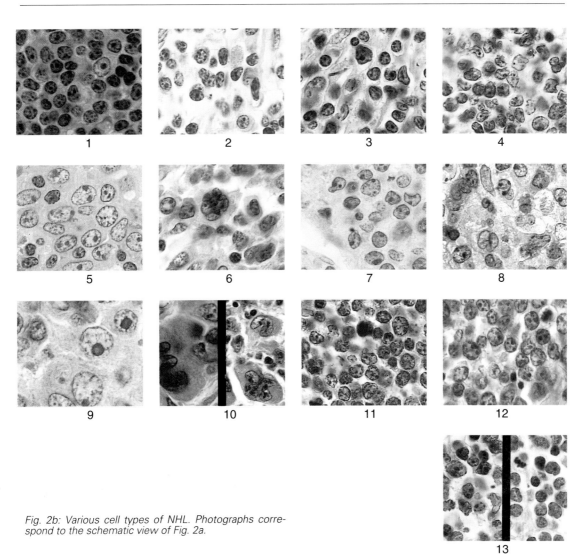

Fig. 2b: Various cell types of NHL. Photographs correspond to the schematic view of Fig. 2a.

other characteristics such as the form and the outline of the nucleus, the chromatin structure, the number and shape of nucleoli, and the abundance and tinctorial affinities of the cytoplasm. Other features must also be described: number of mitoses, reactive cell characteristics, importance of vascularisation, degree of sclerosis, and presence of necrotic areas.

Immunohistology

Immunohistochemical studies

These techniques allow better recognition of the different lymphoid cell populations and are useful for distinguishing non-Hodgkin's lymphomas from other neoplasias. B- and T-cell antigens may be detected by immuno-histochemical methods using specific antibodies conjugated either to a fluorochrome or to an enzyme. This enzyme will be revealed by a colour generated by reaction with its substrate (1-7). These techniques are performed on paraffin-embedded tissues or on frozen sections.

Membrane or cytoplasmic antigens can be demonstrated on frozen sections. Immuno-histochemical studies on frozen sections are the reference method for phenotyping non-Hodgkin's lymphomas. Numerous mono-clonal antibodies have been produced to recognize human leucocyte differentiation antigens which are clustered *(listed in Table 1)*. Moreover, several monoclonal antibodies detect epitopes which are preserved after fixation (8-12), thus allowing determination

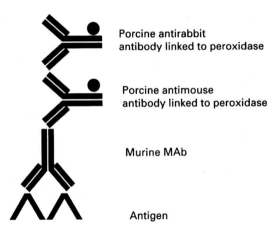

Fig. 3: Three-stage immunoperoxidase indirect method.

of the lineage of NHL on parrafin-embedded tissues. Preservation of a good morphology, and the possibility of retrospective studies and of phenotyping cases in which no frozen sections are available are the advantages of these tech-niques. However, pre-digestion with proteolytic enzymes (trypsin, pronase, etc.) may be necessary to detect and/or enhance the labelling of antigens on "routine" paraffin sections.

Several immunohistochemical techniques can be used on paraffin-embedded and frozen sections. Indirect immunoenzymatic labelling techniques are the most widely used for the study of malignant lymphomas. Indeed, immunofluorescence methods do not allow proper localization of cellular antigens in tissue sections; in addition, the main drawback of direct immunoenzymatic methods is the need for a different conjugated antibody for each antigen.

Three-stage immunoperoxidase technique (fig. 3) (13)

Incubation with a mouse monoclonal antibody for an appropriate period is followed by incubation, for example, with a peroxi-dase-conjugated rabbit antimouse antibody, then with a peroxidase-conjugated porcine antirabbit antibody.

Each incubation is performed for 30 minutes in a moist chamber at room temperature. Monoclonal antibodies are diluted in Tris Buffer Saline (TBS) 0.05 M pH 7.6 with 1 % bovine serum albumin. Secondary and tertiary antibodies are diluted in the same buffer with normal human serum (diluted to 1/3) to decrease non-specific binding. After each incubation, slides are rinsed with TBS and carefully wiped around the smears which must not be allowed to dry. Peroxidase is revealed with a 0.06% diaminobenzidine (DAB) solution in 0.05 M TBS pH 7.6 and hydrogen peroxide. The reaction product is brown. Staining can be enhanced by the use of metallic salts (nickel or cobalt) (14). After washing, slides are slightly counterstained with haematoxylin. Chromogens other than DAB, such as amino-ethylcarbazol, can also be used.

PAP method (fig. 4a) (15)

Three reagents are used in this method: primary and secondary antibody, and "PAP complex" made of the peroxidase enzyme and of anti-peroxidase antibodies. The primary antibody which is specific for the tested antigen can be a mouse monoclonal antibody or a rabbit polyclonal antibody.

APAAP method (16) (fig. 4b)

The principle of this method is similar to that of the PAP method. In the APAAP complex, alkaline phosphatase is used instead of peroxidase. Alkaline phosphatase is usually revealed by incubation in fast red and naphtol AS-TR phosphate solution containing levamisole to block endogenous alkaline phosphatase activity. The reaction product is red.

Avidin-Biotin (17) (fig. 5) and Streptavidin-Biotin (18) methods

This method is based on the ability of avidin or streptavidin molecules to bind 4 molecules of the biotin vitamin by a non-

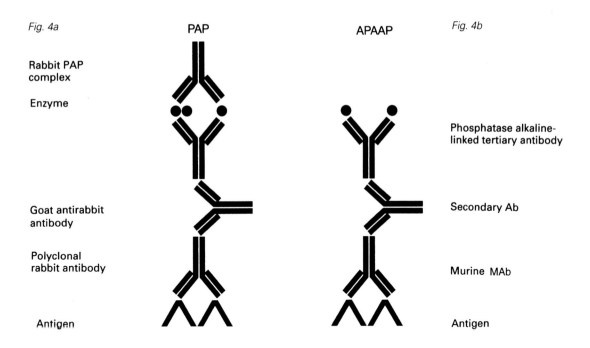

Fig. 4a — PAP

- Rabbit PAP complex
- Enzyme
- Goat antirabbit antibody
- Polyclonal rabbit antibody
- Antigen

APAAP — Fig. 4b

- Phosphatase alkaline-linked tertiary antibody
- Secondary Ab
- Murine MAb
- Antigen

Fig. 4: Soluble enzyme immune complex method preformed complex reacts with secondary antibody. Primary antibody and antibody of enzyme immune complex must be made in the same species. Fig. 4a = PAP method; fig. 4b = APAAP method.

immune reaction. The secondary antibody is conjugated to biotin. The third reagent is a complex of an enzyme (usually peroxidase) conjugated to avidin or streptavidin.

Double labelling (19)

Combination of two of the above methods allows simultaneous detection of different antigens. For example, it is possible to determine the cellular origin of proliferating cells using both a MAb directed against a specific surface determinant and the Ki-67 MAb (which recognizes a nuclear antigen present during the cell cycle) (20). Another example is the simultaneous detection of the cellular and viral antigens in infected cells.

Sensitivity and specificity

Numerous studies have focused on the respective sensitivity of the different immunohistochemical methods. Techniques using amplification of the staining such as PAP, APAAP or avidin (or steptavidin)-biotin methods have a greater sensitivity than other techniques such as direct or indirect two-stage methods. Interestingly, stronger

reactivity can be obtained by repeating the reaction from the secondary antibody binding step after completing a first PAP (or APAAP) procedure (16).

The APAAP immunoalkaline method should be employed rather than immunoperoxidase staining methods for the study of blood smears, bone-marrow preparations and other specimens containing numerous blood cells, since background staining due to endogenous peroxidase is avoided (16).

Difficulties in interpreting immunohistochemical results

Interpretation of the results obtained with the immunoperoxidase technique may give rise to some problems. Thus, if the specimens consist of inflammatory and highly vascularized tissue, the endogenous peroxidase activity of eosinophil granulocytes and the "pseudoperoxidase" activity of red blood cells may cause difficulties in the interpretation of a positive staining.

These false positivities may be decreased by preincubation of the slides in 1% hydrogen peroxide for at least 30 minutes.

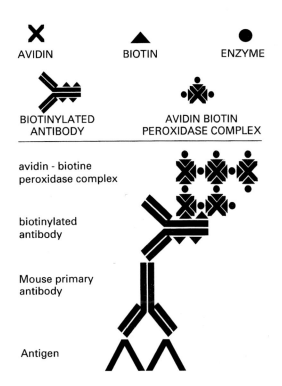

Fig. 5: Avidin-biotin method: preformed avidin-biotin-enzyme complex (ABC) or enzyme-labelled avidin (LAB) reacts with biotinylated secondary antibody.

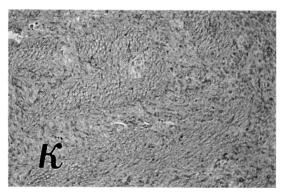

Fig. 6a

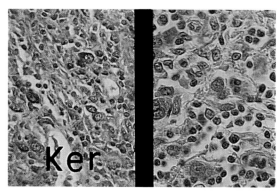

Fig. 6b

Fig. 6a: Non-specific binding of an antikappa antibody on a tissue rich in collagen fibres (indirect immunoperoxidase technique); fig. 6b : immunoperoxidase technique on paraffin-embedded tissues: left, non-specific binding of an anticytokeratin antibody (KL1) on lymphoma cells due to adequate paraffin removal, right: negative staining after adequate paraffin removal.

Diffuse and non-granular background staining may result from a non-specific reaction of the labelled antibodies with components other than the corresponding antigen. It is observed in necrotic areas, in intercellular spaces which contain serum proteins and along collagen fibres which can bind immunoglobulins *(fig. 6)*. Background staining may be decreased by prior trypsin treatment of the slides (0.1% trypsin in TBS pH 7.6 for 10 minutes at 37°C), by preincubation in normal human serum or by using highly diluted primary antibody. Passive adsorption of extracellular immunoglobulins by histiocytes cannot be avoided and may be a source of misinterpretation (suggesting for instance polyclonality in a case of lymphoma). Theoretically, misinterpretation can also be related to non-specific binding of primary antibody on the Fc-receptors of some cells. This can be avoided by the use of F(ab')2 fragments instead of entire immunoglobulins. In fact, this problem is much more often observed on fresh cells than on tissue sections.

Some antigens are not lineage-specific and can be expressed by different cell types. For example, the CD4 antigen is found on a subset of T lymphocytes (T helper cells) and on monocyte-macrophages. CD1 antigen is expressed by thymocytes and also by Langerhans cells and interdigitated cells. Some cross-reactivities of monoclonal antibodies can be due to similar epitopes of apparently non-related antigens on different cells. Thus Leu 4 (anti-CD3) monoclonal antibody recognizes mature T cells but also Purkinje cells in the cerebellum.

Tumour cells often have weaker antigenicity than their normal counterparts. Thus, the absence of demonstration of immunoglobulin production by lymphoma cells does not rule out a diagnosis of B-cell NHL (see below). If a first attempt at antigen demonstration has failed, the use of higher concentrations of primary antibody and/or an amplification technique may be required.

However, tumour cells can fail to express antigens present on their normal counterparts. Thus, in most T-cell NHL, lymphoma cells may not express one or more pan-T antigens. This finding (see below) is frequently used as an indirect marker for clonality in T-cell proliferations.

In addition, if paraffin-embedded tissue specimens are tested, absent or weak expression can be ascribed to the destruction or masking of antigens by the fixative, which is the major limiting factor for immunohistological study on routinely processed paraffin-embedded tissues. To our knowledge, there is no universal fixative which preserves all antigens. Whatever the fixative used, prolonged fixation increases antigen destruction.

Applications of immunohistochemical studies

Immunohistochemical studies can be used for the *in situ* typing, in their natural environment, of normal and neo-plastic B and T lymphocytes, and of accessory cells such as macrophages or "natural killer" cells. Thus they can facilitate diagnosis of malignant lymphomas, and are able in most cases to determine their lineage, even in routine processed tissue specimens.

Schematically (21) *(Table I)*:

- **B lymphocytes** are identified by:

• pan-B differentiation antigens (CD19, CD20, CD21, CD22), others being restricted to some stages of differentiation (CD10, CD23);

• their cytoplasmic or surface immunoglobulins (light and heavy chains).

- **T lymphocytes** are identified by:

• pan-T differentiation antigens (CD2, CD3, CD5, CD7);

• other antigens restricted to some stages of maturation (CD1 = corticothymocytes) or related to a functional differentiation (CD4 = helper, CD8 = cytotoxic/suppressor);

• their specific T-cell receptors (TCR): indeed monoclonal antibodies specific for invariant epitopes of the β chain of TCR-αβ (βF1) (22) and of the δ chain of TCR- δ (TCR-δ1) (23) have been produced that can be used to detect respectively αβ and γδ T cells.

- **Accessory cells** can be recognized by the following markers:

• CD68 is one of the most successful **macrophage markers**;

• CD16 (Leu11), CD57 (HNK-1) and CD56 (NKH-1) are antigens associated with "**natural killer cells**";

• **dendritic reticular cells** can be identified by some specific monoclonal antibodies (R4/23 = DRC1);

• **accessory cells** can also express other antigens, non-lineage-specific, such as C3b receptor (CD35), or S100 protein, which is useful for the detection of interdigitated cells.

- Monoclonal antibodies are also available which do not recognize lineage-associated antigens, but rather other antigens such as:

• **activation antigens** [for example, interleukin-2 receptor antigen (CD25), expressed by activated T cells, or CD30 (Ki-1 antigen) expressed by activated T and B cells, and Reed-Sternberg cells];

• **adhesion molecules**: numerous antigens have recently been recognized which play a major role in different cellular interactions [for example: α (CD11a) and β (CD18) chains of LFA-1, expressed by leucocytes; CD4 and CD8 which act respectively as class II and class I antigen receptors; antigens of the ICAM (ICAM-1 = CD54), the VLA (CDw49) families, ...];

• **cell cycle-associated antigens,** recognized by Ki-67 monoclonal antibody, that can be used as an indicator of proliferative activity;

• products of some **oncogenes** (such as *c-myc, c-ras* or bcl-2);

• **lymphokines**.

Applications of immunohistochemical methods to the study of normal and neoplastic lymphoid tissues are numerous:

- they have allowed better knowledge of normal lymphoid tissue (see "Immunohistology of normal lymph node");

- for the diagnosis of non-Hodgkin's lymphomas, they are useful, and often necessary:

• to differentiate some reactive lymphoid hyperplasias from malignant lymphomas. This distinction can sometimes be very difficult on the basis of routine histology, for example, between some atypical lymphoid follicular hyperplasias and follicular lymphomas; in the latter case, demonstration of light-chain restriction (monotypy) on frozen sections allows diagnosis of follicular lymphoma;

• to differentiate large-cell malignant lymphomas from other poorly differentiated tumours (see below);

• to determine of the B- or T-cell origin of lymphomas.

- Immunohistochemical techniques can also contribute to a better description of the multiple events arising, in situ, during neoplastic transformation (evolution of differentiation or activation markers, oncogene products, etc.).

Despite the development of MAb-recognizing epitopes which are not destroyed during fixation, the respective applications of these methods on routinely processed paraffin-embedded tissue and on frozen tissue specimens remain distinct and must be detailed separately.

Immunohistochemical studies on routinely processed paraffin-embedded tissue (table 2)

Diagnosis of large-cell NHL

Among large-cell tumours, it can be histologically difficult to distinguish between large-cell lymphoma and tumours of other origins, such as carcinoma, melanoma or sarcoma. On routine tissue sections, the diagnosis of lymphoma can be ascertained if the neo-plastic cells are positive with a pan-

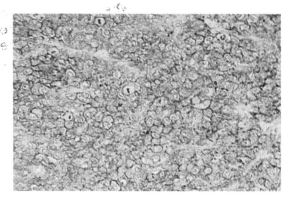

Fig. 7a

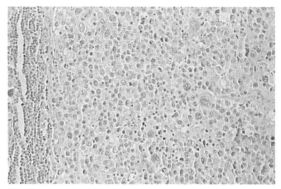

Fig. 7b

Fig. 7: Diagnosis of large-cell NHL on paraffin-embedded tissue: tumour cells express the common leucocyte antigen (CD45) (fig. 7a) but are negative with an anticytokeratin antibody (KL1) (fig. 7b). Three-stage immunoperoxidase technique.

leucocyte antibody (CD45) (8), express neither keratin (present in epithelial cells) (fig. 7), nor protein S100 (present in melanomas) and are usually negative with an anti-vimentin antibody (positive in sarcomas) (24). However, in a few cases of NHL, especially of the anaplastic type, CD45 antigen can be undetectable (25). In such cases, the diagnosis of lymphoma is based on the negativity of the markers of tumours of other origin (i.e. cytokeratin, S100 protein) and on the positivity of other leucocyte-restricted antigen [such as CD20 (L26), CD3, or CD30 (BerH2)].

Determination of tumour-cell lineage

When a diagnosis of lymphoma is made, its B- or T-cell origin can be determined in a great number of cases using a combination of some pan-B and pan-T markers which

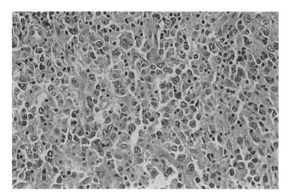

Fig. 8a

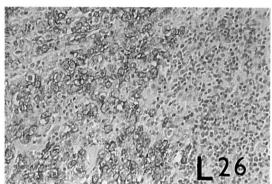

Fig. 8c

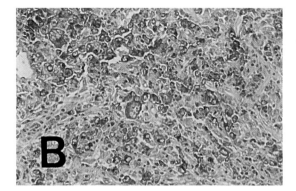

Fig. 8b

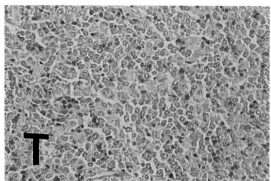

Fig. 8d

have been reported to work well on fixed paraffin-embedded tissue specimens (9-12,26). These are very useful, especially when fresh or frozen tissue is unavailable for analysis. Among the numerous antibodies recently produced *(Table II)*, UCHL1 (CD45R0) and MT1 (CD43) seem to be good pan-T markers, whereas monoclonal antibody L26, which recognizes an intracellular epitope of the B-cell-associated CD20 antigen (27), is a very sensitive and specific marker for B cells, much more than antibodies MB2, LN1 (CDw75), and LN2 (CD74) *(figs. 8 and 9)*. With the exception of L26 (27), most of these antibodies are not highly specific and, for example, react more or less weakly with epithelial cells and histiocytes. MAb reacting with the CD68 cluster, such as Y2/131 (KP1) (28), can recognize macrophages on routinely-processed tissue sections *(fig. 10)* and could be helpful for the diagnosis of the very infrequent true histiocytic lymphomas (29).

Recently, a new strategy has been developed in order to raise monoclonal, or polyclonal

Fig. 8: Staining of a B cell NHL on paraffin-embedded tissue. Fig. 8a = Diffuse large-cell NHL (Hematoxylin-Eosin); fig. 8b = Expression of CW75 antigen (LN1); fig. 8c = Expression of pan-B CD20 antigen (L26); fig. 8d = Only small lymphocytes are stained with a pan-T antibody (UCHL-1, CD45 RO). Three-stage immunoperoxidase technique.

antibodies against synthetic peptide sequences from B- or T-cell antigens. For example, by choosing peptide sequences from the cytoplasmic domain of the CD3 ξ chain, a polyclonal antibody has recently been produced which recognizes epitopes of the CD3 antigen not destroyed by fixation and gives good results on routinely-processed paraffin-embedded tissues (enhanced after digestion with trypsin) (12). A similar strategy could lead to the preparation of other T- or B-cell differentiation antigens. Such specific markers applicable to fixed paraffin-embedded tissues are very helpful in the immunophenotyping of lymphomas, because of the superior morphology of paraffin-embedded tissues and the precision of interpretation of the results *(figs. 11 and 12)*.

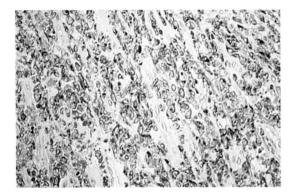

Fig. 9a

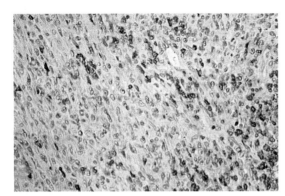

Fig. 9b

Fig. 9: Other example of B-cell NHL study on paraffin-embedded tissue. Tumour cells are stained with the MB2 antibody (fig. 9a) but are negative with anti-CD3 antibody, only rare reactive small T lymphocytes being stained (fig. 9b). APAAP technique.

Diagnosis of clonality

The diagnosis of clonality is usually not possible on routinely processed tissue sections. Indeed, surface immunoglobulins (Ig) are not preserved and cytoplasmic Ig are difficult to detect except in cells where they are highly concentrated. Thus, determination of monotypic light-chain restriction using anti-light-chain antibodies can be essentially performed in cases with plasmacytic differentiation, i.e. plasmocytoma, lymphoplasmacytic proliferations, and immunoblastic B-cell lymphomas.

Diagnosis of Hodgkin's disease and large-cell anaplastic lymphoma

Many studies have shown that Reed-Sternberg cells can be characterized by the expression of CD15 (Hapten X) and CD30 (Ki-1) antigens which can be detected on routinely processed tissue sections respectively by Leu M1 and Ber H2 MAb (30). However, it is now established that these reactivities do not by themselves guarantee the diagnosis of Hodgkin's disease. Indeed, Hapten X (CD15) can be expressed in non-Hodgkin's lymphomas (31) and CD30 is present on normal and neoplastic activated lymphoid cells, especially when they disclose a multilobated "pseudo-Sternberg" morphology (32). Thus, CD30 expression is found on large-cell anaplastic lymphomas *(fig. 13)*. The latter are also often shown to express the Epithelial Membrane Antigen (EMA) normally specific for epithelial cells (33).

Immunohistochemical studies on frozen tissue sections (21)

Until recently, the determination of the B- or T-cell origin of a tumour has been performed on frozen tissue sections, owing to the preservation of cytoplasmic and surface antigens detected by monoclonal antibodies. Thus, immunohistochemistry does allow the demonstration of B- or T-cell origin of nearly all non-Hodgkin's lymphomas.

B-cell lymphomas

B-cell lymphomas are defined by the expression by tumour cells of at least one pan-B antigen (CD19, CD20, CD21, CD22).

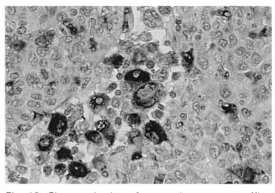

Fig. 10: Characterization of macrophages on paraffin-embedded tissue. In this case of anaplastic large cell NHL, the KP1 (CD68) antibody recognizes the numerous macrophages present in the sinuses but does not bind to tumour cells. APAAP technique.

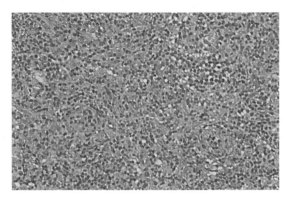

Fig. 11a

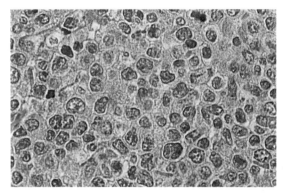

Fig. 12a

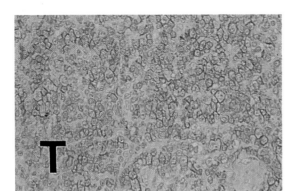

Fig. 11b

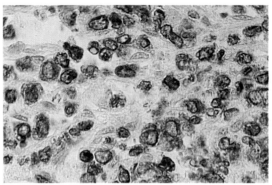

Fig. 12b

Fig. 11: Fig. 11a = Medium-size pleomorphic T-cell NHL (Haematoxylin-Eosin); fig. 11b = Tumour cells express CD45 RO antigen recognized by UCHL-1 antibody. Three-stage immunoperoxidase technique on paraffin-embedded tissue.

Fig. 12: Fig. 12a = Large pleomorphic T cell NHL (Hematoxylin-Eosin); fig.12b = Tumour cells strongly express the CD3 antigen. APAAP technique on paraffin-embedded tissue.

Most of them (about 70 to 80%) clearly disclose immunoglobin light-chain restriction (more often kappa than lambda), which requires predominance of one chain over the other of approximately 90% or greater *(fig.14)*. The μ chain is the heavy chain most frequently expressed, and is sometimes associated with the δ chain. Gamma heavy chain is almost always observed in immunoblastic lymphomas (34-36). This light-chain restriction, called "monotypy", is considered as an immunological marker for clonality (37), which can also bedemons-trated using other techniques [anti-idiotypes, clonal cytogenetic abnormalities, Southern blot analysis *(see chapter "Genotype")*. Thus it has been shown that monotypy correlates with a clonal pattern of rearrangement of heavy-chain (JH) and/or light-chain genes (38-39). Whereas most cases of low-grade lymphomas (follicular

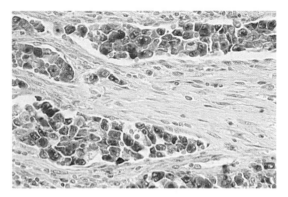

Fig.13: Anaplastic large-cell NHL strongly expressing the CD30 antigen recognized by Ber-H2 antibody. The staining underlines the predominant infiltration of sinuses by tumour cells. APAAP technique of paraffin-embedded tissue.

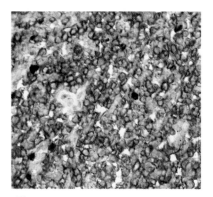

Fig. 14a

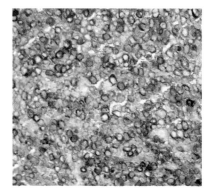

Fig. 14b

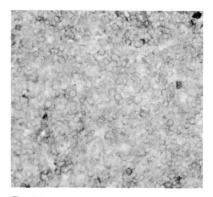

Fig. 14c

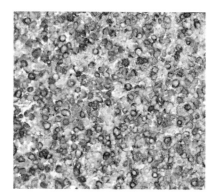

Fig. 14d

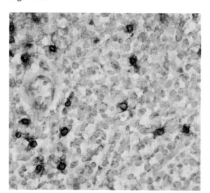

Fig. 14e

Fig. 14: Immunohistochemical characteristics of B-cell NHL (IgM K in this example). Immunoperoxidase technique on frozen tissue. Fig. 14a = staining with an anti-pan-B (CD22) antibody; fig. 14b = with an anti-K antibody; fig. 14c = with an anti- antibody; fig. 14d = with an anti-µ antibody; fig. 14e = with an anti-CD3 antibody.

small cell, mixed-cell type, diffuse small-cell type) show this pattern of light-chain restriction, 20 to 50% of diffuse mixed or diffuse large-cell lymphomas of B-cell type do not show demonstrable light-chain restriction. Cases without demonstrable light-chain restriction (about 20 to 30% of B-non-Hodgkin's lymphomas) correspond:

- to B-cell lymphomas which clearly do not display either Kappa or Lambda chains and are considered Ig light-chain negative; this finding is not technically abnormal since light-chain expression is usually very weak or absent in reactive germinal centres. It seems to arise more frequently in diffuse mixed and diffuse large-cell subgroups, especially in mediastinal large-cell lymphomas (40);

- to uninterpretable light chain cases in which background or equivocal staining prevents definitive determination. Both these Ig light-chain negative and uninter-

pretable lymphomas are regarded as of B-cell origin since tumour cells express one or more pan-B antigens (41,42), and since clonal rearrangement of the Ig heavy-chain genes can be demonstrated (38,39,42);

- to rare cases of bi- or oligoclonal proliferations: indeed, absence of demonstrable monotypy can be related to a bi- or oligoclonal pattern of rearrangement, found in some cases of histological progression from a low-grade lymphoma, or in other cases of NHL arising in HIV-infected patients (39,43,44).

Neoplastic B cells usually express the different antigens present on normal B lymphocytes, such as the different pan-B antigens (CD19, CD20, CD22), the C3b receptor (CR1, CD35), and the MHC class 2 anti-gens (45,46). However, in contrast with the majority of normal B lymphocytes, some "aberrant" antigen expressions have been found in B-lineage lymphomas which can constitute indirect immunohistological diagnostic criteria for lymphomas.

Thus, a pan-B antigen loss is observed in about 25% of cases, and about 10% (almost always of diffuse small-cell type) express the CD5 antigen normally found on most T cells and only on a very minor B-cell subpopulation (21).

Finally, in contrast to normal lymphocytes, a lack of expression of one or two chains of LFA-1 is observed in about 50% of B-lineage lymphomas (21,47).

Antibodies have recently been produced against the bcl-2 protein which can be used on frozen tissue section (48,49), or even on fixed routinely processed paraffin-embedded tissue (49,50). Using these antibodies, it has been demonstrated that the expression of bcl-2 oncogene protein is not specific for the t(14;18) chromosomal translocation (implicating the bcl-2 gene on chromosome 18) frequently observed in follicular lymphomas (49). Indeed, bcl-2 product is found in a variety of lymphoproliferative disorders, and in normal B- and T-lymphoid cells, with the exception of normal germinal centre cells in which bcl-2 protein is undetectable (49). Since expression of bcl-2 protein is found in about 85% of follicular lymphomas (50), anti-bcl-2 antibodies are of great value for distinguishing between follicular lymphomas and reactive follicular hyperplasia, even on conventionally fixed paraffin-embedded material (49,50).

T-cell lymphomas

The immunohistochemical diagnosis of T-cell lymphoma is based on the presence of T-cell membrane antigens, whose expression physiologically correlates with the stage of differentiation, and the functional specialization of T-lymphocytes (21,51). T-cell lymphomas are characterized by their remarkable phenotypic heterogeneity (21,39,51-55). Although its biological significance has not been established, this heterogeneity can be of great help in the immunodiagnosis of T-cell neoplasia, which cannot rely on direct markers of clonality comparable to the Ig light-chain restriction of B-cell malignancies.

T-cell lymphomas are divided into two main groups:

- lymphoblastic lymphomas which are CD1+ in more than 50% of cases and exhibit TdT positivity;

- peripheral T-cell lymphomas (PTCL) which are always CD1-.

Lymphoblastic lymphomas usually strongly express CD7 in addition to CD2, CD3 and CD5 antigens, whereas CD4-/CD8- or CD4+/CD8+ antigen expression is observed in 80% of cases (21,51). TCR $\alpha\beta$, as recognized by βF1 MoAb, is absent in about 40% of cases, whereas very rare cases seem to express the TCR $\gamma\delta$ (56). Thus most CD3+ βF1- lymphoblastic lymphomas may correspond to a stage of thymic differentiation in which CD3 is present in the cytoplasm before surface TCR expression.

In PTCL, the most striking immunological feature is the presence of a pan-T antigen loss which is found in about 80% of cases (21,39,51-55). Indeed, contrasting with the homogenous phenotype (CD2+, CD3+, CD5+, CD7+) of the T-cell population in benign reactive lymphoid processes, neoplastic T cells often lack detectable expression of one or more of the CD2, CD3, CD5 and CD7 pan-T antigens *(fig. 15)*. This has been shown to correlate with the presence of a clonal TCR-β gene rearrangement, and can thus constitute an indirect but suitable marker for clonality (39,51). CD7 and CD5 are the antigens most frequently lost. Considering the T-subset antigen expression,

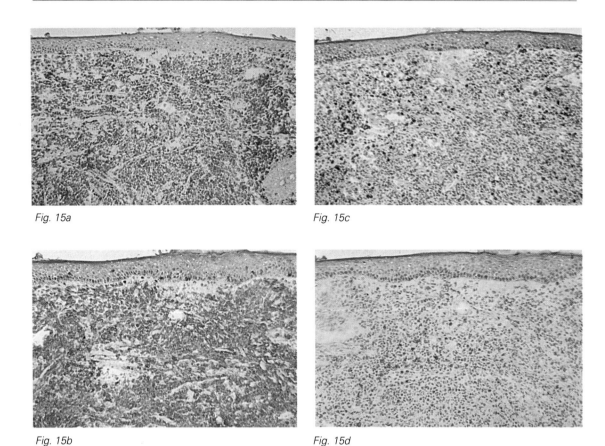

Fig. 15a

Fig. 15c

Fig. 15b

Fig. 15d

Fig.15: Immunohistochemical characteristics of T-cell NHL. Immunostaining on frozen sections with different anti-T antibodies. This pattern is frequently observed: some pan-T antigens are not expressed by neoplastic T cells (loss of expression of CD5 and CD7 in this example). Fig. 15a = anti-CD3 antibody; fig. 15b = anti-CD2 antibody; fig. 15c = anti-CD5 antibody; fig. 15d = anti-CD9 antibody. (Acknowledgments to Dr J.F. Mosnier)

most cases have a normal CD4+ or more rarely a CD8+ phenotype, whereas only 15% of PTCL have an unusual CD4-/CD8- or CD4+/CD8+ phenotype. Recent studies on TCR expression have demonstrated that the majority of PTCL (70%) have a TCR-αβ phenotype like the majority of normal T cells; some cases, however, are γδ proliferations (57,58), whereas a number of others (about 20 to 30%) lack expression of both αβ and γδ TCR (56,58).

Another problem arises when the histological and immunohistological pattern is polymorphous, with a mixture of polyclonal B cells and mature T cells. This is found in some cases of angioimmunoblastic lymphomas, or "granulomatous" proliferations such as lymphomatoid granulomatosis and polymorphic reticulosis. These entities have

recently been recognized in most cases on the basis of immunogenomic studies as clonal T-cell proliferations (59-61).

In conclusion, the main immunophenotypic criteria helpful in the diagnosis of T-cell neoplasia are:

- determination of the T-cell phenotype of the morphologically abnormal cells (the latter sometimes being more easily identified on paraffin sections) *(figs. 11 and 12)*;

- in particular, demonstration of an "abnormal" T-cell phenotype consisting of a deletion of one or more pan-T cell antigens *(fig. 15)*, and/or an abnormal subset antigen expression. Such abnormal phenotypes can be considered as indirect markers of clonality.

Fig.16: Anaplastic large-cell NHL. Few reactive T cells produce IL-2. Demonstration of IL-2-mRNA production by in situ hybridization with a 35S-labelled specific probe.

Lymphoid tumours of uncertain lineage

The number of cases which do not clearly disclose either a B or a T-cell origin ("null-cell" non-Hodgkin's lymphomas) has considerably decreased since the development of cellular markers. These cases corresponded initially to lymphoid proliferations in which tumour cells did not express immunoglobulins, and did not form E rosettes. Extensive immunophenotypic studies using a large panel of monoclonal antibodies directed against B- and T-cell differentiation antigens, as well as recent genomic studies, have demonstrated that most cases are B- or T-cell lymphomas which have lost some or all their lineage-specific antigens (42,62-64). Histologically, these tumours often correspond to large-cell anaplastic lymphomas (32,63). Thus, the diagnosis of so-called true histiocytic lymphomas or malignant histiocytosis should be considered in the rare tumours which do not show expression of any pan-B and pan-T markers, and which do not display clonal rearrangements of the T-cell receptor or immunoglobulin genes. In addition, these histiocytic malignancies should express some specific macrophage/histiocyte antigens, such as CD68 (29,64).

Host-immune response in malignant lymphomas

In any malignant tumour, and especially in NHL, the host develops an immune response against tumour cells (65). At least 4 host-immune pathways may be brought into play to kill the tumour cells: T-cell-mediated cytotoxicity, antibody-dependent cytotoxicity, macrophage cytotoxicity and natural killer cell activity. T lymphocytes infiltrating the tumour (TIL-T) have been demonstrated *in situ* in B-cell NHL. Immunohistochemical studies have described the amounts and the phenotype of TIL-T; these latter cells have mostly a CD3+ CD4+ phenotype (66) associated with a minor subset of CD3+ CD8+ cells (67). The TIL-T express activation markers such as HLA-DR (66), dipeptidylamino-peptidase IV activity (CD26) (68), CD25 (66,69) and T9 (CD71) antigens (69). Polymorphonuclear neutrophils, eosinophils and macrophages are often disclosed in association with TIL-T. NK cells recognized by the CD57 MAb are very rare in tumour tissue and the role of these NK cells in tumour rejection is not clearly determined. It must be pointed out that the number of NK cells *in situ* and of circulating NK cells may be dissociated (70,71).

The question of the precise nature of these cytotoxic cells still remains unanswered. Among T cells, CD4+ (72,73) or CD8 subsets could be cytotoxic and have a role in the proliferation and activation of the polymorphonuclear neutrophils and of the macrophages. In addition, these T cells regulate the proliferation and differentiation of normal and tumour B cells (69,74). Conversely, tumour B cells could inhibit *in vitro* the proliferative response of TIL-T upon recombinant IL-2 (r-IL-2) (69). This latter effect may be direct (soluble factor synthesized by tumour cells) or mediated by suppressor T cells. The pivotal role of T-cell immune response in tumour growth is outlined by spontaneous regression of some ML (67,75). A previous work has demonstrated that 80% of TIL-T proliferate in response to recombinant IL-2, but only 10% are CD25+ and CD71+. B-cell clones have a variable influence on autologous T-lymphocyte proliferation in the presence of recombinant IL-2 with no modification, increase or decrease, of this proliferation. The positive influence of the clone is associated with a favourable prognosis (69). Moreover, *in situ* hybridization methods have demonstrated that IL-2 and IFN-γ are effectively synthesized in the microenvironment of the tumour cells (76,77). These two lymphokines are involved in the activation of cytotoxic cells. Taken together, these data highlight the crucial role of host stromal lymphoid reaction: subsets of TIL-T are indeed involved in the growth control and killing of tumour cells.

TABLE 1

CD Cell Markers

CD	Selection of Assigned Monoclonal Antibodies	Main Cellular Reactivity	Recognized Membrane Component
CD1a	NA1/34; T6; VIT6; Leu6	Thy, DC, B subset	gp49
CD1b	WM-25; 4A76, NUT2	Thy, DC, B subset	gp45
CD1c	L161; M241; 7C6; PHM3	Thy, DC, B subset	gp43
CD2	9.6; T11 ; 35.1	T	CD58 (LFA-3) receptor, gp50
CD2R	T11.3; VIT13; D66	Activated T	CD2 epitopes restr. to activ. T
CD3	T3; UCHT1; 38.1; Leu4	T	CD3-complex (5 chains), gp/p 26,20,16
CD4	T4; Leu3a; 91.D6	T subset	Class II/HIV receptor, gp59
CD5	T1; UCHT2; T101; HH9; AMG4	T, B subset	gp67
CD6	T12; T411	T, B subset	gp100
CD7	3A1; 4A; CL1.3; G3-7	T	gp40
CD8	Alpha-chain: T8; Leu2a; M236; UCHT4; T811 beta chain: T8/2T8-5H7	T subset	Class I receptor, gp32a, /or/ßdimer
CD9	CLB-thromb/8; PHN200; FMC56	Pre-B, M, Plt	p24
CD10	J5, VILA1, BA-3	Lymph.Prog., CALL, Germ Ctr. B, G	Neutral endopeptidase, gp100 CALLA
CD11a	MHM24; 2F12; CRIS-3	Leucocytes, broad	LFA-1, gp180/95
CD11b	Mo1; 5A4.C5; LPM19C	M, G, NK	C3bi receptor, gp155/95
CD11c	B-LY6; L29; BL-4H4	M, G, NK, B sub	gp150/95
CDw12	M67	M, G, Plt	(p90-120)
CD13	MY7, MCS-2, TUK1, MOU28	M, G	Aminopeptidase N, gp150
CD14	Mo2, UCHM1, VIM13, MoP15	M, (G), LHC	gp55
CD15	My1, VIM-D5	G, (M)	3-FAL, X-Hapten
CD16	BW209/2; HUNK2; VEP13; Leu11c	NK, G, Mac.	FcRIII, gp50-65
CDw17	GO35, Huly-m13	G, M, Plt	Lactosylceramide
CD18	MHM23; M232; 11H6; CLB54	Leucocytes, broad	ß-chain to CD11a,b,c
CD19	B4; HD37	B	gp95
CD20	B1; 1F5	B	p37/32, Ion channel?
CD21	B2; HB5	B subset	C3d/EBV-Rec. (CR2),p140
CD22	HD39; S-HCL1; To15	Cytopl. B./surface B subset	GP135, homology to myelin assoc. gp (MAG)
CD23	Blast-2, MHM6	B subset, act.M, Eo	FceRII, gp45-50
CD24	VIBE3; BA-1	B, G	gp41/38?
CD25	TAC; 7G7/B6; 2A3	Activated T, B, M	IL-2Rßchain, gp55
CD26	134-2C2; TS145	Activated T	Dipeptidylpeptidase IV, gp120
CD27	VIT14; S152; OKT18A; CLB-9F4	T subset	p55(dimer)
CD28	9.3; KOLT2	T subset	gp44
CD29	K20; A-1A5	Broad	VLAß-,integrin ß1-chain,Plt GPIIa
CD30	Ki-1; Ber-H2; HSR4	Activated T, B, Reed-Sternberg	gp120, Ki-1
CD31	SG134; TM3; HEC-75; ES12F11	Plt, M, G, B, (T)	gp140, Plt, GPIIa
CDw32	CIKM5; 41H16; IV.3	M, G, B	FcRII, gp40
CD33	My9; H153; L4F3	M, Prog., AML	gp67
CD34	My10, BI-3C5, ICH-3	Prog	gp105-120
CD35	TO5, CBO4, J3D3	G, M, B	CR1
CD36	5F1, CIMeg1; ESIVC7	M, Plt, (B)	gp90, Plt GPIV
CD37	HD28; HH1; G28-1	B, (T,M)	gp40-52
CD38	HB7; T16	Lymph.Prog., Pc, Act. T	p45
CD39	AC2; G28-2	B subset, (M)	gp70-100
CD40	G28-5	B, carcinomas	gp50, Homology to NGF-Receptor
CD41	PBM 64; CLB-thromb/7; PL273	Plt	Plt GPIIb/IIIa complex and GPIIb
CD42a	FMC25; BL-H6; GR-P	Plt	Plt GPIX, gp23
CD42b	PHN89; AN51; GN287	Plt	Plt GPIb, gp135/25

CD43	OTH 71C5; G19-1; MEM-59	T, G, brain	Leucosialin, gp95
CD44	GRHL1; F10-44-2; 33-383; BRIC35	T, G, brain, RBC	Pgp-1, gp80-95
CD45	T29/33; BMAC 1; AB 187	Leucocytes	LCA, T200
CD45RA	G1-15; FB-11-13; 73.5	T subset, B, G, M	Restricted T200, gp220
CD45RB	PTD/26/16	T subset, B, G, M	Restricted T200
CD45RO	UCHL1	T subset, B, G, M	Restricted T200, gp180
CD46	HULYM5; 122-2; J4B	Leucocytes, broad	Membrane co-factor protein (MCP) gp66/56
CD47	BRIC 126; CIKM1; BRIC 125	Broad	gp 47-52, N-linked glycan, Rh assoc.
CD48	WM68; LO-MN25; J4-57	Leucocytes	gp41, PI-linked
CDw49b	CLB-Throm/4; Gi14	Plt, cultured T	VLA-alpha2-chain, Plt GPIa
CDw49d	B5G10; HP2/1; HP1/3	M, T, B, (LHC), Thy	VLA-alpha4-chain, gp150
CDw49f	GoH3	Plt, (T)	VLA-alpha6-chain, Plt GPIc
CDw50	101-1D2; 140-11	Leucocytes, broad	gp180/108, PI-linked
CD51	13C2; 23C6; NKI-M7; MKI-M9	(Plt)	VNR alpha-chain
CDw52	097; YTH66.9; Campath-1	Leucocytes	Campath-1, gp21-28
CD53	MEM-53; HI29; HI36; HD77	Leucocytes	gp32-40, PI-linked
CD54	RR1/7F7; WEHI-CAMI	Broad, Activ.	ICAM-1
CD55	143-30; BRIC 110; BRIC 128; F2B-7.2	Broad	DAF (decay accelerating factor),
CD56	Leu19; NKH1; FP2-11.14, L185	NK, activ. lymphocytes	gp220/135, NKH1, isoform of N CAM
CD57	Leu7; L183; L187	NK, T, B sub, Brain	gp110, HNK1
CD58	TS2/9; G26; BRIC5	Leucocytes, Epithel	LFA-3, gp40-65
CD59	Y53.1; MEM-43	Broad	gp18-20
CDw60	M-T32; M-T21; M-T41; UM4D4	T sub	NeuAc-NeuAc-Gal-
CD61	Y2/51; CLB-thromb/1; VI-PL2; BL-E6	Plt	Integrinß3-, VNRß-chain, PltGPIIIa
CD62	CLB-thromb/6,; CLB-thromb/5; RUU-SP1.18.1	Plt activ.	GMP-140 (PADGEM), gp140
CD63	RUU-SP2.28; CLB-gran/12	Plt activ., M, (G, T, B)	gp53
CD64	Mab32.2; Mab22	M	FcRI, gp75
CDw65	VIM2; HE10; CF4; VIM8	G, M	Ceramide-dodecasaccharide 4c
CD66	CLB gran/10; YTH71.3	G	Phosphoprotein pp180-200
CD67	B13.9; G10F5; JML-H16	G	p100, PI-linked
CD68	EBM11; Y2/131; Y-1/82A; Ki-M7; Ki-M6	Macrophages	gp100
CD69	MLR3; L78; BL-Ac/p26; FN50	Activated B, T	gp32/28, AIM
CDw70	Ki-24; HNE 51; HNC 142	Activated B,-T, Reed-Sternberg cells	Ki-24
CD71	138-18; 120-2A3; MEM-75; VIP-1; Nu-TfR2	Proliferating cells, Mac.	Transferrin receptor
CD72	S-HCL2; J3-109; BU-40; BU-41	B	gp43/39
CD73	1E9.28.1; 7G2.2.11; AD2	B subset, T subset	ecto-5'-nucleotidase, p69
CD74	LN2; BU-43; BU-45	B, M	Class II assoc. invariant chain, gp41/35/33
CDw75	LN1; HH2; EBU-141	Mature B, (T subset)	p53?
CD76	HD66; CRIS-4	Mature B, T subset	gp85/67
CD77	38.13(BLA); 424/4A11; 424/3D9	Restr. B	Globotriaosylceramide (Gb3)
CDw78	antiBa; LO-panB-a; 1588	B, (M)	?

Agreement on designation of human leucocyte differentiation antigens obtained at the Fourth International Workshop on Human Leucocyte Differentiation Antigens (Vienna, 1989).

Abbreviations : Thy = thymocytes, DC = dendritic cells, B = B cells, T = T cells, M = monocytes, G=granulocytes, Plt = platelets, Prog = progenitor cells, Germ.Ctr.B. = germinal centre B-cells, NK = NK-cells, Mac = macrophages, cyto = cytoplasmic, LHC = epidermal Langerhans cells

From W KNAPP, B DORKEN, P RIEBER, RE SCHMIDT, H STEIN, AEGKr VON DEM BORNE, CD Antigens 1989 Blood, 1989, 74, 1448-1450

TABLE II

Main antibodies commonly used for the immunophenotyping of lymphomas in routinely fixed paraffin-embedded tissues

Antibody	CD	Main cellular Reactivity	Recognized membrane component	Diagnostic value
2BV11+PD7/26	45	leucocytes	leucocyte common antigen, T200	haematopoietic tumours of white cell origin
UCHL1	45 RO	Most T cells occasionally B, G, M	Restricted T200, gp180	Most T-cell lymphomas, rare B-cell lymphomas
MT1/DFT1	43	T-cells, occasionally B, G, M	Leucosialin, gp95	Most T-cell lymphomas, rare B-cell lymphomas
Poly-CD3	3	T-cells	CD3 antigen (Σ chain)	T-cell lymphomas
β-F1 +		T-cells	ß chain of T-cell receptor	T-cell lymphomas
MB2°		B-cells, macrophages,		Most B-cell lymphomas rare T-cell lymphomas
LN1°	w75	Mature B-cells, T-cell subset, macrophages		Most B-cell lymphomas, rare T-cell lymphomas
LN2°/MB3	74	B-cells, T-cell subset, macrophages	HLA invariant chain	Most B-cell lymphomas, rare T-cell lymphomas
L26°°	20	B-cells		B-cell lymphomas
Ber-H2/Ki1	30	Activated T, B, Reed-Sternberg cells	Ki-1 (gp 120)	Hodgkin's disease, anaplastic large-cell lymphoma
Leu M1	15	Myeloid cells, macrophages, Reed-Sternberg cells	X-hapten	Hodgkin's disease
KP1	68	Macrophages, myeloid cells		True histiocytic lymphomas
E11	35	Follicular dendritic reticulum cells, G, M, B		Follicular lymphomas
BCL-2		Lymphoid cells, except reactive germinal centre cells	BCL-2 gene product	Follicular lymphomas, versus lymphoid follicular hyperplasia

+ Better results on frozen sections; on paraffin sections, to be used after proteolytic digestion;
° not leucocyte-restricted; °° better results after formalin fixation

Abbreviations: *see Table 1*

References

1. POLAK JM, VAN NOORDEN S

   Immunocytochemistry, practical applications in pathology and biology.
   John Wright and Sons, Bristol, 1983.

2. POLAK JM, VAN NOORDEN S

   An introduction to immunocytochemistry: current techniques and problems.
   Oxford University Press Royal Microscopical Society, 1984.

3. TAYLOR CR.

   Immunoperoxidase techniques: practical and theoretical aspects.
   Arch Pathol Lab Med, 1978; 102: 113-121.

4. TAYLOR CR, KLEDZIK G

   Immunohistologic techniques in surgical pathology. A spectrum of new special stains.
   Hum Pathol, 1981; 12: 590-596.

5. FALINI B, TAYLOR CR

   New developments in immunoperoxidase techniques and their application.
   Arch Pathol Lab Med, 1981; 107: 105-117.

6. MASON DY, BIBERFELD P

   Technical aspects of lymphoma histology.
   J Histochem Cytochem, 1980; 28: 731-745.

7. MASON DY, ERBER WN, FALINI B, STEIN H, GATTER KC

   Immunoenzymatic labelling of haematological samples with monoclonal antibodies.
   In PCL Beverley, ed 1986. Methods in haematology: monoclonal antibodies. London, Churchill Livingstone, 145.

8. WARNKE RA, GATTER KC, FALINI B et al.
Diagnosis of human lymphoma with monoclonal anti-leukocyte antibodies.
N Engl J Med, 1983; 309: 1275-1281.

9. TAYLOR CR
Monoclonal antibodies and "routine" paraffin sections.
Arch Pathol Lab Med, 1985; 109: 115-116.

10. MASON DY, GATTER KC
The role of immunocytochemistry in diagnostic pathology.
J Clin Pathol, 1987; 40: 1042-1054.

11. DAVEY FR, GATTER KC, RALFKIAER E, PULFORD K, KRISSANSEN GW, MASON DY
Immunophenotyping of non-Hodgkin's lymphomas using a panel of antibodies on paraffin-embedded tissues.
Am J Pathol, 1987; 129: 54-63.

12. MASON DY, CORDELL J, BROWN M et al.
Detection of T cell in paraffin wax embedded tissue using antibodies against a peptide sequence from the CD3 antigen.
J Clin Pathol, 1989; 42: 1194-1200.

13. MASON DY, SAMMONS RE
The labelled-antigen method of immunoenzymatic staining.
J Histochem Cytochem, 1979; 27: 832-840.

14. GREEN MA, SVILAND L, MALCOM AJ, PEARSON ADJ
Improved method for immunoperoxidase detection of membrane antigens in frozen sections.
J Clin Pathol, 1989; 42: 875-880.

15. STERNBERGER LA, HARDY PH, CUCULIS JJ, MEYER HG
The unlabelled antibody enzyme method immunohistochemistry. Preparation and properties of soluble antigen-antibody complex (horseradish peroxidase-antihorseradish peroxidase) and its use in identification of spirochetes.
J Histochem Cytochem, 1970; 18: 315-333.

16. CORDELL JL, FALINI B, ERBER WN et al.
Immunoenzymatic labelling of monoclonal antibodies using immune complexes of alkaline phosphatase and monoclonal anti-alkaline phosphatase (APAAP complexes).
J Histochem Cytochem, 1984; 32: 219-229.

17. HSU SM, RAINE L, FANGER H
Use of avidin-biotin-peroxidase complex (ABC) in immunoperoxidase techniques: a comparison between ABC and unlabelled antibody (PAP) procedures.
J Histochem Cytochem, 1981; 29: 577-580.

18. BONNARD C
The streptavidin-biotin bridge technique: application in light and electron microscope immunocytochemistry in immunolabelling for electron microscopy.
Ed. Polak JM and Varndell IM, Elsevier Scientific Publishers, Amsterdam, 1984.

19. FALINI B, ABDULAZIZ Z, GERDES J et al.
Description of sequential staining procedure for double immunoenzymatic staining of pairs of antigens using monoclonal antibodies.
J Immunol Methods, 1986; 93: 265-273.

20. GERDES J, SCHWARTING R, STEIN H
High proliferative activity of Reed-Sternberg-associated antigen Ki-1 positive cells in normal lymphoid tissue.
J Clin Pathol, 1986; 39: 993-997.

21. PICKER LJ, WEISS LM, MEDEIROS LJ, WOOD GS, WARNKE RA
Immunophenotypic criteria for the diagnosis of non-Hodgkin's lymphoma.
Am J Pathol, 1987; 128: 181-201.

22. BRENNER MB, MC LEAN J, SCHEFT M, WARNKE RA, JONES N, STROMINGER JL
Characterization and expression of the human αβ T-cell receptor using a framework monoclonal antibody.
J Immunol, 1987; 138: 1502-1507.

23. BAND H, HOCHSTENBACH F, MC LEAN J, KRANGEL MS, BRENNER MB
Immunochemical proof that a novel rearranging gene encodes the T-cell receptor gamma subunit.
Science, 1987; 238: 682-685.

24. POSTON RN, SIDNU YS
Diagnosis of tumors on routine surgical sections by immunohistochemistry: use of cytokeratin, common leukocyte antigens, and other markers.
J Clin Pathol, 1986; 39: 524-529.

25. FALINI B, PILERI S, STEIN H et al.
Variable expression of leucocyte-common (CD45) antigen in CD30 (Ki1)-positive anaplastic large-cell lymphoma. Implications for the differential diagnosis between lymphoid and non-lymphoid malignancies.
Hum Pathol, 1990; 21: 624-629.

26. CARTUN RW, BRUCE COLES F, PASTUSZAK WT
Utilization of monoclonal antibody L26 in the identification and confirmation of B-cell lymphomas. A sensitive and specific marker applicable to Formalin-and B5-fixed, paraffin-embedded tissues.
Am J Pathol, 1987; 129: 415-421.

27. MASON DY, COMAANS-BITTER WM, CORDELL JL, VERHOEVEN MAJ, VAN DONGEN JMM
Antibody L26 recognizes an intracellular epitope on the B-cell-associated CD20 antigen.
Am J Pathol, 1990; 136: 1215-1222.

28. PULFORD KAF, RIGNEY EM, MICKLEM KJ et al.
KP1: a new monoclonal antibody that detects a monocyte / macrophage associated antigen in routinely processed tissue sections.
J Clin Pathol, 1989; 42: 414-421.

29. RALFKIAER E, DELSOL G, O'CONNOR NTJ et al.

Malignant lymphomas of true histiocytic origin. A clinical, histological, immunophenotypic and genotypic study.

J Pathol, 1990; 160: 9-17.

30. CHITTAL SM, CAVERIVIERE P, SCHWARTING R et al.

Monoclonal antibodies in the diagnosis of Hodgkin's disease: the search for a rational panel.

Am J Surg Pathol, 1988; 12: 9-21.

31. KORNSTEIN MJ, BONNER H, GEE B, COHEN R, BROOKS J

Leu M1 and S 100 in Hodgkin's disease and non-Hodgkin's lymphomas.

Am J Clin Pathol, 1986; 85: 433-437.

32. STEIN H, MASON DY, GERDES J et al.

The expression of the Hodgkin's disease-associated antigen Ki-1 in reactive and neoplastic lymphoid tissue: evidence that Reed-Sternberg cells and histiocytic malignancies are derived from activated lymphoid cells.

Blood, 1985; 66: 848-858.

33. DELSOL G, AL SAATI T, GATTER KC et al.

Coexpression of epithelial membrane antigen (EMA), Ki-1 and interleukin-2 receptor by anaplastic large-cell lymphomas. Diagnostic value in so-called "Malignant Histiocytosis".

Am J Pathol, 1988; 130: 59-70.

34. TUBBS RR, FISHLEDER A, WEISS RA, SAVAGE RA, SEBEK BA, WEICK JK

Immunohistologic cellular phenotypes of lymphoproliferative disorders. Comprehensive evaluation of 564 cases including 257 non-Hodgkin's lymphomas classified by the International Working Formulation.

Am J Pathol, 1983; 113: 207-221.

35. KVALEY S, LANGHOLM R, KAALHUS O, MARTON PF, HOST H, GODALT T

Immunologic subsets in B-cell lymphomas defined by surface immunoglobulin isotype and complement receptor. Their relationship to survival.

Scand J Haematol, 1985; 145: 67-74.

36. SCHURMAN HJ, VAN BAARLEN J, HUPPES W et al.

Immunophenotyping of non-Hodgkin's lymphoma. Lack of correlation between immunophenotype and cell morphology.

Am J Pathol, 1987; 129: 140-151.

37. LEVY R, WARNKE RA, DORFMAN RF, HAIMOVICH J

The monoclonality of human B-cell lymphomas.

J Exp Med, 1977; 145: 1014-1028.

38. AISENBERG AC, WILKES BM, JACOBSON JO, HARRIS NL

Immunoglobulin gene rearrangements in adult non-Hodgkin's lymphoma.

Am J Med, 1987; 82: 738-743.

39. HENNI T, GAULARD PH, DIVINE M et al.

Comparison of genetic probe with immunophenotypic analysis in lymphoproliferative disorders: a study of 87 cases.

Blood, 1988; 72: 1937-1942.

40. MOLLER P, MOLDENHAUER G, MOMBURG F et al.

Mediastinal lymphoma of clear cell type is a tumor corresponding to terminal steps of B-cell differentiation.

Blood, 1987; 69: 1087-1094.

41. BOROWITZ MJ, BOUSUAROS A, BRYNES RK et al.

Monoclonal antibody phenotyping of B-cell non-Hodgkin's lymphomas. The Southeastern cancer study group experience.

Am J Pathol, 1985; 121: 514-521.

42. KNOWLES DM, DODSON L, BURKE JS et al.

SIg-E- ("Null-cell") non-Hodgkin's lymphomas. Multiparametric determination of their B- or T-cell lineage.

Am J Pathol, 1985; 120: 356-364.

43. SIEGELMAN MH, CLEARY ML, WARNKE RA, SKLAR J.

Frequent biclonality and Ig gene alterations among B-cell lymphomas that show multiple histologic forms.

J Exp Med, 1985; 161: 850-859.

44. PELICCI PG, KNOWLES DM, ARLIN ZA et al.

Multiple clonal B-cell expansions and c-myc oncogene rearrangements in acquired immune deficiency syndrome-related lymphoproliferative disorders.

J Exp Med, 1986; 164: 2049-2060.

45. STEIN H, LENNERT K, FELLER AC, MASON DY.

Immunohistological analysis of human lymphoma. Correlation of histological and immunological categories.

Adv Cancer Res, 1984; 42: 67-147.

46. KRAJEWSKI AS, GUY K, DEWAR AE, COSSAR D.

Immunohistochemical analysis of human MHC class II antigens in B-cell non-Hodgkin's lymphomas.

J Pathol, 1985; 145: 185-194.

47. INGHIRAMI G, WIECZOREK R, ZHU BY, SILBER R, DALLA-FAVERA R, KNOWLES DM

Differential expression of LFA-1 molecules in non-Hodgkin's lymphoma and lymphoid leukemia.

Blood, 1988; 72: 1431-1441.

48. NGAN BY, CHEN-LEVY Z, WEISS LM, WARNKE RA, CLEARY ML

Expression in non-Hodgkin's lymphoma of the bcl-2 protein associated with the t(14;18) chromosomal translocation.

N Engl J Med, 1988; 318: 1638-1644.

49. PEZZELA F, TSE A, CORDELL JL, PULFORD KAF, GATTER KC, MASON DY

Expression of the bcl-2 oncogene protein is not specific for the 14;18 chromosomal translocation.

Am J Pathol, 1990; 137: 225-232.

50. GAULARD P, D'AGAY MF, PEUCHMAUR M et al.

Expression of the bcl-2 gene product in follicular lymphoma.

Am J Pathol, 1992 (in press).

51. KNOWLES DM

Immunophenotypic and antigen receptor gene rearrangement analysis in T-cell neoplasia.

Am J Pathol, 1989; 134: 761-785.

52. WEISS LM, CRABTREE GS, ROUSE RV, WARNKE RA

Morphologic and immunologic characterization of 50 peripheral T-cell lymphomas.

Am J Pathol, 1985; 118: 316-324.

53. GROGAN TM, FIELDER K, RANGEL C et al.

Peripheral T-cell lymphomas: aggressive disease with heterogeneous immunotypes.

Am J Clin Pathol, 1985; 120: 356-370.

54. HORNING SJ, WEISS LM, CRABTREE GS, WARNKE RA

Clinical and phenotypic diversity of T-cell lymphomas.

Blood, 1986; 67: 1578-1590.

55. COIFFIER B, BERGER F, BRYON PA, MAGAUD JP

T-cell lymphomas: immunologic, histologic, clinical and therapeutic analysis of 63 cases.

J Clin Oncol, 1988; 6: 1584-1591.

56. PICKER LJ, BRENNER MB, MICHIES S, WARNKE RA

Expression of T-cell receptor δ chain in benign and malignant T-lineage lymphoproliferations.

Am J Pathol, 1988; 132: 401-405.

57. FARCET JP, GAULARD P, MAROLLEAU JP et al.

Hepatosplenic T-cell lymphoma : sinusal/sinusoidal localization of malignant cells expressing the T-cell receptor γδ.

Blood, 1990; 75: 2213-2219.

58. GAULARD P, BOURQUELOT P, KANAVAROS P et al.

Expression of the alpha/beta and gamma/delta T-cell receptors in 57 cases of peripheral T-cell lymphomas. Identification of a subset of γδ T-cell lymphomas.

Am J Pathol, 1990; 137: 617-628.

59. WEISS LM, STRICKLER JG, DORFMANN RF, HORNING SJ, WARNKE RA, SKLAR J

Clonal T-cell populations in angioimmunoblastic lymphadenopathy, and angioimmunoblastic lymphadenopathy-like lymphoma.

Am J Pathol, 1986; 122: 392-403.

60. GAULARD P, HENNI T, MAROLLEAU JP et al.

Lethal midline granuloma (polymorphic reticulosis) and lymphomatoid granulomatosis: evidence for a monoclonal T-cell lymphoproliferative disorder.

Cancer, 1988; 62: 49-57.

61. LIPFORD EH, MARGOLICK JB, LONGO DL, FAUCI A, JAFFE ES

Angiocentric immunoproliferative lesions: a clinicopathologic spectrum of post-thymic T-cell proliferations.

Blood, 1988 ; 72 : 1674-1681.

62. WEISS LM, TRELA MJ, CLEARY ML, TURNER RR, WARNKE RA, SKLAR J

Frequent immunoglobulin and T-cell receptor rearrangements in "histiocytic" neoplasms.

Am J Pathol, 1985; 121: 369-373.

63. KADIN ME, SAKO D, BERLINER N et al.

Childhood Ki-1 lymphoma presenting with skin lesions and peripheral lymphadenopathy.

Blood, 1986; 68: 1042-1049.

64. VAN DER VALK P, VAN OOSTVEEN JW, STEL HV, VAN DER KWAST TH, MELIEF CJF, MEIJER CJLM

Phenotypic and genotypic analysis of large-cell lymphomas, formerly classified as true histiocytic lymphoma: identification of an unusual group of tumors.

Leukemia Res, 1990; 14: 337-346.

65. AL SAATI T, CAVERIVIERE P, BROUSSE N et al.

Cells associated with the malignant clone in non-Hodgkin's lymphoma.

In: Ed. S. Karger, Basel, 1980: pp 61-72.

66. JARRY A, BROUSSE N, SOUQUE A, BARGE J, MOLAS G, POTET F

Lymphoid stromal reaction in gastrointestinal lymphomas: immuno-histochemical study of 14 cases.

J Clin Pathol, 1987; 40: 760-765.

67. AGNARSSON BA, KADIN ME

Host response in lymphomatoid papulosis.

Hum Pathol, 1989; 20: 747-752.

68. COZZI M, GLOGHINI A, SULFARO S, VOLPE R, CARBONE A

Dipeptidylaminopeptidase IV activity in T-lymphocyte subsets in B-cell non-Hodgkin's lymphomas.

Hum Pathol, 1989; 20: 987-993.

69. JACOB MC, PICCINI MP, BONNEFOIX T et al.

T-lymphocytes from invaded lymph nodes in patients with B-cell-derived non-Hodgkin's lymphoma: reactivity toward the malignant clone.

Blood, 1990; 75: 1154-1162.

70. VOSE BM, MOORE M

Human tumor-infiltrating lymphocytes: a marker of host response.

Semin Hematol, 1985; 22: 27-33.

71. KLEIN G, KLEIN E

    Evolution of tumours and the impact of molecular oncology.

    Nature, 1985; 315: 190-191.

72. SPITS H, YSSEL H, TEERBORST C et al.

    Establishment of human T-lymphocyte clones highly cytotoxic for an EBV-transformed B cell-line in serum-free medium: isolation of clones that differ in phenotype and specificity.

    J Immunol, 1982; 128: 95-101.

73. YSSEL H, SPITS H, DE VRIES JE

    A cloned human T-cell-line cytotoxic for autologous and allogenic B lymphoma cells.

    J Exp Med, 1984; 160: 239-241.

74. HIROHATA S, LIPSKY E

    T-cell regulation of human B-cell proliferation and differentiation. Regulatory influences of CD45R+, and CD45R+, cell subsets.

    J Immunol, 1989; 142: 2597-25.

75. DROBYSKI WR, QAZI R

    Spontaneous regression in non-Hodgkin's lymphoma: clinical and pathogenetic considerations.

    Am J Hematol, 1979; 31: 138-141.

76. PEUCHMAUR M, EMILIE D, CREVON MC, SOLAL-CELIGNY P et al.

    IL-2mRNA expression in Tac-positive malignant lymphomas.

    Am J Pathol, 1990; 136: 383-390.

77. PEUCHMAUR M, EMILIE D, CREVON MC et al.

    IL-2 and IFN-γ expression in follicular lymphoma.

    Am J Clin Pathol, 1991; 95: 55-62.

Genotype

F. REYES

The genotype approach has recently been proposed in order to overcome some limitations of immunohistological techniques in establishing the phenotype and clonality of malignant cells, especially in the case of T-cell neoplasms. This approach is based on the study of the DNA rearrangements which assemble the genes for antigen-receptors in B- or T- cells (1). The organisation of genes encoding Ig and TCR and the processes of DNA recombination which take place during B- or T-cell differentiation have been described above (see pp. 19-30). DNA recombinations, or rearrangements, create genotypic markers unique to each individual cell, hence allowing recognition of a clonal expansion and, theoretically, of its B- or T-cell derivation. The identification of Ig and TCR gene rearrangements is based on a hybridization technique using DNA-specific probes. DNA is extracted from tissue biopsy samples, digested with restriction endonucleases, subjected to electrophoresis in agarose gel, transferred onto a nitrocellulose filter by the Southern method and hybridized to ^{32}P-labelled DNA probes (2-4).

Ig gene rearrangements

The organisation of the κ light-chain locus, both in its germ-line and rearranged configuration, is shown in fig. 5 on p. 24. Restriction sites for a widely used endonuclease, termed BamHI, are also shown. As a result of the VJ rearrangement which takes place during B-cell differentiation, the position of some restriction sites is modified; DNA digestion will then generate fragments whose length differs from that observed in the germ-line configuration.

Thus, rearrangements of the κ locus can be detected by using an appropriate restriction endonuclease (BamHI) and DNA probe (Cκ). In the case of a polyclonal B-cell population, the multiple rearrangements generate multiple fragments of different lengths, resulting in a smear upon electrophoresis. Conversely, in the case of a monoclonal B-cell population, the unique rearrangement of one (or both) κ locus (loci) will be detected as one (or two) non-germ-line band(s), together with a decreased (or absent) germ-line signal.

Finally, rearrangements of the κ locus can be detected with a Cκ probe which reveals a 12 kb BamHI germ-line band. Rearrangements of the heavy-chain locus are usually analyzed with a J_H probe (fig. 6, p. 25) which reveals an 18 kb BamHI or a 19 kb EcoRI (another endonuclease) germ-line band. Endonucleases HindIII or BglII can also be used, since corresponding restriction sites are located 5' (upstream) of the switch (S) sequence and are thus not affected by the heavy chain isotype switching of maturing B cells. The study of rearrangements of the λ locus is made difficult by the polymorphism of the C subsegments.

TCR gene rearrangements

These are also detected by using appropriate restriction endonucleases and specific DNA probes. However, the method described above is not suitable for analyzing rearrangements of the TCR-α locus, since the very large size of the Jα region *(see fig. 8, p. 26)* would require the use of a large number of Jα probes. Rearrangements of the TCR-ß locus are detected by a Cß probe which hybridizes to both highly homologous Cß1 and Cß2 subsegments *(fig. 7, p. 26)*. This probe reveals a 24 kb germ-line band after BamHI digestion; two 11 and 4 kb germ-line bands after Eco-RI digestion; three 3.5, 6.5 and 8 kb germ-line bands after HindIII digestion. In BamHI-digested DNA, depending whether one or two alleles are involved, the VDJ rearrangement of either the Cß1 or Cß2 region of the ß locus results in the presence of one (or two) additional non-germ-line band(s), together with an absence or a decreased intensity of the 24 kb band. As shown in *fig. 7 on p. 26*, the assignment of such a rearrangement to either Cß1 or Cß2 is based on the patterns oberved after EcoRI and HindIII digestion, respectively. Theoretically, Cß1 rearrangements result in additional EcoRI bands and a germ-line HindIII configuration. Cß2 rearrangements generate additional HindIII fragments and the deletion of the 11 kb EcoRI band. It should be noted that the 4 kb EcoRI germ-line band is never altered in either rearrangement.

Rearrangements of the TCR-γ locus *(fig. 9, p. 27)* are usually analysed by a Jγ1 probe which detects all VJ combinations. Moreover, the assignment of rearrangements to a given V and J subsegment can be effected by comparing the size of the bands observed after BamHI, EcoRI, HindIII and KpmI digestion [reviewed in (5)].

Rearrangements of the TCR-δ locus *(fig. 8, p. 26)* have recently been studied. According to current findings the use of two probes, Jδ1 and Jδ2, detects the vast majority of the rearrangements of this locus in HindIII and BamHI-digested DNA (4).

Sensitivity of the Southern blot assay

The genotypic patterns described above were first established in cell suspensions containing virtually 100% malignant clonal cells, e.g circulating leukaemic cells or established cell lines. In these cases, in addition to the rearranged bands, the disappearance of the germ-line band, as a result of a bi-allelic rearrangement or of a gene deletion (such as the deletion of the δ locus in T cells rearranging the α locus), is easily recognized. Similarly, a mono-allelic rearrangement results in a 50% decrease of the germ-line band intensity. However, other samples under study - such as those with partial infiltration of the marrow by malignant cells or most of the tissue biopsy samples from malignant lymphomas - contain sizeable amounts of "contaminating" non-malignant cells including non-T or non-B cells. The latter account for the persistence of a germ-line signal, even when malignant cells have rearranged or deleted on both alleles. Non-germ-line rearranged fragments are still recognized, however, even when malignant cells are present as a minor population accounting for as little as 5% of the total cells in a tissue sample (6,7).

Contribution of the genotypic study for the determination of clonality and lineage in malignant lymphoma

That DNA analysis by the Southern blot assay for Ig and TCR genes provides a reliable marker for clonality is well established (1). However, comparative phenotypic and genomic studies have established that in most cases of malignant lymphoma, gene-rearrangement assays are not essential to the diagnostic procedure since an accurate immunohistological study of biopsy samples is conclusive by detecting either an Ig monotypy or a pan-T antigen loss (CD7, CD5, CD2): Ig monotypy or pan-T antigen loss have been shown to correlate with a clonal process as revealed by DNA analysis

(3). Some cases remain, however, in which DNA analysis provides a critical support in identifying a clonal population within tumour cells (3). First, a few T-cell lymphoma specimens do not display pan-T antigen loss. Second, in some rare cases, large anaplastic lymphoma cells may not express either B- or T-differentiation antigens. Third, the partial infiltration of a node biopsy or the polymorphism of the cellular infiltrate seen in occasional cases makes it impossible to determine accurately the phenotype of tumour cells. Finally, DNA analysis is the only way to detect the presence of more than one clone, as revealed by at least three non-germ-line bands, within individual tumours. Such a so-called oligoclonal process is observed in the setting of histological conversion of low-grade into high-grade lymphomas, as well as in AIDS-related lymphomas (8, 9).

It should be noted that DNA analysis *per se* does not allow the assignment of malignant cells to the T-cell or the B-cell series. Indeed, uncharacteristic rearrangements exist, e.g. lymphoma cells may display a rearrangement of both Ig and TCR genes whereas they retain a completely characteristic B or T phenotype. This has been observed in 5 to 10% of malignant lymphomas (3,10). The same has been largely described in 25-50% of B- or T-cell leukaemias (5). It is generally assumed that such rearrangements result from a recombinase "mistake" since the heptamer/nonamer recombination signals that flank V,D and J segments in B- or T-cells are remarkably similar (11). Thus, the lineage specificity of clonal DNA rearrangements is not absolute and a conclusive definition requires an immunophenotypic study demonstrating that such rearrangements are productive.

References

1. KORSMEYER SJ

   Antigen receptor genes as molecular markers of lymphoid neoplasms.

   J Clin Invest, 1987; 79: 1291-1296.

2. LOISEAU P, DIVINE M, LE PASLIER D et al.

   Phenotypic and genotypic heterogeneity in large granular lymphocyte expansion.

   Leukemia, 1987; 205: 1-7.

3. HENNI T, GAULARD PH, DIVINE M et al.

   The respective contribution of the immunophenotypic and immunogenotypic methods for the determination of clonality and lineage in lymphoproliferative disorders. A study of 87 cases.

   Blood, 1988; 72: 1937-1943.

4. FARCET JP, GAULARD PH, MAROLLEAU JP et al.

   Hepatosplenic T-cell lymphoma: sinusal/sinusoidal localisation of malignant cells expressing the T-cell receptor γδ.

   Blood, 1990; 75: 2213-2219.

5. LEFRANC MP

   Organization of the human T-cell receptor genes.

   Eur Cytokine Net, 1990; 1: 121-130

6. CLEARLY ML, CHAO J, WARNKE R, SKLAR J

   Immunoglobulin gene rearrangement as a diagnostic criterion of B-cell lymphoma.

   Proc Natl Acad Sci USA, 1984; 81: 593-596.

7. AISENBERG AC, WILKES BM, JACOBSON JO, HARRIS NL

   Immunoglobulin gene rearrangements in adult non-Hodgkin's lymphoma.

   Am J Med, 1987; 82: 738-742.

8. SIEGELMAN MM, CLEARLY ML, WARNKE R, SKLAR J

   Frequent biclonality and Ig gene alterations among B-cell lymphomas that show multiple histologic forms.

   J Exp Med, 1985; 161: 850-856.

9. PELICCI PG, KNOWLES II DM, ARLIN ZA et al.

   Multiple monoclonal B-cell expansions and c-myc oncogene rearrangements in acquired immune deficiency syndrome-related lymphoproliferative disorders.

   J Exp Med, 1986; 164: 2049-2054.

10. PELICCI PG, KNOWLES II DM, DALLA FAVERA R

    Lymphoid tumors displaying rearrangements of both immunoglobulin and T-cell receptor genes.

    J Exp Med, 1985; 162: 1015-1028.

11. YANCOPOULOS GD, BLACKWELL TK, SUH H, HOOD L, ALT FN

    Introduced T-cell receptor variable region gene segments recombine in pre-B cells: evidence that B and T cells use a common recombinase.

    Cell, 1986; 44: 251-259.

3.

NODAL NON-HODGKIN'S LYMPHOMAS

edited by

N. Brousse, P. Solal-Céligny

The normal lymph node: structure and function

N. BROUSSE, J.Y. SCOAZEC

Lymph nodes, located along the lymphatic vessels, are peripheral lymphoid organs containing a great diversity of cell populations involved in the immune response, including various functional subpopulations of B and T lymphocytes, and several types of specialized antigen-presenting cells (dendritic cells) and antigen-processing cells (phagocytic histiocytes). Lymph nodes play three main roles: **(a)** concentration and filtration of the antigens, **(b)** contribution to the induction of B-and T-cell-mediated immune reactions, and **(c)** control of lymphocyte recirculation in the body. Knowledge of the normal structure and function of the lymph node is essential for the understanding of current classifications of non-Hodgkin's lymphomas, based on the assumption that neoplastic lymphoid populations have their counterparts in the normal immune system.

Lymph node architecture and organization

Lymph nodes are ovoid formations presenting both a convex and a concave face, the latter constituting the hilum (1). They are covered by a thin fibrous capsule, which sends numerous fibrous trabeculae throughout the lymphoid tissue. The fibrous structure of the lymph node is best visualized using reticulin stainings.

The overall structure of the lymph node is polarized. On its convex face, it receives afferent lymphatic vessels which penetrate the capsule. The hilum situated on the opposite face is the point by which efferent lymphatic vessels leave the lymph node. Between afferent and efferent vessels, the lymph circulates in sinuses through which it enters into contact with immune cells. Beneath the capsule is the marginal or subcapsular sinus from which numerous branches penetrate the lymphoid tissue. These sinuses are interconnected and progressively fuse into larger structures, best visible near the hilum. The sinuses of the lymph node contain macrophages, variable numbers of small lymphocytes, and a few plasma cells. They also contain a distinctive subset of B cells, the so-called monocytoid B cells or immature sinus histiocytes (2). These cells have round or oval nuclei and a moderate amount of pale staining cytoplasm. While morphologically similar to monocytes, they express the pan-B differentiation antigens. They are more prominent in certain reactive conditions [such as *Toxoplasma gondii* infections (3)].

Morphologically, the lymph node may be divided into two main zones *(fig. 1)*: the cortex and the medulla. The cortex constitutes the periphery of the lymph node. It comprises a dense lymphoid tissue containing a typical structure: the follicle, i.e. a discrete nodular aggregate of lymphoid cells. The distribution of follicles is uneven. On this basis, the cortex may be further subdivided into an outer cortex, containing the lymphoid follicles separated by

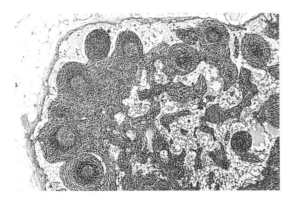

Fig. 1: **Normal lymph node.** *The overall structure shows the capsule, the marginal sinus and the two main zones: the cortex and the medulla.*

the interfollicular tissue, and an inner cortex, or paracortex, devoid of follicles. The medulla constitutes the perihilar region of the lymph node. It contains large sinuses separated by broad aggregates of lymphoid cells known as the medullary cords.

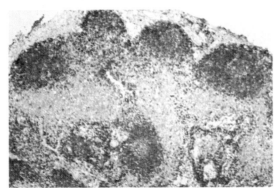

Fig. 2a

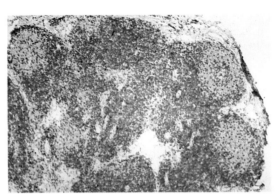

Fig. 2b

Fig. 2: **Normal lymph node.** *Immunoperoxidase staining using monoclonal antibodies directed against anti-pan-B (CD22) (fig. 2a) and anti-pan-T (CD3) (fig. 2b): the B-cell compartment is constituted by the lymphoid follicles and the T-cell compartment by the paracortex.*

Functionally, the lymph node may be divided into B- and T-lymphocyte regions or compartments. This distinction, suggested by earlier physiological experiments, then confirmed and detailed by immunohistochemical studies (4-7), is most obvious in the cortex. This zone comprises a B-lymphocyte compartment constituted by the lymphoid follicles of the outer cortex and a T-cell compartment corresponding to the interfollicular tissue and to the paracortex *(fig. 2)*. In each compartment, distinctive subsets of antigen-presenting cells are associated with the lymphoid cells (8). In contrast to cells of the monocyte-macrophage lineage, specialized antigen-presenting cells are incapable of phagocytosis and therefore lack most of the enzymatic equipment characteristic of typical tissue macrophages (9). The medulla lacks specific compartments for B and T cells, which are closely mixed, and is devoid of specialized antigen-presenting cells.

We will successively analyze the morphological and immunological characteristics of each of these compartments.

The B-cell compartment: the lymphoid follicles

Lymphoid follicles are evolutive structures whose number and morphological aspects closely depend on the degree of antigenic stimulation of the lymph node. Two types of lymphoid follicles are usually distin-

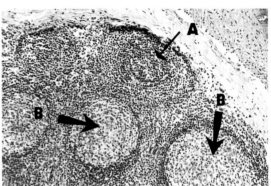

Fig. 3: Primary (—> A) and secondary (—> B) **lymphoid follicles** *located in the cortex.*

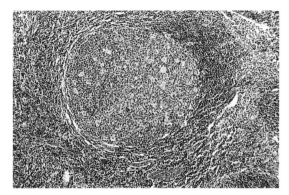

Fig. 4: **Secondary lymphoid follicle.** The mantle zone of the follicle, constituted by small lymphocytes, surrounds the germinal centre. Macrophages are easily seen in the germinal centre.

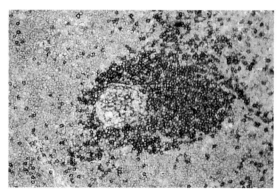

Fig. 6a

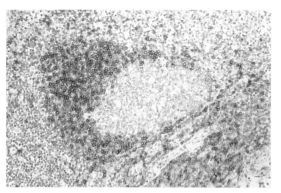

Fig. 6b

Fig. 6: **Normal lymph node.** Immunoperoxidase staining using monoclonal antibodies directed against anti-IgM (fig. 6a), staining mantle cells and germinal-centre network and anti-IgD (fig. 6b) staining only mantle cells.

guished: the primary follicles, corresponding to resting structures, and the secondary follicles, which appear after antigenic stimulation *(figs. 3 and 4)* (1). Primary lymphoid follicles are discrete nodular aggregates of small lymphocytes. Cells constituting primary follicles have a regular or slightly indented nucleus. Their cytoplasm is scanty and usually not visible on routine preparations. Immunohistochemically, lymphoid cells of primary follicles constitute a distinctive subpopulation of B lymphocytes, characterized by the coexpression of membrane IgM and IgD *(fig. 6)*, and the presence of C3b receptors. These B cells stain for alkaline phosphatase.

Secondary lymphoid follicles consist of two distinct regions *(fig. 4)*: a peripheral mantle and a germinal centre. The mantle consists of

B-cells morphologically and immunohistochemically identical to those of primary follicles, from which they are thought to derive. In this zone, the normal ratio between kappa and lambda chains is approximately 2:1 *(fig. 7)*. The germinal centre is polymorphous *(fig. 5)* (10). It is made up of two main cell-types: centrocytes and centroblasts. Centrocytes are small-to-medium-sized lymphoid cells characterized by indented nuclei, containing dispersed chromatin with small nucleoli. Their cytoplasm is pale staining and usually scanty. Centroblasts are large lymphoid cells, with a rounded nucleus, whose fine chromatin contains several large nucleoli frequently fixed to the nuclear membrane. Their cytoplasm is relatively abundant and usually moderately basophilic. Typical germinal centres are polarized. Centrocytes concentrate in the so-called pale region, opposite

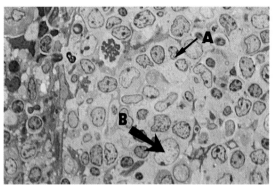

Fig. 5: **The germinal centre of the secondary lymphoid follicle** is polymorphous, constituted by lymphoid cells (small cleaved cells or centrocytes) (—> A) and large cells or centroblasts (—> B)), and non-lymphoid cells (macrophages, dendritic reticulum cells). Mitoses are numerous.

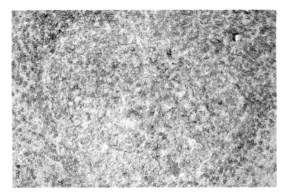

Fig. 7a

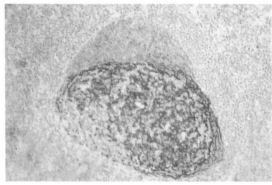

Fig. 9a

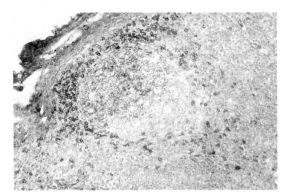

Fig. 7b

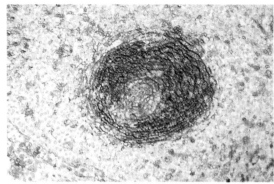

Fig. 9b

Fig. 7: **Normal lymph node.** Immunoperoxidase stain-ing using monoclonal antibodies directed against anti-kappa (fig. 7a) and anti-lambda (fig. 7b) light chains.

Fig. 9: **Normal lymph node.** Immunoperoxidase stain-ing using monoclonal antibodies directed against anti-dendritic reticulum cells (DRC1) (fig. 9a) and anti-C3bR (CD35) (fig. 9b).

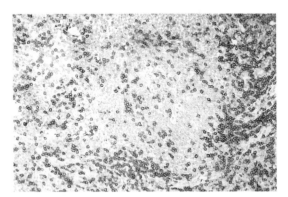

Fig. 8: **Normal lymph node.** Immunoperoxidase stain-ing using monoclonal antibody directed against anti-pan-T (CD3, Leu4): T cells are located in the paracortex and in the secondary follicles.

the capsule. Centroblasts are more numerous in the so-called dark region, at the opposite pole of the germinal centre. In this zone, mitoses are numerous and lymphoid cells are interspersed with tingible macrophages.

Lymphoid cells of the germinal centre are mainly B cells, expressing all the pan-B cell differentiation antigens (10). They exhibit a distinctive phenotype characterized by the expression of the CD10 antigen, of comple-ment receptor CR3 for C3d fragment (CD21 antigen), and of HLA-DR antigens. In addi-tion, centrocytes and centroblasts express low levels of membrane and/or cytoplasmic immunoglobulins. When detectable, these immunoglobulins are mainly of the IgM class. Unequivocal demonstration of cellu-lar immunoglobulins in germinal centres is often difficult since anti-Ig antibodies give intense extracellular labelling in this region. It is likely to be due to non-specific binding of antibodies on the Fc receptor for Ig expressed on the antigen-presenting cells associated with secondary follicles. Immu-nohistochemistry has revealed that sec-ondary follicles contain an unexpectedly high number of T cells (fig. 8) (4), unde-

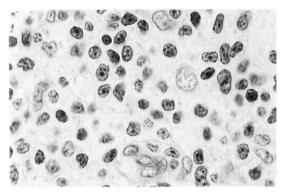

Fig. 10: **Normal lymph node.** Morphological aspect of the paracortex: pleomorphic lymphoid cells, interdigitating cells and post-capillary venule.

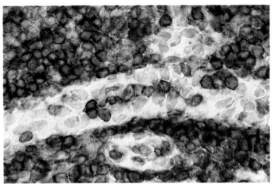

Fig. 11: **Normal lymph node.** Recirculating lymphocytes are visible amongst endothelial cells of the post-capillary venule of the paracortex (anti-CD3, Leu 4).

tectable on routine histological preparations. Indeed, follicular T cells, predominantly of the CD4 phenotype (95% of follicular T cells), may account for 5 to 30% of all lymphoid cells of secondary follicles.

Lymphoid follicles contain a specialized type of antigen-presenting cell: the dendritic reticulum cell (DRC). DRCs are not easily recognized on routine histological preparations. Their morphology has been revealed by electron microscopy (9). Ultra-structurally, DRCs are characterized by long and narrow cellular processes closely associated with B cells. Immunohistochemistry has greatly improved knowledge of this cell subset. Indeed, DRCs may be easily visualized using antibodies against complement receptors (including CR3 for the C3d fragment) or against specific differentiation antigens, such as R4/23 (DRC1) *(fig. 9)* (11). In addition, DRCs are strongly HLA-DR positive and express large numbers of Fc receptors for immunoglobulins. Using

immunohistochemistry, DRCs have been shown to constitute an organized network throughout the germinal centres, from which they send processes within the peripheral mantle (11). They are also present, although in lower numbers, within primary follicles.

The T-cell compartment interfollicular tissue and paracortex

Morphologically, interfollicular tissue and paracortex consist of a pleomorphic lymphoid population *(fig. 10)*. The majority of these cells are small to medium-sized. Their nuclei are irregular or indented. Their cytoplasm is scanty. In addition, variable proportions of plasma cells and immunoblasts may be observed. These cells are more prominent in cases of antigenic stimulation.

Histologically, the most characteristic feature of the T-cell compartment is the presence of particular vessels: the post-capillary venules. Post-capillary venules are small vessels lined by tall, turgescent endothelial cells, bound by a dense basal lamina, which is PAS+. Lymphoid cells are often visible amongst endothelial cells, migrating from blood to lymphoid tissue. Indeed, post-capillary venules represent the route used by recirculating lymphocytes for entry into the lymph node *(fig. 11)*.

As emphasized above, most lymphoid cells in interfollicular tissue and paracortex are of T-cell phenotype. In the normal state, CD4+ cells outnumber CD8+ cells; the ratio is about 2:1 *(fig. 12)* (4). A few B cells are also present. A distinctive type of antigen-presenting cell is present in the T-cell compartment; the interdigitating cell (IDC). Like DRCs, IDCs are not easily visible on routine histological preparations. Their morphology has been demonstrated using electron microscopy (9). In contrast to DRCs, IDCs lack long cellular processes. They present relatively short expansions, insinuating between adjacent lymphoid T cells. IDCs display an immunohistochemical phenotype clearly distinct from that

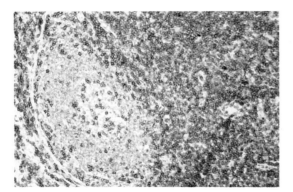

Fig. 12a

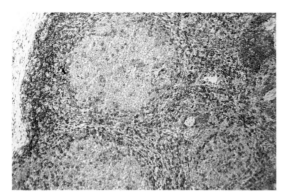

Fig. 12b

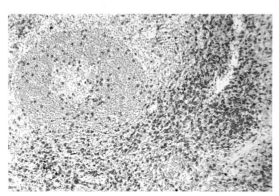

Fig. 12c

Fig. 12: **Normal lymph node.** Immunohisto-chemical study of the T.cell of the paracortex using anti-pan-T antibodies (CD5, Leu 1) (fig. 12 a), anti helper T cell antibodies (CD4, Leu 3) (fig. 12 b) anti suppressive T cell antibodies (CD8, Leu 2) (fig. 12 c).

of DRCs. They are rich in S100 protein, lack C3d receptor and the specific differentiation antigens of DRCs (12,13). CD1 reactivity has been reported on occasions (12,13). Most of these characteristics resemble those of the Langerhans cell, a distinctive CD1+ antigen-presenting cell characteristic of epidermis (13). It is likely that IDCs and Langerhans cells belong to the same subset of specialized antigen-presenting cells.

IDCs must be distinguished from the phagocytosing macrophages present in the T-cell compartment. These tissue macrophages, devoid of the specific immunological phenotype of IDCs, are most prominent in reactive paracortical hyperplasias, such as in viral lymphadenitis.

The medulla

In contrast to the cortex, the medulla is rich in large, easily visible sinuses. Between the sinuses, lymphoid cells are organized in cords. These cords contain numerous plasma cells, tissue macrophages and an admixture of small B and T lymphocytes.

Morphological variations related to site

Resting axillary and inguinal lymph nodes are constituted of large amounts of adipose tissue surrounded by a thin rim of lymphoid cells containing a few follicles. Usually, inguinal lymph nodes are distorted by large bands of fibrous tissue resulting from previous inflammations. Resting mesenteric lymph nodes are characterized by a very large medulla surrounded by a poorly developed cortex, with only few follicles.

Blood vascularization

Blood vessels of lymph nodes comprise:

- one or two arteries which penetrate the lymph node via the hilum, cross the medulla and the cortex, and divide and end in subcapsular capillaries;

- capillaries which form a dense network in the subcapsular areas, less dense in the central part of the cortex and denser in the medullary cords; and

- post-capillary venules in the paracortex, formed from 4 to 5 capillaries joining into veins which emerge through the hilum.

Relations between structure and function

Role of the lymph node in immune reactions

The lymph node plays a critical role in B-cell stimulation. This process involves the lymphoid follicles. Exposure of the organism to foreign antigens induces dramatic alterations in the aspect of cortical follicles. Germinal centres appear within a few hours and lymphoid B cells rapidly proliferate and differentiate (10). There is some controversy regarding the sequence of morphological events. According to Lennert (14), the resting B lymphocyte first transforms into a centroblast, then into a centrocyte. According to Lukes (15), the transformation of the small B lymphocyte of the primary follicle first produces a small cleaved cell (equivalent to the centrocyte), then a large cleaved cell. This large cleaved cell in turn gives a small non-cleaved cell (resembling the neoplastic cell characteristic of Burkitt's lymphoma) and finally, a large non-cleaved cell (equivalent to the centroblast). It is generally accepted that this differentiation process finally leads to production of B memory cells. Its role in the formation of plasma cells remains controversial. Indeed, plasma cells are observed in exceptional cases within secondary follicles. Moreover, plasma cells may differentiate in the absence of lymphoid follicles. Initiation of the differentiation process of B cells within secondary follicles is due to presentation of the antigen by the specialized dendritic reticulum cells. It is likely that the antigen presented has been primarily processed by the "conventional" tissue and sinusoidal macrophages present in large amounts within the lymphoid tissue. Interaction between DRCs and germinal B cells requires complement C3 (16).

The role of the lymph node in T-cell stimulation is less well established. It is, however, likely that IDCs may function as antigen-presenting cells capable of inducing proliferation of resting T cells and their differentiation into T memory cells.

Role in the recirculation of lymphocytes

The lymph node is one of the main sites for recirculation of lymphocytes between blood and lymph. Circulating lymphocytes enter the lymph node via the hilum, following the arterial supply. They leave the blood circulation in the specialized post-capillary high endothelial venules of paracortex and interfollicular tissue. Part of the molecular process allowing the passage of emigrating lymphocytes through the endothelial lining of post-capillary venules has now been elucidated.

Endothelial cells of post-capillary venules express cell surface adhesion molecules, or addressins (17), which specifically interact with a corresponding structure on lymphocyte membrane. Three distinct, tissue-specific addressins have so far been characterized: one in peripheral lymph nodes (18-20), another in mucosal lymphoid tissue (21), and the last in synovium (22). Addressins actually function as homing receptors conducting the traffic of distinct lymphocyte subpopulations towards their various targets within peripheral lymphoid tissues.

References

1. HAM AW, AXELRAD AA, CORMACK DH
   Blood cell formation and the cellular basis of immune responses.
   JB Lippincott Company, Philadelphia, 1979.

2. STEIN H, LENNERT K, MASON DY, et al.

Immature sinus histiocytes. Their identification as a novel B-cell population.

Am J Pathol, 1984; 15: 330-335.

3. SHEIBANI K, FRITZ RM, WINBERG CD, BURKE JS, RAPPAPORT H

Monocytoid cells in reactive follicular hyperplasia with and without multifocal histiocytic reaction: an immunohistochemical study of 21 cases of toxoplasmic lymphadenitis.

Am J Clin Pathol, 1984; 27: 453-458.

4. HSU SM, COSSMAN J, JAFFE ES

Lymphocyte subsets in normal human lymphoid tissues.

Am J Clin Pathol, 1983; 80: 21-30.

5. MASON DY

Immunohistology of lymphoid tissue.

In: Histochemistry in Pathology, FILIPE MI, LAKE BD Eds; 1983, Churchill Livingstone, Edinburgh.

6. STEIN H, BONK A, TOLKSDORF G, LENNERT K, RODT H, GERDES J

Immunohistologic analysis of the organization of normal lymphoid tissue and non-Hodgkin's lymphomas.

J Histochem Cytochem, 1980; 28: 746-760.

7. DELSOL G, AL-SAATI T, CAVERIVIERE P, VOIGT JJ, ANCELIN E, RIGAL-HUGUET F

Etude en immunoperoxydase du tissu lymphoïde normal et pathologique. Intérêt des anticorps monoclonaux.

Ann Pathol, 1984; 4: 165-183.

8. RALFKIAER E, PLESNER T, WANTZIN G, THOMSEN K, NISSEN NI, HOU-JENSEN K

Immunohistochemical identification of lymphocyte subsets and accessory cells in human hyperplastic lymph nodes.

Scand J Haematol, 1984; 32: 536-543.

9. TEW JG, THORBECKE GJ, STEINMAN RM

Dendritic cells in the immune response: characteristics and recommended nomenclature.

J Reticulendothel Soc, 1982; 31: 371-380.

10. STEIN H, GERDES J, MASON DY

The normal and malignant germinal centre.

Clin Haematol, 1982; 11: 531-559.

11. NAIEM M, GERDES J, ABDULAZIZ Z, STEIN H, MASON DY

Production of a monoclonal antibody reactive with human dendritic reticulum cells and its use in the immunohistological analysis of lymphoid tissue.

J Clin Pathol, 1983; 36: 167-175.

12. RALFKIAER E, STEIN H, PLESNER T, HOU-JENSEN K, MASON DY

In situ *immunological characterization of Langerhans cells with monoclonal antibodies: comparison with other dendritic cells in skin and lymph nodes.*

Virchows Arch (Pathol Anat), 1984; 403: 401-412.

13. WOOD GS, TURNER RR, SHIURBA RA, ENG L, WARNKE RA

Human dendritic cells and macrophages. In situ immunophenotypic definition of subsets that exhibit specific morphologic and microenvironmental characteristics.

Am J Pathol, 1985; 119: 73-82.

14. LENNERT K

Malignant lymphomas other than Hodgkin's disease.

Springer Verlag, Berlin, 1978.

15. LUKES RJ, PARKER JW, TAYLOR CR, TINDLE BH, CRAMER AD, LINCOLN T

Immunologic approach to non-Hodgkin lymphomas and related leukemias. Analysis of the results of multiparameter study of 425 cases.

Semin Hematol, 1978; 15: 322-351.

16. KLAUS GGB, HUMPHREY JH

The generation of memory cells. I. The role of C3 in generation of B memory cells.

Immunology, 1977; 33: 31-40.

17. BERG EL, GOLDSTEIN LA, JUTILA MA, NAKACHE MM, PICKER LJ, STREETER PR, WU NW, ZHOU D, BUTCHER EC

Homing receptors and vascular addressins: cell adhesion molecules that direct lymphocyte traffic.

Immunol Rev, 1989; 108: 5-18.

18. SIEGELMAN M, BOND MW, GALLATIN WM, ST-JOHN T, SMITH HT, FRIED VA, WEISSMAN IL

Cell surface molecule associated with lymphocyte homing is a ubiquinated branched-chain glycoprotein.

Science, 1986; 231: 823-850.

19. BOWEN BR, NGUYEN T, LASKY LA

Characterization of a human homologue of the murine lymph node homing receptor.

J Cell Biol, 1989; 109: 421-427.

20. BERG EL, ROBINSON MK, WARNOCK RA, BUTCHER EC

The human peripheral lymph node vascular addressin is a ligand for LECAM-1, the peripheral lymph node homing receptor.

J Cell Biol, 1991; 114: 343-349.

21. NAKACHE M, BERG EL, STREETER PR, BUTCHER EC

The mucosal vascular addressin is a tissue-specific endothelial cell adhesion molecule for circulating lymphocytes.

Nature, 1989; 337: 179-181.

22. JALKANEN S, STEERE A, FOX E, BUTCHER E

A distinct endothelial cell recognition system that controls traffic into inflamed synovium.

Science, 1986; 233: 556-558.

Histological classification of non-Hodgkin's lymphomas

N. BROUSSE

Historical account

In 1832, Thomas Hodgkin described the tumours of lymph nodes and, among them, 7 cases of a tumour of lymph nodes and spleen which have a different course. Hodgkin's disease (the name proposed by Wilks in 1865) was distinguished from other lymph node neoplasia. Sternberg in 1898 and Reed in 1902 described more precisely their morphological aspects, especially the giant cells which now carry their name. In 1893, Kundrat first used the term of lymphosarcoma for all primitive neoplasia of lymph nodes. Among lymphosarcomas, Oberling, in 1928, distinguished the group of reticulosarcomas, tumours considered as originating from lymph-node reticulo-endothelial cells. Concomitantly, Brill and Symmers distinguished the "giganto-follicular" forms of lymphosarcoma because of their more indolent course.

In 1956, Rappaport, taking these data together with his own studies, proposed the first morphological classification of lymphosarcomas, progressively improved until the final report in 1966 (1) *(Table I)*. The major contribution of this classification resides in the importance given to the architecture of lymph node proliferation and to its cytological characteristics. Its usefulness has been largely confirmed by multiple clinico-pathological studies (2) and by the prognostic and therapeutic significance of the separate entities (3). Rappaport's classification has been widely used for 15 years. However, Rappaport's classification had 2 major disadvantages:

TABLE I

Rappaport classification

Nodular and/or diffuse
Well differentiated lymphocytic
Poorly differentiated lymphocytic
Mixed
Histiocytic
Undifferentiated

- a group of so-called "histiocytic" lymphomas was distinguished but it was further shown by morphological and immunological criteria that most of them were of lymphoid origin; and

- several sub-groups of NHL such as Burkitt's lymphoma, lymphoblastic lymphomas and some cutaneous T-cell lymphomas were not distinguished.

From 1974 to 1982, because of the description of new clinico-pathological entities, and of the huge increase in knowledge of the immune system and its relationships with lymphoid proliferations (4-10), several new classifications of NHL were proposed. Some used only morphological criteria such as Dorfman's classification (11); others used both morphological and immunological criteria such as Lukes-Collins' classification (12,13) and Kiel's first (or Lennert's) classification (14,15) *(Table II)*.

TABLE II

First Kiel classification (1978)

Low-grade malignancy	Lymphocytic	1) B-CLL
		2) T-CLL
		3) Hairy cell leukaemia
		4) Mycosis fungoides and Sézary syndrome
		5) T-zone
	Lymphoplasmacytic Immunocytoma	1) Lymphoplasmacytic subtype
		2) Lymphoplasmacytoid subtype
		3) Polymorphic subtype
	Plasmacytic (plasmacytoma)	
	Centrocytic	1) Small-cell subtype
		2) Large-cell subtype
	Centroblastic-centrocytic	(follicular; follicular and diffuse; diffuse)
		1) Small-cell subtype
		2) Large-cell subtype

High-grade malignancy	Centroblastic	Primary
		   1) Monomorphic (pure) subtype
		   2) Polymorphic subtype
		Secondary
		   1) Purely centroblastic variant
		   2) Immunoblastic variant
		   3) Large anaplastic centrocytic variant

	Lymphoblastic	B-lymphoblastic lymphoma
		   1) Burkitt-type
		   2) Other than Burkitt-type
		T-lymphoblastic lymphoma
		   1) Convoluted cell type
		   2) Without convoluted nuclei
		Unclassified, including null-lymphoblastic lymphomas

	Immunoblastic	Variants or subtypes
		1) Immunoblastic with plasmablastic or plasmacytic
		   differentiation (B cell)
		2) Purely immunoblastic without plasmacytic or
		   plasmacytic differentiation (B- or T-cell origin)

Nathwani (16) compared these different classifications and pointed out the similarities and differences. There are many similarities between the classifications of Lukes-Collins and Dorfman.

On the other hand, Kiel's classification differs from the other classifications since some leukaemias such as chronic lymphocytic leukaemia are included in the NHL entity, some subgroups such as immunocytoma are isolated and Burkitt's and lymphoblastic lymphomas are considered as a single entity. Some classifications (such as the Rappaport, Lukes-Collins and Dorfman classifications) use both architectural and cytological

TABLE III

Working Formulation of Non-Hodgkin's Lymphomas for Clinical Usage

Low-grade	A. Malignant lymphoma Small lymphocytic	consistent with CLL plasmacytoid
	B. Malignant lymphoma, follicular Predominantly small cleaved cell	diffuse areas sclerosis
	C. Malignant lymphoma, follicular Mixed, small cleaved and large-cell	diffuse areas sclerosis
Intermediate-grade	D. Malignant lymphoma, follicular Predominantly large-cell	diffuse areas sclerosis
	E. Malignant lymphoma, diffuse Small cleaved cell	sclerosis
	F. Malignant lymphoma, diffuse Mixed, small and large-cell	sclerosis epithelioid cell component
	G. Malignant lymphoma, diffuse Large cleaved cell, non-cleaved cell	sclerosis
High-grade	H. Malignant lymphoma Large-cell, immunoblastic	plasmacytoid clear cell polymorphous epithelioid cell component
	I. Malignant lymphoma Lymphoblastic	convoluted cell non-convoluted cell
	J. Malignant lymphoma Small non-cleaved cell Burkitt's	sclerosis Follicular areas
Miscellaneous	Composite Mycosis fungoides Histiocytic Extramedullary plasmacytoma Unclassifiable Other	

TABLE IV

Updated Kiel classification of non-Hodgkin's lymphomas

	B	*T*
Low grade	Lymphocytic-chronic lymphocytic and prolymphocytic leukaemia; hairy-cell leukaemia	Lymphocytic-chronic lymphocytic and prolymphocytic leukaemia Small, cerebriform cell mycosis fungoides, Sézary syndrome
	Lymphoplasmacytic (cytoid) (LP immunocytoma)	Lymphoepithelioid (Lennert's lymphoma)
	Plasmacytic	Angioimmunoblastic (AILD, LgX)
	Centroblastic centrocytic - follicular ± diffuse - diffuse	T-zone
	Centrocytic	Pleomorphic, small-cell (HTLV-1±)
High grade	Centroblastic	Pleomorphic, medium- and large-cell (HTLV-1±)
	Immunoblastic	Immunoblastic (HTLV-1±)
	Large-cell anaplastic (Ki-1+)	Large-cell anaplastic (Ki-1+)
	Burkitt lymphoma	
	Lymphoblastic	Lymphoblastic
Rare types		

criteria, whereas Kiel's classification relies primarily upon cytological criteria, architecture being considered as a subordinate criterion.

During the years 1980-1982, experts in these classifications met to study their reproducibility and concordance (17). They concluded that discrimination between follicular and diffuse architecture was the most reproducible criterion (concordance in 95% of cases) (18). On the other hand, reproducibility of the cell-type analysis was lower (from 53% to 93% (18)).

Before 1982, each group used either its own classification or a classification of its choice. Schematically, Rappaport and Lukes-Collins classifications were most widely used in the USA and Kiel's classification in Europe. Other classifications (such as the WHO classification, Dorfman's classification) were not extensively used. None of these classifications was clearly superior to the others, and their multiplicity, the absence of a common terminology, and the variation in histological criteria precluded comparison between clinical and therapeutic studies, especially European and American.

Working Formulation for Clinical Usage

On the initiative of the National Cancer Institute, an international cooperative study was conducted in 4 reference centres from 1976 to 1980 to improve agreement between the major NHL classifications. Each of the 1175 cases studied was classified on the basis of the clinical and histological data. The experts proposed some recommendations which were simple and as uniformly accepted as possible. The "Working Formulation for Clinical Usage" *(Table III)* was initially proposed to facilitate communication between classifications and so to make understanding of and comparison between clinico-pathological studies easier (18). In fact, the Working Formulation has been increasingly used as a reference classification for international reports. The Working Formulation for Clinical Usage is a classification relying upon strictly morphological criteria. It proved useful for B-cell non-Hodgkin's lymphomas, the most frequent cell types in Europe and in USA. However, classification of T-cell non-Hodgkin's lymphomas is much more difficult. In Japan where T-cell NHL are more frequent, other classifications are more widely used (19).

- rely on precise morphological criteria;

- allow the classification of almost all NHL cases;

- be easy to understand and to learn;

- be accurate according to the latest findings of lymphoid cell biology;

- be reproducible from pathologist to pathologist; and

- categorize NHL into groups characterized by different prognoses.

Several studies have confirmed that the classifications proposed by Rappaport or Lukes-Collins and Kiel allowed between distinction of groups of patients with different prognoses. For instance, in one study of 1,127 cases, Brittinger et al. (21) confirmed the prognostic value of the 2 groups of low and high malignancy of the first classification. The prognostic significance of the Working Formulation for Clinical Usage with its 3 malignancy groups has been proved by the initial study of 1,175 cases (18) and by others (22-24). Prospective studies with large groups of patients with all grades of NHL treated under the most recent chemotherapy regimens are in progress.

Updated Kiel classification of non-Hodgkin's lymphomas

In 1988, an updated Kiel classification of NHL was published (20) *(Table IV)* in which B- and T-cell NHL were separated, although this classification remains morphological. Two grades of malignancy - low and high - have been adopted. A new entity, large-cell anaplastic (Ki-1+) NHL has been included in T- and B-NHL classes.

Prognostic value of NHL classifications

Rappaport (2) outlined the characteristics of an ideal classification of NHL. Such a classification must:

References

1. RAPPAPORT H

   Tumors of the hematopoietic system.

   In: Atlas of tumor pathology, section III, fasc. 8, Washington D.C. U.S. Armed Forces Institute of Pathology, 1966: p. 97-161.

2. JONES SE, FUKZ Z, BULL M, et al.

   Non-Hodgkin's lymphomas. IV. Clinicopathologic correlations in 450 cases.

   Cancer, 1977; 31: 806-823.

3. ROSENBERG SA

   Non-Hodgkin's lymphomas. Selection of treatment on the basis of histologic type.

   N Engl J Med, 1981; 301: 925-928.

4. BERARD CW, JAFFE ES, BRAYLAN RC, MANN RB, NANBA K

Immunologic aspects and pathology of the malignant lymphomas.

Cancer, 1978; 42: 911-921.

5. COSSMAN J, BERARD CW

Malignant lymphomas. The role of immunologic markers in diagnosis, subclassification and management.

Hum Pathol, 1980; 11: 309-312.

6. LUKES RJ, PARKER JW, TAYLOR CR, TINDLE BH, CRAMER AD, LINCOLN TL

Immunologic approach to non-Hodgkin's lymphomas and related leukemias. Analysis of the results of multiparameter studies of 425 cases.

Sem Hematol, 1978; 15: 322-351.

7. LUKES RJ, COLLINS RD

New approaches to the classification of the lymphomata.

Br J Cancer, 1975; 31 suppl. 2: 1-28.

8. AISENBERG AC

Cell surface markers in lymphoproliferative disease.

N Engl J Med, 1981; 304: 331-336.

9. WHITESIDE TL, ROWLANDS Jr DT

T-cell and B-cell identification in the diagnosis of lymphoproliferative disease.

Am J Pathol, 1977; 88: 754-790.

10. MANN RB, JAFFE ES, BERARD CW

Malignant lymphomas. A conceptual understanding of morphologic diversity.

Am J Pathol, 1979; 94: 105-165.

11. DORFMAN RF

Classification of non-Hodgkin's lymphomas.

Lancet, 1974; 1: 1295-1296.

12. LUKES RJ, COLLINS RD

Lukes-Collins classification and its significance.

Cancer Treat Rep, 1977; 61: 971-979.

13. LUKES RJ, COLLINS RD

Immunological characterization of human malignant lymphomas.

Cancer, 1974; 34: 1488-1503.

14. GERARD MARCHANT R, HAMLIN I, LENNERT K, et al.

Classification of non-Hodgkin's lymphomas.

Lancet, 1974; 2: 406-408.

15. LENNERT K, MOHRI N

Malignant lymphomas other than Hodgkin's disease.

New York-Springer Verlag, 1978.

16. NATHWANI BN

A critical analysis of the classifications of non-Hodgkin's lymphomas.

Cancer, 1979; 44: 347-384.

17. *N.C.I. non-Hodgkin's classification project writing committee. Classification of non-Hodgkin's lymphomas. Reproducibility of major classification systems.*

Cancer, 1985; 55: 91-95.

18. *The non-Hodgkin's lymphomas pathologic classification project. National Cancer Institute sponsored study of classifications of non-Hodgkin's lymphomas.*

Cancer, 1982; 49: 2112-2135.

19. SUCHI T, LENNERT K, TU LY, et al.

Histopathology and immunohistochemistry of peripheral T-cell lymphomas: a proposal for their classification.

J Clin Pathol, 1987; 40: 995-1015.

20. STANSFELD AG, DIEBOLD J, KAPANCI Y, et al.

Updated Kiel classification for lymphomas.

Lancet, 1988; 1: 293-294.

21. BRITTINGER G, BARTELS H, COMMON H, et al.

Clinical and prognostic relevance of the Kiel classification of non-Hodgkin's lymphomas. Results of a prospective multicenter study by the Kiel lymphoma study group.

Hematol Oncol, 1984; 2: 269-306.

22. ERSBOLL J, SCHULTZ HB, HOUGAARD P, NISSEN NI, HOU-JENSEN K

Comparison of the Working Formulation of non-Hodgkin's lymphoma with the Rappaport, Kiel and Lukes-Collins classifications.

Cancer, 1985; 55: 2442-2458.

23. LIEDERMAN PH, FILIPPA DA, STRAUS DJ, THALER HT, CIRRINCIONE C, CLARKSON BD

Evaluation of malignant lymphomas using 3 classifications and the Working Formulation.

Am J Med, 1986; 81: 365-380.

24. SIMON R, DURRLEMAN S, HOPPE RT, et al.

The Non-Hodgkin's Lymphoma Pathologic Classification Project. Long-term follow-up of 1153 patients with non-Hodgkin's lymphoma.

Ann Intern Med, 1988; 109: 939-945.

Staging of non-Hodgkin's lymphomas

P. SOLAL-CÉLIGNY

When NHL has been diagnosed in a patient, the aims of staging are various (1,2):

(a) to assess the extent of disease in order to determine the treatment;

(b) to look for involvement sites of prognostic significance such as bone marrow, central nervous system etc.;

(c) to estimate the tumour burden by determining the extent of the disease and the size (with measurement, if possible, of all 3 dimensions, or if not, of the largest diameter) of the most significant lymph node or extranodal involvement sites; and

(d) to document response to treatment.

General symptoms must be looked for:

- weight loss (significant if equal to or more than 10% of body weight over the previous 6 months);

- night sweats; and

- fever (significant if greater than 38° C for at least 15 days without any documented infection).

Initial staging must include a semi-quantitative estimation of the patient's performance status on either the Karnofsky scale *(Table I)* or on the scale proposed by the Eastern Cooperative Oncology Group *(Table II)*. The latter appears to be easier to reproduce in the same patient and from patient to patient.

Lymph node involvement must be looked for in major areas as well in "accessory" areas such as epitrochlear, occipital or popliteal sites more often involved than in Hodgkin's disease. If the involvement is doubtful, especially on inguinal lymph nodes, confirmation may be obtained by needle aspiration. Mediastinal lymph node enlargement may be visible on routine chest radiography. However, thoracic CT scan should be regularly employed especially in patients with normal or doubtful chest X-rays or those who have no visible extrathoracic spread (3,4). Thoracic CT scan is superior to radiography for determining the extent of mediastinal lymphadenopathy, and the presence of any chest wall, pericardial or paracardial invasion. Conversely, there is no clear advantage of magnetic resonance imaging over CT scan (5,6).

Lymphangiography probably has a slight advantage over CT scan in detecting retroperitoneal lymph node involvement (4) because of the ability of the former to discern disease in lymph nodes which are normal in size or slightly enlarged (7). But lymphangiography does not allow the study of lymph nodes in the mesentery or in the splenic and hepatic hila, which are frequently involved in NHL and have to be studied by CT scan. The sensitivity of ultrasonography in detecting abdominal lymph nodes is lower than that of CT scan (8). Most authors therefore suggest performing only a CT scan to detect the involvement of abdominal lymph nodes.

TABLE I

Karnofsky Performance Scale

Activity status	Point	Description
Normal activity	10	Normal, with no complaints or evidence of disease
	9	Able to carry on normal activity but with minor signs or symptoms of disease present
	8	Normal activity but requiring effort; signs and symptoms of disease more prominent
Self-care	7	Able to care for self, but unable to work or carry on other normal activities
	6	Able to care for most needs but requires occasional assistance
	5	Considerable assistance required, along with frequent medical care; some self-care still possible
Incapacitated	4	Disabled and requiring special care and assistance
	3	Severely disabled; hospitalization required but death from disease not imminent
	2	Extremely ill; supportive treatment, hospitalized care required
	1	Imminent death
	0	Dead

Lymphangiography may also be performed on rare patients who have a normal abdomen CT scan and whose treatment is intended to be limited to supradiaphragmatic radiotherapy.

Clinical examination of Waldeyer's ring must be performed systematically. It is regularly completed by lateral radiography, or, if, by CT scan, of the post-nasal space. If any involvement is suspected, a confirmatory biopsy must be done since enlargement of the soft tissue of the post-nasal space may be related to other causes than NHL. Whether or not a routine biopsy of this region is useful remains questionable.

In one study, Albada et al. (9) reported an 18% incidence of histologically proven Waldeyer's ring involvement in 55 patients who had no clinical manifestation. But all the positive specimens were observed in patients who had other extranodal involvement and diagnosis of Waldeyer's ring involvement had no direct therapeutic implication.

A bone-marrow iliac crest trephine biopsy must be routinely performed (1,2) whatever the histological type of NHL. If a first biopsy is negative, a contralateral iliac crest biopsy may increase the incidence of bone-marrow involvement by 5 to 20% (10,11). Bilateral biopsies must then be done:

- in patients with limited disease who are scheduled to be treated only by radiotherapy, especially if they have a low-grade NHL;

TABLE II

Eastern Cooperative Oncology Group scale of performance status

0	No symptoms
1	With symptoms but continued ambulatory ability
2	Bedridden status less than 50% of the day
3	Bedridden status greater than 50% of the day
4	Chronic bedridden status requiring assistance for daily maintenance

-in patients in whom an autologous bone-marrow transplantation is scheduled.

Examination of a buffy coat can be useful in documenting peripheral blood involvement.

Laboratory tests and CT scan are helpful in identifying liver involvement only in a minority of patients. If systematic liver biopsies are performed (percutaneously or during peritoneoscopy), the incidence of liver involvement is greatly increased (12), especially in patients with low-grade NHL. But such biopsies have rarely to be done, since liver involvement is almost always associated with other extranodal sites (especially bone marrow). In such cases, documenting liver involvement does not modify the staging or treatment programme (2). Ultrasonography and CT scan allow optimal study of the size and homogeneity of the spleen.

Routine examination of a cerebro-spinal fluid buffy coat should be carried out in patients with high-grade NHL. Cerebral CT scan is usually performed only in patients with symptoms suggestive of CNS involvement.

Digestive tract examination, either by endoscopy or by radiography, is performed only in symptomatic patients or in patients who have NHL involvement frequently associated with digestive involvement such as head-and-neck [especially tonsils (13)] or lungs, i.e. involving the Mucosa-Associated Lymphoid Tissue.

^{99}Technetium scintigraphy is most useful in documenting bone involvement. It must be performed in symptomatic patients or in patients who have hypercalcaemia or isolated increased serum alkaline-phosphatase levels. Because of their lack of specificity, all radionuclide scan abnormalities must be confirmed by radiography and, if necessary, biopsy.

Staging laparotomy is no longer carried out for the following reasons (12):

- new non-invasive imaging techniques, such as CT scan, have greatly increased the yield of abdominal involvement documentation;

- most patients, even with localized supradiaphragmatic disease, are treated with chemotherapy and abdominal pathological staging would not modify the treatment schedule.

The Ann Arbor classification (14), initially proposed for Hodgkin's disease, is usually applied to NHL (Table 3). But its prognostic value is less than in Hodgkin's disease since:

(a) a much greater proportion of patients have extranodal involvement (from 50% in high-grade NHL to 80% in low-grade NHL);

(b) disease stage has no major prognostic significance; and

(c) the treatment programme is often the same for stage II to IV patients.

Other tests must be performed at initial presentation of the patient because of their prognostic significance:

TABLE III

Ann Arbor staging classification

Stage	Definition
I	Involvement of a single lymph node region (I) or a single extranodal organ or site (I_E)
II	Involvement of two or more lymph node regions on the same side of the diaphragm (II) or localized involvement of an extralymphatic organ or site in addition (II_E)
III	Involvement of lymph node regions on both sides of the diaphragm (III), which may also be accompanied by involvement of the spleen (III_S) or by localized involvement of an extralymphatic organ or site (III) or both (III_{SE})
IV	Disseminated involvement of one or more extralymphatic organs or tissues, with or without associated lymph node involvement

The absence or presence of fever (At least 38° C for 15 consecutive days without documented infection), or night sweats or unexplained loss of at least 10% of body weight in the preceding 6 months are denoted by the suffixes A or B respectively.

- HIV serological testing;

- serum LDH level, which is a useful indicator of tumour burden (15-17);

- serum beta 2-microglobulin, one of the HLA class I antigen components expressed by lymphoid cells, and which is related, at least in some studies, to tumour burden and prognosis (18,19); and

- serum and urine calcium levels.

References

1. CHABNER BA, FISHER RI, YOUNG RC, DE VITA VT
   Staging of non-Hodgkin's lymphomas.
   Sem Oncol, 1980; 7: 285-291.

2. CROWTHER D, RANKIN EM
   Staging patients with non-Hodgkin's lymphomas.
   Br J Haematol, 1982; 52:357-364.

3. KHOURY MB, GODWIN JD, HALVORSEN R, HANUN Y, PUTMAN CE
   Role of Chest CT in non-Hodgkin's lymphomas.
   Radiology, 1986; 158: 659-662.

4. MARGLIN SI, CASTELLINO RA
   Selection of imaging studies for newly presenting patients with non-Hodgkin's lymphomas.
   Semin Ultrasound, CT and MR, 1986; 7 : 2-8.

5. GAMSU G, SOSTMAN D
   Magnetic resonance imaging of the thorax.
   Am Rev Resp Dis, 1989; 139: 254-274.

6. DOOMS GC, HRICACK H, CROOKS LE, HIGGINS CB
   Magnetic resonance imaging of the lymph-nodes: comparison with CT.
   Radiology, 1984; 153: 719-728.

7. CLEMENT JF, TILLY H, DIOLOGENT B, MONCONDUIT M, PIGUET H
   Apport de la tomodensitométrie dans le bilan initial des lymphomes hodgkiniens et non hodgkiniens.
   Sem Hop Paris, 1986; 62: 239-242.

8. NEUMANN CH, ROBERT NJ, ROSENTHAL D, CANELLOS G
   Clinical value of ultrasonography for the management of non-Hodgkin's lymphoma patients as compared with abdominal computed tomography.
   J Comput Assist Tomogr, 1983; 7: 666-669.

9. ALBADA J, HORKIJK GJ, VAN UNNIK JAM, DEKKER AW
   Non-Hodgkin's lymphoma of Waldeyer's ring.
   Cancer, 1985; 56: 157-166.

10. COLLER BS, CHABNER BA, GRALNICK HR
    Frequencies and patterns of bone-marrow involvement in non-Hodgkin's lymphomas: observations on the value of bilateral biopsies.
    Am J Hematol, 1977; 3: 105-119.

11. BRUNNING RD, BLOOMFIELD CD, MCKENNA RW, PETERSON L
    Bilateral trephine bone marrow biopsies in lymphoma and other neoplastic diseases.
    Ann Intern Med, 1975; 82; 365-366.

12. CHABNER BA, JOHNSON RE, YOUNG RC, et al.

    Sequential non-surgical and surgical staging of non-Hodgkin's lymphomas.

    An Intern Med, 1976; 85: 149-154.

13. BANFI A, BONADONNA G, RICCI SB, et al.

    Malignant lymphomas of Waldeyer's ring: natural history and survival after radiotherapy.

    Br Med. J., 1972; 56: 768-776.

14. CARBONE PP, KAPLAN HS, MUSSHOFF K, SMITHERS DW, TUBIANA M

    Report of the committee on Hodgkin's disease staging classification.

    Cancer Res, 1971; 31: 1860-1861.

15. FERRARIS AM, GIUNTINI P, GAETANI GF

    Serum latic dehydrogenase as a prognostic tool for non-Hodgkin's lymphomas.

    Blood, 1979; 54: 928-932.

16. SCHNEIDER RJ, SEIBERT K, PASSE S, et al.

    Prognostic signifiance of serum lactate dehydrogenase in malignant lymphoma.

    Cancer, 1980; 46: 139-143.

17. HAGBERG H, SIEGBAHN A

    Prognostic value of serum lactate dehydrogenase in non-Hodgkin's lymphomas.

    Scand J Haematol, 1983; 31: 49-56.

18 HAGBERG H, KILLANDER A, SIMONSSON B

    Serum beta-2-microglobulin in malignant lymphoma.

    Cancer, 1983; 51: 2220-2225.

19. CONSTATINIDES IP, PATHOULI C, KARVOUNTZIS G

    Serum beta 2-microglobulin in malignant lymphoproliferative disorders.

    Cancer, 1985, 55: 2384-2389.

Analytical study of the different subtypes of non-Hodgkin's lymphoma: clinical, histological and immunohistochemical aspects

M. Peuchmaur, J.Y. Scoazec, P. Gaulard, P. Solal-Céligny, N. Brousse

We shall present the clinical, histological and immunohistochemical characteristics of the different subtypes of NHL in the order adapted by the Working Formulation for Clinical Use (1,2) *(see Table III, p. 97)* and the updated Kiel classification (3), taking into account the B- or T-cell phenotype and separating follicular lymphomas from diffuse lymphomas. Correspondences between the two classifications are shown in *Table I, p. 140.*

Table II on p. 141 gives correlations between histology and phenotype.

B-cell NHL

Follicular NHL

Follicular NHL (F-NHL) represent a homogeneous group of NHL in terms of clinical, histological and immunohistochemical characteristics. They originate from B cells in normal germinal centres (4-6). This is why they are often grouped with their diffuse counterparts under the term of centrofollicular NHL. Their frequency has been estimated to be as high as 35% of all NHL (7-8). In France, they repre-sent approximately 20% of NHL (Groupe d'Etude des Lymphomes). They are very unusual in patients less than 20 years old. The median age of patients is about 55 years.

Clinical aspects

Follicular NHL are most often systemic diseases involving superficial and deep lymph node sites, and extranodal sites, such as bone marrow (60-70%), spleen (50%), liver (50%) and Waldeyer's ring (see the chapters dedicated to each of these locations). On the other hand, gastrointestinal involvement is rare, and CNS involvement is very uncommon. Skin involvement has been described (9). Localized stages (Ann Arbor stages I and II) represent less than 10% of cases of F-NHL.

The clinical course of F-NHL is slow and diagnosis is often performed several weeks to several months after the onset of the first lymph node involvements. Systemic symptoms are infrequent (15%) but unfavourable in prognosis. About 10% of patients have hyperlymphocytosis ("lymphosarcoma cell leukaemia") with small cleaved cells, either at the time of diagnosis or during the course of the disease.

Histological aspects

Follicular NHL are characterized by the presence in the lymph node of nodules formed by lymphoma cells. These nodules are distributed throughout the lymph node, in the cortical zone and in the medullary zone *(fig. 1)*. Their size is variable, often small, and approximately equal from one nodule to another. Their limits are ill-defined and no mantle zone can usually be discerned. Four types can be distinguished on the basis of the degree of follicularity (7):

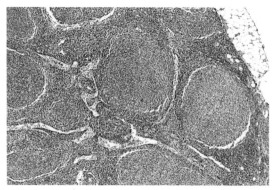

Fig. 1: **Follicular lymphoma**, intrafollicular type. Low magnification: multiple follicles, without mantle or germinal centre.

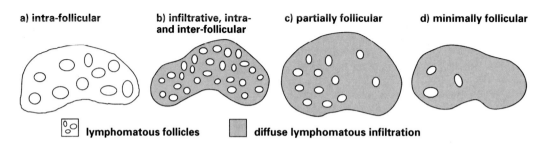

Fig. 2: Four main histological types of **follicular lymphoma** described by Lukes (7) classified on the basis of the degree of nodularity.

- the intrafollicular type: lymphoma cells are located only inside tumoral nodules *(fig. 3)*;

- the infiltrative or intra- and interfollicular type (the most frequent) in which lymphoma cells also infiltrate the interfollicular areas; and

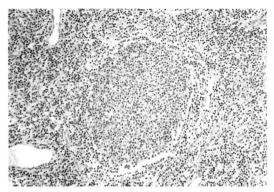

Fig. 3: **Follicular lymphoma**, intra-follicular type: lymphoid proliferation is limited to the follicles.

- the partially and minimally follicular types which associate one zone with a follicular pattern and another with a diffuse pattern. The latter prevails in the minimally follicular type.

The nodular architecture is outlined by an increased reticulin network between the follicles and in rare cases, especially in retroperitoneal lymph nodes, by dense interfollicular sclerosis (10).

The tumoral proliferation of follicular NHL is composed of variable amounts of two cell-types: small cleaved cells and large cells, either cleaved or non-cleaved.

The small cleaved cell (also called centrocyte in Kiel's classification) (11,12) can be characterized by the form of nucleus and other cytological criteria. Its diameter is 6 to 12 μ. The nucleus is oblong, has irregular outlines and is cleaved, notched or deeply indented. The chromatin is dense, usually without any visible nucleolus, occasionally with one or more small, barely distinct, nucleoli. Cytoplasm is scanty.

Large cells are approximately 20 μm in diameter. Non-cleaved large cells (also called centroblasts in Kiel's classification) have a regular ovoid nucleus, with a thin membrane, a fine chromatin and 2 to 3 small-sized nucleoli, close to the nuclear membrane. The cytoplasm is quite abundant and strongly basophilic. Large cleaved cells (also called large centrocytes in Kiel's classification) are marked off by the irregular, indented or cleaved form of their nucleus. The chromatin is fine, without any nucleolus. Large cleaved cells are usually fewer in number than the other cell types.

Depending upon the respective proportions of these 2 cell types, the Working Formulation for Clinical Use (1) distinguishes 3 types of follicular NHL: predominantly small cleaved cell *(fig. 4a)*, mixed, small cleaved and large-cell *(fig. 4b)* and predominantly large-cell *(fig. 4c)* types. There is no agreement upon the cytological and quantitative criteria to be used in distinguishing the 3 subtypes. The following criteria can be used:

- less than 5% of large cells in the predominantly small-cell type;
- from 5% to 50% of large cells in the mixed-cell type; and
- more than 50% of large cells in the predominantly large-cell type.

The number of mitoses must also be taken into account to distinguish the small-cell type from the mixed type (16).

There are some problems in the reproducibility of follicular NHL classification (13). In particular, there is no definitive consensus upon the percentage of large cells in each subtype nor upon the correct method for the evaluation of this percentage (13-15). Finally, it has to be emphasized that correct diagnosis of follicular NHL can only be performed on the basis of a lymph node biopsy.

It seems - although it has not been uniformly accepted - that the more follicular the NHL, the better the prognosis (17,18). But the cytological subtype probably has greater prognostic significance (19,20). In the Wor-

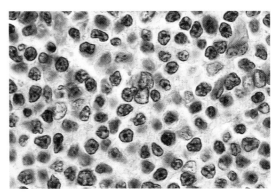

Fig. 4a

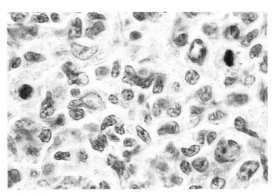

Fig. 4b

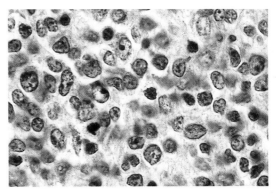

Fig. 4c

Fig. 4: Cytological types of **follicular lymphomas:** predominantly small cleaved cell (4a), mixed, small cleaved and large-cell (4b), predominantly large-cell (4c).

king Formulation, small-cell and mixed-cell types are considered to be NHL of low-grade malignancy whereas large-cell follicular NHL are included in the intermediate-grade group (21).

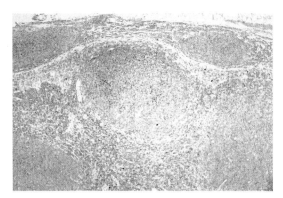

Fig. 5a

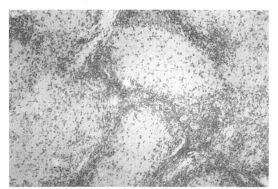

Fig. 5b

*Fig. 5: Immunohistochemical aspects of **follicular lymphoma**: immunoperoxidase staining using monoclonal antibodies directed against pan-B antigen (CD22) (5a) and pan-T antigen (CD3) (5b): the lymphomatous follicles are composed of B cells. The interfollicular areas are rich in T cells.*

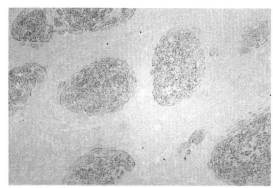

Fig. 6a

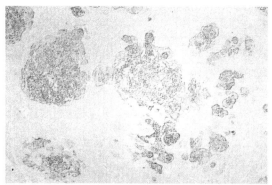

Fig. 6b

Fig. 6: Dendritic reticulum cell (DRC) network. Immunoperoxidase staining using monoclonal antibody directed against DRC. The network is either regular and homogeneous (6a) or loose and dissociated (6b).

However, apart from follicular NHL with predominantly large cells, which have an aggressive course, no definitive histological criteria allow prediction of the prognosis of follicular NHL and especially of the risk of relapse. From a clinical point of view, tumour burden and response to chemotherapy are the most reliable prognostic factors (8,22).

During their course, approximately 15 to 20% of follicular NHL evolve towards a more aggressive histological type, either by an increase in the amount of large cells, with the architectural pattern remaining follicular, or by transformation into a diffuse NHL, with the same or different cell type (23-25). The possible occurrence of such transformation warrants performing a new lymph node biopsy at each clinical outbreak of a follicular NHL.

Immunohistochemical aspects

Tumoral nodules are composed of monoclonal B cells. Between these nodules, the interfollicular tissue is rich in reactive T cells *(fig.5)* (26-29). Tumoral nodules are similar to normal lymph node follicles. Dendritic reticulum cells (DRC) form a network of normal follicles which differ from one follicle to another (30). In some cases, DRC are present in the whole follicle: they form a fairly dense homogeneous network *(fig. 6a)*. Usually, the network is loose, disjoined, heterogeneous and has disappeared in certain more or less extensive zones of the follicles *(fig. 6b)*. Unlike normal germinal centres, this network usually does not bind anti-immunoglobulin antibodies and the disappearance of this extracellular binding has been considered as characteristic of lymphomatous follicles (27-29). Together with the dendritic reticulum network,

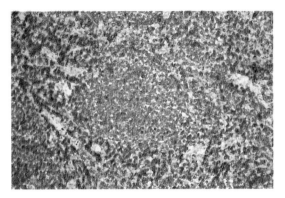

Fig. 7a

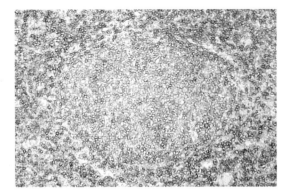

Fig. 7b

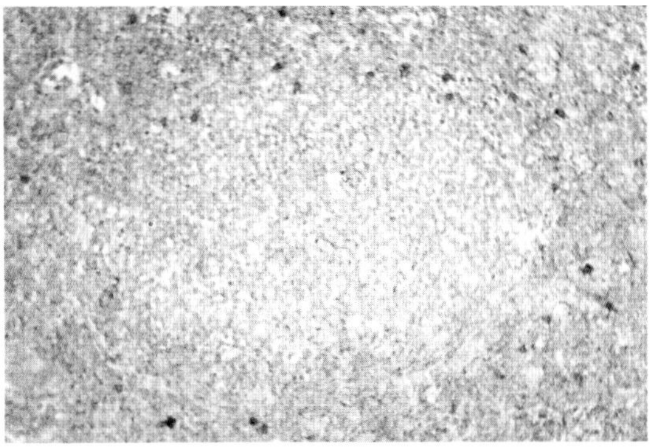

Fig. 7c

Fig. 7: **Follicular lymphoma** IgM kappa phenotype. Immunoperoxidase staining using monoclonal antibodies directed against IgM (7a), kappa (7b) and lambda (7c).

laminin and type IV collagen are produced in both normal germinal centres and in tumoral follicles (31). Generally, lymphomatous follicles are devoid of any man-

tle zone. However, if such a mantle zone is present, it is either polyclonal or monoclonal with exactly the same light-chain restriction as intrafollicular malignant lymphoid cells (28). The phenotype of malignant B cells is similar to that of B cells of normal germinal centres (29-32). They have membrane Igs, more often of μ/kappa isotypes than of μ/lambda (fig. 7), C3b (CD35) and C3d (CD21) receptors and express HLA-DR antigens. But in approximately 10% of follicular NHL, no light-chain restriction can be demonstrated using immunohistochemical techniques on frozen sections (33). They express pan-B antigens such as CD19, CD20, CD22 and CD24; they also express CD10 (CALLA) antigen. Immunoglobulin gene rearrangement studies have confirmed the monoclonality of follicular NHL (34-36).

Besides neoplastic B cells, tumour follicles also contain some reactive or residual polyclonal B cells (fig. 7c) and T-cells. T cells (fig.8) are mainly located in interfollicular areas. Their location is similar to that of reactive follicular hyperplasias but differs in the distribution of T-cell subtypes (18,20,22,23). The total amount of intrafollicular T cells may be higher in lymphomatous follicles than in reactive follicles (28,37-39). This high number is related to the high number of CD8+ cells, while the number of CD4+ cells is decreased. In other studies, such a distribution has not been confirmed and is considered in follicular NHL to be similar to that of T cells in normal lymph nodes (27). In interfollicular areas, the CD4/CD8 ratio is similar to that of normal paracortical zones. CD4+ T cells have a tendency to aggregate around lymphomatous follicles. In one study from Stanford (40), a relationship between a high density of CD4+ lymphocytes in the interfollicular areas and the occurrence of spontaneous regressions has been observed. In the normal state, NK cells are found mainly inside the follicles (22). In follicular lymphomatous lymph nodes, their number is increased and they are found both in the follicles and in interfollicular zones (27,41). The increased number of T cells in follicular NHL has been considered to be a response of the host directed against the malignant proliferation. Most of these reactive T cells express CD25 (p55 chain of the IL-2

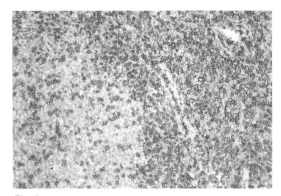

Fig. 8a

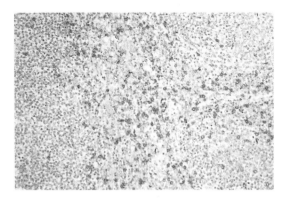

Fig. 8b

*Fig. 8: **Follicular lymphoma**. T cells are shown by immunoperoxidase staining using monoclonal antibodies directed against CD4 (8a) and CD8 (8b): CD4+ T cells predominate in the inter-follicular areas.*

receptor), while tumour cells usually do not (43-45). Recently it has been demonstrated that some of these T cells synthesize IL-2 and INF γ mRNA, two cytokines which participate in the recruitment and activation of cytotoxic T cells (46). The precise role of these reactive T cells remains unknown. They may limit the proliferation to the follicles either by blocking their dissemination or by inducing a differentiation level such that tumour cells remain located in areas where they are found in the normal state (38,46).

In an attempt to establish a reliable prognostic index, several studies have been carried out (20,58) to assess the proliferative rate of tumour cells using semi-quantative measurement of Ki-67 expression (47) or cytofluorometry (48). They failed to demonstrate any significant difference between the various histological subtypes of follicular NHL (49).

At present, several monoclonal antibodies recognizing fixative-resistant epitopes allow demonstration of the B-cell phenotype of follicular NHL on paraffin-embedded tissue sections. Follicular tumour cells express CD74 (LN2), CDw75 (LN1), CD20 (L26) and MT2 (49-51). Reactive T cells can be demonstrated using an anti-CD45RO antibody (UCHL1) and an anti-CD3 antibody. Bcl2 protein can be detected both in paraffin-embedded tissue samples and in cryostat sections; this oncogene is overexpressed in follicular lymphoma, in contrast with normal germinal centres (33,52,52bis) *(fig. 9)*.

Diagnosis

Nodal follicular reactive hyperplasias must be distinguished from follicular NHL. The most useful histological *(fig. 10)* and immunohistochemical *(fig. 11)* criteria are summarized in *Table III* and *Table IV* respectively.

The main criteria for ascertaining a diagnosis of follicular NHL are (53):
- the uniform and regular distribution of follicles throughout the lymph node;
- their back-to-back arrangement with minimal interfollicular tissue;
- the absence of a perifollicular mantle zone;
- their different cell composition with absence of macrophages; and
- the presence in interfollicular areas of cells with the same cytological characteristics as lymphoma cells in the follicles.

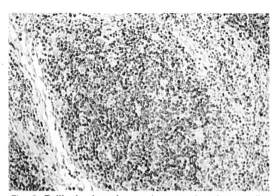

*Fig. 9: **Follicular lymphoma**. Immunophosphatase alkaline staining using monoclonal antibody directed against bcl2. Centrofollicular tumoral cells express this oncogene.*

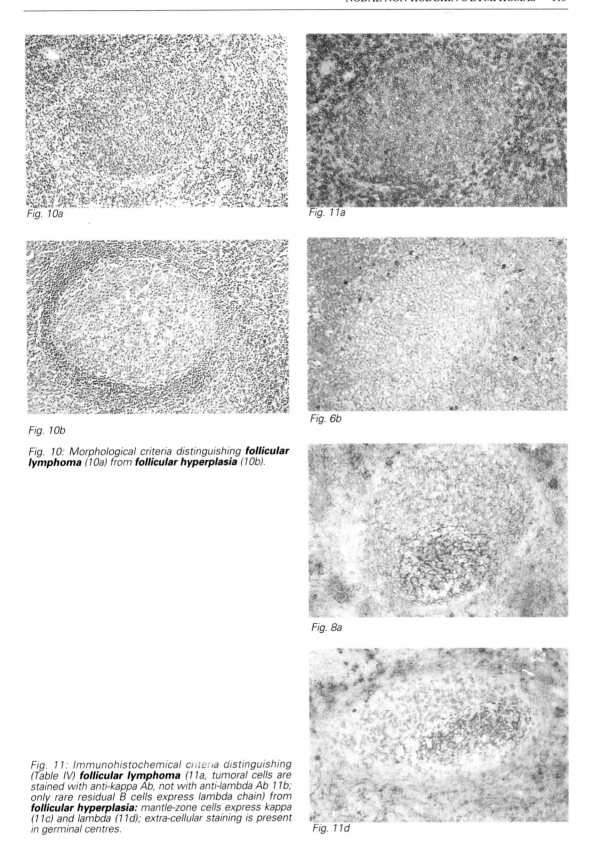

Fig. 10a

Fig. 10b

Fig. 10: Morphological criteria distinguishing **follicular lymphoma** (10a) from **follicular hyperplasia** (10b).

Fig. 11a

Fig. 6b

Fig. 8a

Fig. 11: Immunohistochemical criteria distinguishing (Table IV) **follicular lymphoma** (11a, tumoral cells are stained with anti-kappa Ab, not with anti-lambda Ab 11b; only rare residual B cells express lambda chain) from **follicular hyperplasia:** mantle-zone cells express kappa (11c) and lambda (11d); extra-cellular staining is present in germinal centres.

Fig. 11d

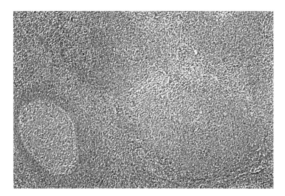

Fig. 12a

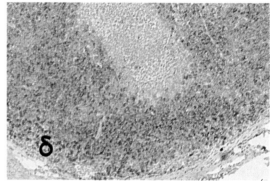

Fig. 13a

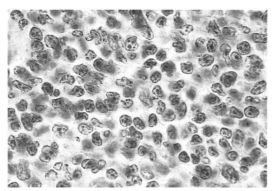

Fig. 12b

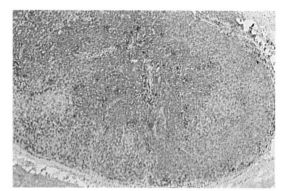

Fig. 13b

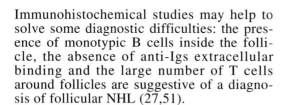

Fig. 12: **Mantle-zone lymphoma:** persistence of germinal centres (12a) at low magnification; cytological aspects of the tumoral cells (12b) at high magnification.

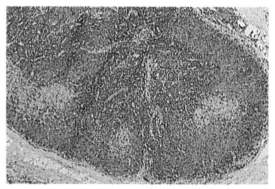

Fig. 13c

Fig. 13: **Mantle-zone lymphoma: IgD CD5** phenotype. Immunoperoxidase staining using monoclonal antibodies directed against IgD (13a), CD3 (Leu 4) (13b), CD5 (Leu 1) (13c). Tumour cells express IgD and CD5. T cells are stained by CD3 and CD5.

Immunohistochemical studies may help to solve some diagnostic difficulties: the presence of monotypic B cells inside the follicle, the absence of anti-Igs extracellular binding and the large number of T cells around follicles are suggestive of a diagnosis of follicular NHL (27,51).

Follicular NHL are associated with a translocation (14;18) involving the bcl-2 gene (52,54-56). Using an antibody directed against the bcl-2 protein, Ngan et al. (33) were able to demonstrate an overexpression of bcl-2 gene associated with the occurrence of a t(14;18) on tissue sections. This technique could be very useful for distinguishing a reactive follicular hyperplasia from a follicular NHL (33).

Other follicular NHL

Mantle-zone lymphomas *(fig. 12)* are neoplastic proliferations of lymphoid cells with

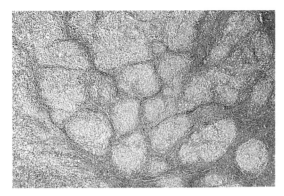

Fig. 14a

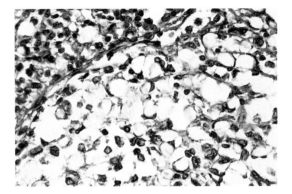

Fig. 14b

Fig. 14: **Signet ring-cell follicular lymphoma** (14a) with lymphoid cells containing large intra-cytoplasmic vacuoles (14b).

tle-zone lymphomas must be distinguished from interfollicular small lymphocytic lymphomas (62).

In **signet ring-cell follicular NHL** *(fig. 14)*, lymphoma cells contain large cytoplasmic vacuoles resulting from intracellular storage of immunoglobulins (63).

Follicular NHL with sclerosis are characterized by abundant collagen fibre sclerosis of interfollicular areas. Their prognosis would seem to be especially good (64).

In **follicular NHL with plasma cell differentiation,** the intrafollicular B cell proliferation is associated with a monoclonal interfollicular plasma cell infiltration. The latter belongs most probably to the same malignant clone as the former but at a different stage of differentiation (65,66).

Diffuse B-cell NHL

Diffuse NHL form a morphologically and immunohistochemically heterogeneous group.

They include small lymphocytic NHL, consistent with chronic lymphocytic leukaemia and plasmacytoid small lymphocytic NHL.

Diffuse small lymphocytic NHL

Clinical aspects

an indented and irregular nucleus, forming a ring around non-malignant germinal centres which are either normal, hyperplastic or atrophic (57). The phenotype *(fig. 13)* of tumour cells is similar to that of normal lymphoid cells in the mantle: B cells which express membrane IgM and IgD (58,59); they express CD5 but not CD10 (CALLA). It has been suggested that mantle-zone NHL are a malignant proliferation of a peculiar lymphoid subpopulation, called lymphocyte of the marginal zone (60). They are considered to be the follicular equivalent of intermediate diffuse NHL (57,58). Although there are very few anatomo-clinical studies, their prognosis and course seem similar to that of usual follicular NHL. However, rare cases of leukaemic evolution are unfavourable in prognosis (61). These man-

Patients with diffuse small lymphocytic NHL most often present with disseminated lymph-node involvement, bone-marrow infiltration and sometimes spleen enlargement. Blood infiltration, at presentation or during the course of the disease, is especially frequent and the distinction between small lymphocytic NHL and chronic lymphocytic leukaemia (CLL) is somewhat arbitrary (67). Cases without increased blood lymphocytes are usually called small lymphocytic NHL whereas cases with a lymphocyte count greater than 4.5×10^9 are called CLL, whatever the tumour burden.

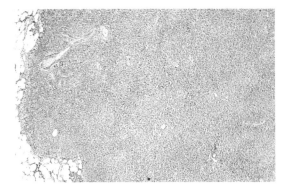

Fig. 15: **Diffuse small lymphocytic lymphoma,** at low magnification.

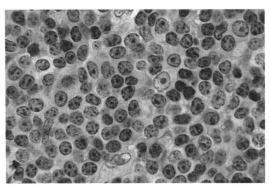

Fig. 16: **Diffuse small lymphocytic lymphoma:** at high magnification the proliferation is monomorphous with small lymphoid cells with round and regular nucleus. Absence of mitoses.

Morphological aspects

The proliferation always has a diffuse architecture *(fig. 15)*. Lymph-node involvement may be partial, sparing the sinuses and the capsule. At the onset of the disease, infiltration may be limited to the medullary zone (11,12,67,68).

A malignant proliferation is composed of a uniform sheet of monomorphic cells, whose size is equal to or slightly greater than normal peripheral blood lymphocytes *(fig. 16)*. They have a round and regular nucleus, with a dense heterochromatin and no nucleolus. Cytoplasm is very scanty. Mitoses are

Fig. 17: **Diffuse small lymphocytic lymphoma,** IgG kappa phenotype. Immunoperoxidase staining using monoclonal antibody directed against IgG (17a), IgM (17b), kappa (17c) and lambda (17d). Tumoral cells express IgG kappa; rare residual cells express IgM lambda.

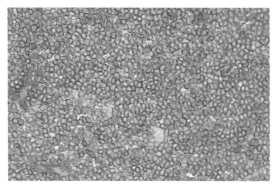

Fig. 17a

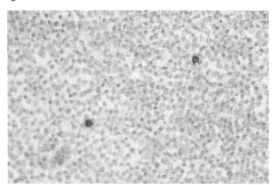

Fig. 17b

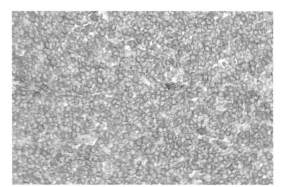

Fig. 17c

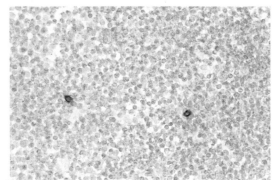

Fig. 17d

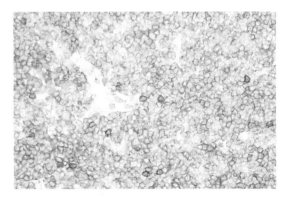

Fig. 18a

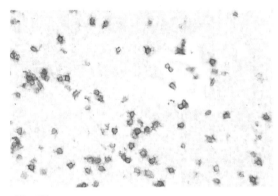

Fig. 18b

Fig. 18: **Diffuse small lymphocytic lymphoma.**
Immunoperoxidase staining using monoclonal antibody directed against CD5 (Leu 1) and CD3 (Leu 4): the B-tumoral
cells express CD5; the T-reactive cells are stained
intensely by CD5 and CD3.

uncommon. Amongst these small cells there
are always some larger cells. Some are prolymphocytes: medium-size cells with a regular nucleus containing one central and
large nucleolus, and a basophilic cytoplasm.
Other cells are identica to large non-cleaved
cells or to immunoblasts but their cytoplasm
is not, or only very slightly, basophilic.
These large cells may be scattered amongst
the proliferation of small lymphocytes or,
more often, they gather to form clusters
called "proliferation centres", mimicking
follicles. This pseudofollicular pattern must
be distinguished from follicular NHL.

In approximately 10 to 15% of cases, diffuse
small lymphocytic NHL evolve towards a
more aggressive histological type
(11,12,67,69). Such a histological transformation was initially called Richter's syndrome (70). When transformed, the histo-

logical pattern is that of a diffuse non-
cleaved large cell NHL or a diffuse large-
cell immunoblastic NHL (71). It is generally
agreed that the histologically transformed
NHL belongs to the same clone as the initial
small lymphocytic NHL. Several items of
cytogenetic and immunological data support
this hypothesis (72). Nevertheless, in some
cases, the secondary tumour belongs to
another clone, expressing either another
light chain isotype or different immunoglobulin gene rearrangements (73).

Immunohistochemical aspects

Approximately 95% of small lymphocytic
NHL are B-cell proliferations, with, amongst
these B cells, very few reactive T cells
(11,12,74) (figs. 17 and 18). They have a
peculiar immunological phenotype. They
express low amounts of surface immunoglobulins, most often of the μ chain isotype
(with or without coexpression of the δ
chain), and more rarely of the γ chain isotype (74-76). These amounts are lower than
those of surface immunoglobulin for normal
peripheral blood lymphocytes and
of other lymphoma cells (77). There is a
correlation in clinical outcome with the
degree of surface immunoglobulin (sIg)
expression (78). Tumour cells carry C3d
receptors (CD21) and rarely C3b receptors
(CD35). They are also HLA-DR+. In addition, they carry CD19, CD20 and CD22,
and are CD10-negative. They almost always
react with anti-CD5 antibodies which are
directed against an antigen found on normal
blood T cells (fig. 18) (79). But the reactivi-

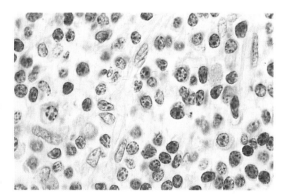

Fig. 19: **Diffuse small lymphocytic lymphoma with
plasma cell differentiation:** polymorphous proliferation
consisting of lymphocytes, plasma cells and lymphoplasmacytic cells. High magnification.

ty is lower than that of normal T cells (80). Such a peculiar phenotype makes the determination of their normal counterpart difficult. It could be either a minority subpopulation of normal perifollicular mantle B cells (81) or immature B cells (82). The proliferative rate, estimated using the Ki-67 antibody, is usually very low, with the exception of "proliferation centres" (47).

Diffuse small lymphocytic NHL with plasma cell differentiation or lymphoplasmacytic/cytoid NHL or immunocytoma

Clinical aspects

Patients with small lymphocytic NHL with plasma cell differentiation present either with disseminated lymph node involvement or bone-marrow infiltration, with or without blood involvement, or spleen enlargement. There is no clinical or histological difference from the histological pattern of lymphnode and bone-marrow Waldenström's macroglobulinaemia (67). The name of Waldenström's macroglobulinaemia is usually reserved for cases with a serum IgM component.

Morphological aspects

The tumour cell proliferation is heterogeneous, comprising lymphocytes, plasma cells and lymphoplasmacytic cells (11,12,83) *(fig. 19)*. Plasma cells are easily recognizable. These are medium-size cells, with an eccentric nucleus containing a mottled chromatin and with an abundant and basophilic cytoplasm. Lymphoplasmacytic cells have an intermediate morphological aspect between small lymphocytes and plasma cells: their cytoplasm is scanty but basophilic and their nucleus is slightly eccentric but mottled. Some eosinophilic, PAS+ inclusions may be found in the cytoplasm or in the nucleus, giving evidence of the production of immunoglobulins. Some large immunoblastic cells may be found among these cells.

In the updated Kiel classification (3), this histological group of NHL has been designated as "immunocytomas". It has been subdivided into 3 categories: the lymphoplasmacytic type, with numerous plasma cells; the

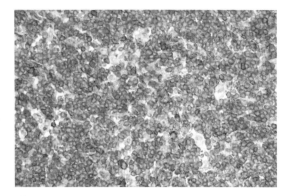

Fig. 20a

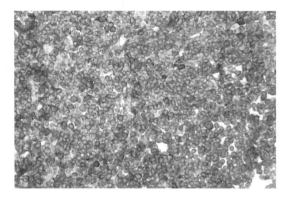

Fig. 20b

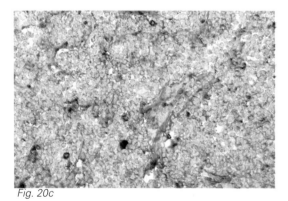

Fig. 20c

Fig. 20: **Diffuse small lymphocytic lymphoma** *IgM kappa phenotype.Immunoperoxidase staining using monoclonal antibody directed against IgM (20a), kappa (20b) and lambda (20c): the tumoral cells are stained with anti-IgM and anti-kappa. Few residual cells and extra-cellular matrix of collagen fibres are stained with anti-lambda monoclonal antibody.*

lymphoplasmacytoid type, with numerous "lymphoplasmacytic" cells and the polymorphic type, with many immunoblasts, small cleaved cells and large non-cleaved cells. In the Working Formulation for Clinical Use, the latter subtype is included in the diffuse mixed group and considered as an intermediate-grade NHL whereas the two former are low-grade NHL (1).

Immunohistochemical aspects

All small lymphocytic NHL with plasma cell differentiation are of B-cell origin. They are characterized by the presence of intracytoplasmic immunoglobulins. Reactive T cells are numerous. Malignant B cells have a different phenotype related to their cell differentiation stage. Membrane and cytoplasmic immunoglobulins more often have a kappa than lambda light chain isotype. In order of decreasing frequency, their heavy chain class is μ,γ or α (84-86) *(fig. 20)*. If lymphoplasmacytic cells are numerous, they are HLA-DR, CD19 and CD20 positive. If plasma cells are numerous, they are HLA-DR, CD19 and CD20 negative, but CD38, PC-1 or PCA-1 positive (69,70).

Small cleaved-cell NHL

Within the framework of the Working Formulation for Clinical Use, diffuse small cleaved-cell NHL represent the diffuse equivalent of follicular small cleaved-cell NHL (1). Diffuse small-cleaved NHL may be primary or secondary to the transformation of a follicular small cleaved-cell NHL. They are included in the intermediate-grade group of the Working Formulation and in the B low-grade group of the updated Kiel classification.

Morphological aspects

The proliferation is homogeneous, and is composed of small lymphoid cells which are morphologically very similar to the malignant cells of follicular small cleaved-cell (FSC) NHL *(fig. 21)*. Mitoses are more numerous. There may be a minority of cleaved or non-cleaved large cells.

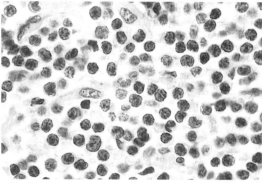

Fig. 21a

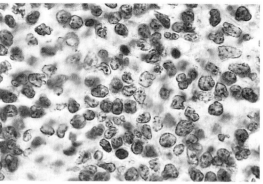

Fig. 21b

Fig. 21: **Diffuse small cleaved-cell lymphoma.** *Cytological aspects at low (21a) and high (21b) magnification. Rare mitoses are present.*

Immunohistochemical aspects

Lymphoid cell proliferation is composed of monoclonal B cells admixed with variable amounts of reactive T cells. In approximately 75% of cases, loose networks of dendritic reticulum cells may be seen (84,87). The phenotype of neoplastic B cells is slightly different from that of malignant B cells of FSC-NHL (29,82,88,89). They also express surface immunoglobulins, most often of the μ class (with or without δ chains), more rarely of the γ class. They are HLA-DR+, CD19, CD20, CD22 positive, but they lack expression of CD10 (CALLA) and rarely express C3b (CD35) and C3d (CD21) receptors. Approximately 50% of cases are CD5 positive, whereas FSC-NHL are usually not (28,79). They may express CD25 (37,38). The percentage of Ki-67 positive tumour cells is usually lower than in follicular NHL (47).

The amounts of T cells are variable. They usually represent approximately 10% of all cells, a proportion lower than in follicular NHL. Most of them are CD4+ (38). NK cells are rare or absent (41). In some cases, mostly diffuse small cleaved-cell NHL resulting from the histological transformation of follicular small cleaved-cell NHL, reactive T cells are numerous (90). This might suggest an erroneous diagnosis of T-cell NHL secondary to a follicular B-cell NHL (91).

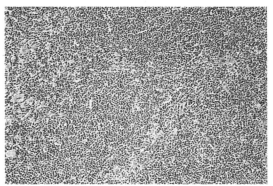

Fig. 22: **Diffuse intermediate lymphoma** at low magnification.

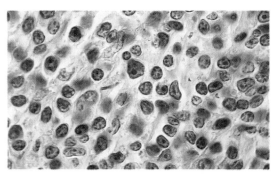

Fig. 23: **Diffuse intermediate lymphoma**. Cytological aspect at a high magnification demonstrating the association of small lymphocytic cells and small cleaved cells.

Diffuse intermediate NHL

The name of intermediate NHL is at present used in the meaning given by C.W. Bérard, i.e. a diffuse NHL *(fig. 22)* with morphological and immunological characteristics intermediate between those of diffuse small lymphocytic and diffuse small cleaved-cell NHL (92-94). This histological subtype has not been distinguished in the Working Formulation (1). Three cell types may be seen: small lymphocytes, small cleaved cells and larger cells with a round and irregular but non-cleaved nucleus *(fig. 23)* (94,94a). Mitoses are not frequent.

The malignant B cells carry surface immunoglobulins, either kappa or lambda, with μ and δ heavy chains. They are also CD10+ and CD5+ (88). Ki-67 expression is higher than that observed in diffuse small lymphocytic NHL. They express CD74 (LN2) but not CDw75 (LN1) on paraffin sections (59,95). They express CD20 (L26). Their immunological and cytochemical properties (alkaline phosphatase activity) (96) suggest that diffuse intermediate NHL originate from a B-cell subpopulation of the normal mantle zone and are the diffuse equivalent of mantle-zone NHL.

Differential diagnosis

Diffuse small cleaved-cell NHL must be distinguished from lymphoblastic NHL, which they superficially resemble in size and in the irregular shape of the nucleus. The chromatin features, the absence of nucleus cleavage and, above all, the presence of numerous mitoses allow establishment of a diagnosis of lymphoblastic lymphoma.

Diffuse small cleaved cell NHL must be distinguished from T-cell NHL with "intermediate-size cells" described by Japanese pathologists (97,98). This histological subtype accounts for 10 to 15% of T-cell NHL in Japan (99) and in western countries (100). If frozen sections are not available, the use of CD45 (UCHL-1) and CD3 (101)

Fig. 24: **Diffuse mixed lymphoma**. Double staining with immunoperoxidase (anti pan-B Ab) and immunophosphatase alkaline (anti pan-T Ab) showing the two B- and T-lymphoid populations: it corresponds to a diffuse B-cell lymphoma associated with a T-cell stromal reaction.

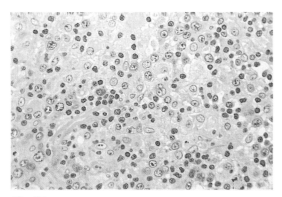

Fig. 25a

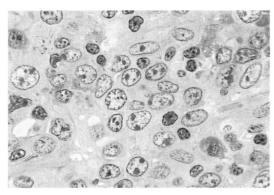

Fig. 25b

Fig. 25: **Diffuse mixed lymphoma**. In fact, it corresponds to a non-cleaved large-cell lymphoma, B-cell phenotype associated with small reactive T cells. Low magnification 25a, high magnification 25b.

monoclonal antibodies is useful in demonstrating their T-cell phenotype in contrast with the B-cell phenotype of intermediate NHL.

Diffuse mixed B-cell NHL

Diffuse mixed B-cell NHL are rare, accounting for less than 10% of all NHL (GELF protocol, France) and their frequency has probably been overestimated (1).

Most cases considered as mixed cell type are in fact large B-cell NHL associated with a significant T-cell reaction *(fig. 24)* (102-104). The T-cell reaction may be considerable and may hamper the identification of the malignant B-cell clone. Real diffuse mixed B-cell NHL have been described. They are either the diffuse counterpart of follicular mixed cell NHL, or polymorphic immunocytomas (11,12). The former occurs either directly or by transformation of an initially follicular NHL. The malignant proliferation includes small cleaved cells and a variable proportion of large cells, either cleaved or non-cleaved *(fig. 25)*. The maximum proportion of large cells for a diagnosis of diffuse mixed NHL to be admissible varies between 25 and 70% (6,105,106). A figure of 50% seems a practical and adequate limit. Phenotypically, the proliferation includes a majority of monoclonal B cells associated with a variable proportion of small reactive T cells. There is often an irregular network of dendritic reticulum cells (30,84).

Large B-cell NHL

The large-cell group corresponds to the "histiocytic" lymphomas of Rappaport's classification. This term should no longer be used since almost all cases are of B-cell origin. This histological type is especially frequent, and accounts for 25 to 45% of all NHL (1,8,12). Their morphological aspects are variable and several subclassifications have been proposed (107,108). The distinction suggested in the Working Formulation between centrofollicular large-cell NHL and immunoblastic large-cell NHL relied upon a difference in prognosis as suggested by past clinical studies (107,108). Such a distinction no longer seems justified since differences in prognosis have been eradicated with the use of modern and aggressive chemotherapy programmes (12,109-111). Tumour mass, bone-marrow involvement and seric LDH are of greater value prognostic than the histological subtype.

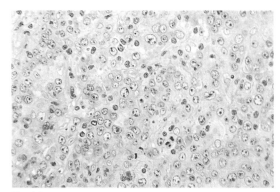

Fig. 26a

Cleaved or non-cleaved large-cell NHL

Morphological aspects

This histological type is characterized by the prevailing presence of large cells, either cleaved or non-cleaved *(fig. 26)* [corresponding to large centrocytes and centroblasts, respectively, in Kiel's classification (3)]. Most cases are quite monomorphic. Some are more heterogeneous, associating variable proportions of large cleaved and non-cleaved cells. There is also a significant proportion of immunoblasts in cases called centroblastic polymorph in Kiel's classification (3). Such cases may represent a transition from centrofollicular large-cell NHL to immunoblastic large-cell NHL. A more precise classification may be difficult.

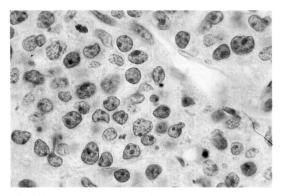

Fig. 26b

Multilobated large-cell NHL have been described by G.S. Pinkus *(fig. 27)*. Initially, because of the predominantly mediastinal involvement and of the pathological features, they were considered T-cell NHL (112). Meanwhile, some histological criteria such as the concomitant presence of large non-cleaved cells (centroblasts) have suggested the B-cell origin which was confirmed by the immunohistochemical studies (113,114). Mitoses are numerous. Necrotic cells and, in some cases, many phagocytic cells may be found. Fibrosis is often present, especially in axillary, mediastinal, mesenteric and retroperitoneal localizations (115). Such fibrosis may be pro-

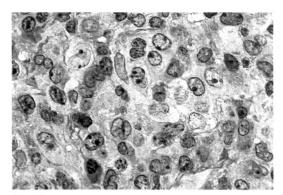

Fig. 26c

Fig. 26: **Diffuse large cell lymphoma**. Low magnification (26a): numerous mitoses; high magnification: comparison of non-cleaved large cells (26b) and cleaved large cells (26c).

minent, either with pericellular reticulin bands forming compartmentalization patterns *(fig. 28)*, or with thick collagen bands. Unlike follicular NHL, such fibrosis

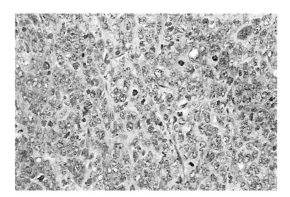

Fig. 27a

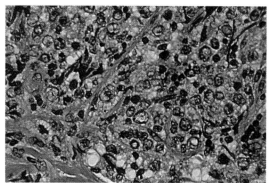

Fig. 28: **Diffuse large-cell lymphoma with fibrosis.**
The fibrosis forms pericellular bands with compartmentalization patterns.

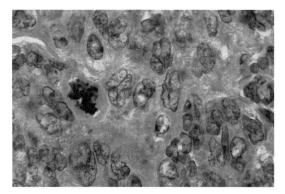

Fig. 27b

Fig. 27: **Diffuse multilobated large-cell lymphoma**
(Pinkus). Cytological aspects at low (27a) and high (27b)
magnification.

Immunoblastic large-cell NHL

In the Working Formulation, the term
"immunoblast" is used to designate any
"transformed" lymphoid cell, i.e. any cell
whose morphological characteristics are
similar to those of stimulated lymphoid
cells. This term is not limited to a large
basophilic cell in the definition used by
many authors (116). Immunoblastic large-
cell NHL may have a B- or T-cell origin and
there is no strict relationship between
the morphological pattern and the immunological phenotype.

Morphological aspects

does not seem to have a prognostic
influence.

In the Working Formulation, besides the
monomorphic type, four other subtypes are
distinguished: immunoblastic NHL with
plasma-cell differentiation, clear-cell,
polymorphic immunoblastic NHL and
immunoblastic NHL with epithelioid component (1).

Immunohistochemical characteristics

The cell proliferation includes malignant
B cells and variable amounts of reactive
T cells. The phenotype of malignant
B cells may be heterogeneous. They usually express membrane or cytoplasm
immunoglobulin, most often μ kappa. They
rarely express the receptor for C3b (CD35)
and C3d (CD21). They are HLA-DR positive. Most of them are CD19 and CD20
positive but CD5 and CD10 negative
(29,76). They are never simultaneously sIg
and CD19/CD20 negative, with the result
that their B-cell origin can always be
shown.

Immunoblastic NHL with plasma-cell differentiation are characterized by the presence of large cells 30 to 60 μ in diameter
(117). The nucleus is very large, ovoid,
with regular outline and a thick nuclear
membrane. The chromatin is fine, with a
bulky, and usually central, nucleolus
(fig. 29). The cytoplasm is abundant and

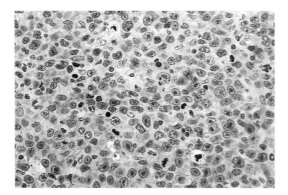

Fig. 29a

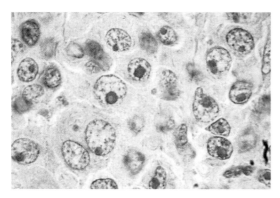

Fig. 29b

Fig. 29: **Diffuse immunoblastic large-cell lymphoma,** *with plasma cell differentiation. Cytological aspect at low (29a) and high (29b) magnification.*

basophilic. Some cells have plasma cell characteristics, being of smaller size and having an eccentric nucleus, and a more abundant and more basophilic cytoplasm. Mitoses are numerous.

The three other morphological types have similar characteristics. These three variant types usually have a T-cell immunopheno-type, as shown by immunohistochemical studies, and are described in the T-cell NHL chapter.

Immunohistochemical aspects

Approximately 60% of immunoblastic NHL have a B-cell and 30% a T-cell phenotype (118-120). As previously mentioned, there

is no strict relationship between the morphological pattern and the immunological phenotype (121-123). Nevertheless, almost all immunoblastic NHL with plasma-cell differentiation have a B-cell origin while most other subtypes have a T-cell origin (117,122). Approximately 50 to 60% of B-cell immunoblastic NHL express membrane and/or cytoplasmic Ig. They are usually HLA-DR positive. Almost all of them express pan-B-cell antigens (76,120,124).

Diffuse non-cleaved small-cell NHL

Burkitt's lymphomas

Clinical manifestations differ between the African endemic form and sporadic forms in Europe and North America.

Burkitt's lymphoma is endemic in Africa (between latitude 10° North and 10° South) and in Papua - New Guinea. In Eastern and Western Africa (125,129,130), Burkitt's lymphoma is very rare before the age of one. Frequency reaches a peak between 5 and 7 years of age, then falls abruptly after the age of 12. In a series of 430 cases, initial presentation was a cheek tumour in 39.3% of patients, an abdominal mass in 38.6% and both cheek and abdomen involvement in 20.3% (129). Other initial pre-sentations are very rare (130). Cheek tumours develop from dental alveoli and progressively spread to maxillae and orbit. Abdominal masses are usually huge, multiple, and associated with a peritoneal effusion in some cases. They are most often retroperitoneal and may be responsible for paraplegia either by spinal-cord compression or by vascular ischaemia. Renal, ovarian and testicular involvement is also frequent. CNS involvement is frequent at relapse (131). The prognosis of Burkitt's NHL with facial involvement is better than that with abdominal or multifocal involvements (125,129,132).

In Europe and North America, median age differs among series: 11 years (133), 8.5 years (134), 17 years (135). In almost all these series, there is a large male predo-

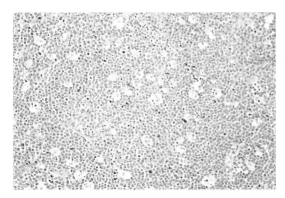

*Fig. 30: **Diffuse non-cleaved small-cell lymphoma, Burkitt-like.** The "starry sky" pattern is shown at a low magnification.*

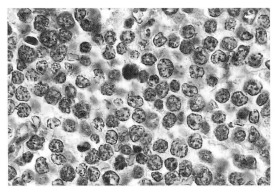

*Fig. 31: **Burkitt's lymphoma.** Numerous mitoses and cell necrosis.*

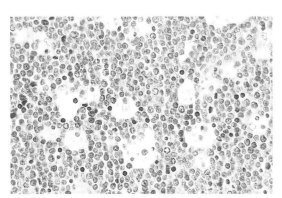

*Fig. 32: **Burkitt's lymphoma.** The "starry sky" pattern is due to the presence of numerous macrophages.*

minance. In approximately 70 to 90% of cases, the initial presentation is an abdominal mass, involving principally the ileocaecal region and, more rarely, the ovaries. Peripheral lymph nodes are involved in 20% of cases, and bone marrow in 15 to 25% at initial presentation, more often in relapse (134). In a group of 64 sporadic cases in the United States (136), 15 (23%) had CNS involvement during the course of the disease, 9 at presentation and 6 at relapse. Several staging classifications for Burkitt's NHL have been proposed. The most widely used is shown in *Table V.*

Morphological characteristics

The morphological pattern is distinctive. The proliferation is diffuse *(fig. 30)* and follicular only in very rare cases (126,128). Malignant cells are monomorphic, of intermediate size (15 to 20 μ in diameter), with a round and regular nucleus. The chromatin is reticular and contains 2 to 4 well-defined nucleoli. The cytoplasm is scarce and very basophilic. Mitoses are numerous *(fig. 31)*. Many macrophages are scattered among malignant cells, forming a pattern described as "starry sky". However, this aspect is neither constant nor specific *(fig. 32)*.

Immunological characteristics

Malignant cells have a B-cell phenotype and express cytoplasmic and membrane μ chains, associated or not associated with a light chain. They probably derive from a germinal-centre B-cell subpopulation (6,125-128).

Burkitt-like small non-cleaved NHL

This histological type is morphologically heterogeneous (126). Some differ from typical Burkitt's lymphoma by the variable size of their malignant cells and nucleus shape, which has single large nucleoli. The "starry sky" pattern is variable *(fig. 33)*. Other cases are similar to immunoblastic NHL, with smaller malignant cells: approximately 85% have a B-cell origin and 15% a T-cell origin (137).

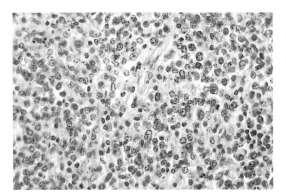

Fig. 33a

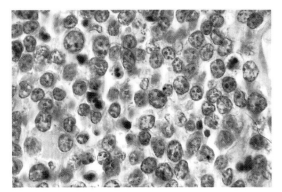

Fig. 33b

Fig. 33: **Diffuse non-cleaved small-cell lymphoma, Burkitt-like.** *Cytological aspect at low (33a) and high (33b) magnification.*

Lymphoblastic lymphomas

Lymphoblastic lymphomas are essentially of T phenotype. The B-lymphoblastic lymphomas reveal the same morphology as those of T-lymphoblastic lymphomas. They are described with the T-lymphoblastic lymphomas.

Other B-Cell NHL

1. B-cell NHL which originate from mucosa-associated lymphoid tissues (**MALT**) are described *on pp. 171-177.*

2. Monocytoid B-cell NHL. This histological subtype has recently beeen described (138-141). They form a proliferation of intermediate-size cells, with a clear abundant cytoplasm and an ovoid nucleus. The proliferation predominates in interfollicular areas and sinuses. Malignant cells have a B-cell phenotype. They are of low-grade malignancy (142).

3. Mediastinal NHL are described *on pp. 227-230.* They are formed of large cells, clear in some cases, and often associated with fibrosis. They have a B-cell phenotype.

4. "Malignant angioendotheliomatosis" or angiotropic large cell NHL. This lymphoma is rare and of very unfavourable prognosis. It presents multiple sites, most often skin and CNS. The malignant cells are large, pleomorphic and located in small-vessel lumina. Immunohis-tochemical and genetic studies demonstrate their B-cell clonality, eliminating the possibility of their endothelial origin. The term *malignant angioendotheliomatosis* could be replaced by that of *angiotropic large-cell NHL* (143-152).

T-cell NHL

T-cell NHL are not covered individually in the Working Formulation for Clinical Use, but are described separately in the updated Kiel classification (3). If there are nosological relationships between B-cell and T-cell NHL, the latter usually raise problems of specific diagnosis, prognosis and treatment. We shall therefore describe T-cell NHL separately following the updated Kiel classification (3). We shall first describe the common clinical characteristics of the peripheral T-cell NHL, then the specific characteristics of both peripheral T-cell and T-lymphoblastic NHL.

Clinical characteristics

Patients with peripheral T-cell NHL usually present with peripheral lymphadenopathies (85%) (153-159) but generally have stage IV involvement. Among extranodal sites, which

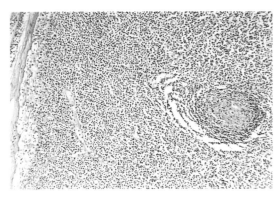

Fig. 34: **T-cell lymphoma**. At low magnification, the lymphoid proliferation is located in the paracortical area with sparing of a lymphoid follicle.

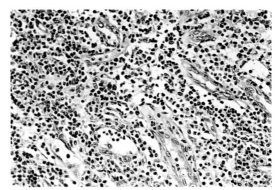

Fig. 35: **T-cell lymphoma**. Post-capillary venule hyperplasia.

may reveal the disease (159-161,163), cutaneous involvement is found in 50% of patients. Liver (50%), pleuropul-monary (20%) and bone-marrow (30%) involvement are also frequently observed (161,162). Blood involvement (30%) may be found especially in patients with skin involvement. Around 15% of patients have a previous history of dysimmune or autoimmune disorders such as Hashimoto's thyroiditis, Sjögren's disease, of coeliac disease (153,154).

HTLV1-associated adult T leukaemia/lymphomas have specific clinical characteristics previously described on p.27. At presentation or during the course of the disease patients often have skin, liver and spleen, lymph-node and bone-marrow involvement. Hypercalcaemia is frequently observed. Neuromeningeal and lung involvement are frequent. Bone-marrow involvement is almost constant and a leukaemic process is frequent either at once or during the course of the disease.

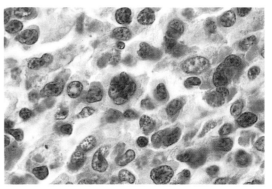

Fig. 36a

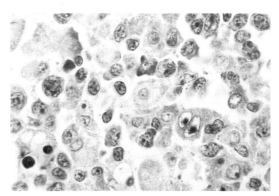

Fig. 36b

Fig. 36: **T-cell lymphoma**. Pleomorphous lymphoid proliferation (36a) with some cells resembling Reed-Sternberg cells (36b) (Giemsa staining).

Morphological characteristics

Some cytological and morphological patterns are suggestive of, but not specific to, T-cell NHL (98,100,153,155,157,159,164). Among these patterns, the most important are:

- initial involvement of paracortical zones with sparing of follicles and sinuses *(fig. 34)* and post-capillary venule hyperplasia *(fig. 35)*;

- pleomorphic aspects of tumor cells, with nuclei of variable size, often irregular, lobulated and variable amounts of clear cytoplasm sometimes associated with Reed-Sternberg-like cells *(fig. 36)*;

- an important associated reactive-cell proliferation composed of lymphocytes, plasma

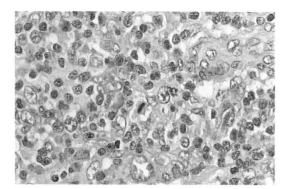

Fig. 37: **T-cell lymphoma.** Beside the T-tumoral cells, numerous reactive cells can be seen, including eosinophils.

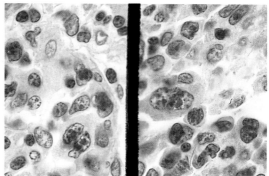

Fig. 38a

cells, eosinophil granulocytes and interdigitating cells *(fig. 37)*;

- in some cases, epithelioid cells, which may be numerous;

- compartmentalization of malignant cells by a thin reticulin or collagen network.

Although these morphological characteristics may suggest a diagnosis of T-cell NHL, they can also raise difficult diagnostic problems, especially with Type-3 mixed cellularity Hodgkin's disease. Normal appearance of small lymphoid cells, absence of hypervascularization, presence of characteristic Reed-Sternberg cells, of "mummified" cells, suggest Hodgkin's disease. Immunohistochemical study *(fig. 38)* is helpful for the diagnosis. Absence of aberrant T-cell expression by the small lymphoid cells and expression of CD30 by Reed-Sternberg cells suggest Hodgkin's disease. However, in some cases of T-cell NHL, tumour cells may express the same antigens, especially CD30, as those expressed by Reed-Sternberg cells.

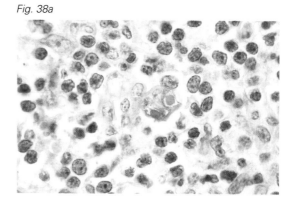

Fig. 38b

Immunohistochemical characteristics

Immunohistochemical stainings (34, 100, 154, 156-159, 164-168) show the characteristic pattern of peripheral (or post-thymic) T cells CD1- and CD3+, but with a variable

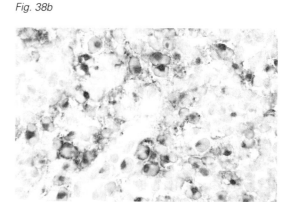

Fig. 38c

Fig. 38: **T-cell lymphoma** (38a) compared to Hodgkin's disease (38b). Immunoperoxidase staining using monoclonal antibodies directed against CD30 (Ki1): tumoral cells of T-cell lymphoma (38c) and Reed-Sternberg cells of Hodgkin's disease express CD30 (38d).

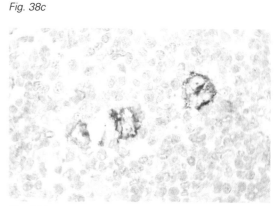

Fig. 38d

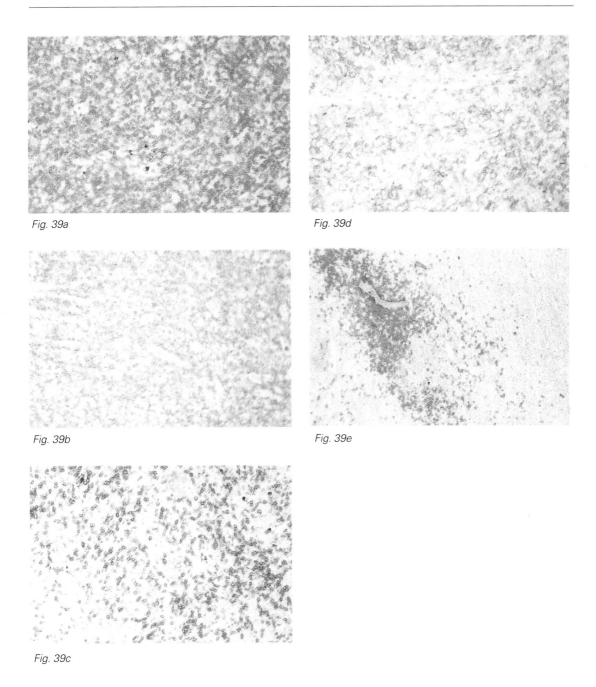

Fig. 39a

Fig. 39d

Fig. 39b

Fig. 39e

Fig. 39c

Fig. 39: **T-cell lymphoma.** Immunoperoxidase staining using monoclonal antibodies directed against CD3 (Leu 4, fig. 39a), CD2 (Leu 5, fig. 39b), CD5 (Leu 1, fig. 39c), CD7 (Leu 9, fig. 39d) and CD22 (pan B, fig. 39e): there is a loss of two T-cell antigens: tumoral cells express CD3 and CD2 but not CD5 nor CD7. Some B cells are visible around vessels.

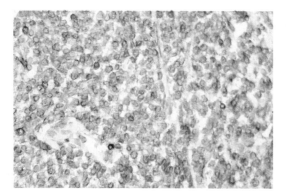

Fig. 40a

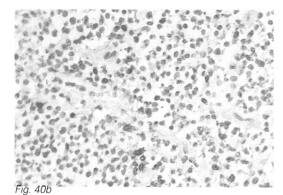

Fig. 40b

Fig. 40: CD4 **T-cell lymphoma**. *Immunoperoxidase staining using monoclonal antibodies directed against CD4 (Leu 3a, fig. 40a) and CD8 (Leu 2a, fig. 40b). Tumoral cells express CD4 but not CD8.*

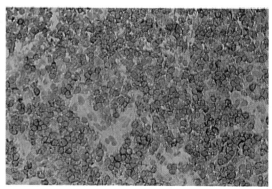

Fig. 41: **T-cell lymphoma**. *Immunoperoxidase staining using monoclonal antibodies directed against βF1 (β chain of the TCR): tumoral cells express βF1.*

expression of pan-T antigens (CD2, CD3, CD5, CD7) *(fig. 39)*. There is a clear dissociation in the expression of these CD2, CD3, CD5, CD7 antigens in 80% of T-cell NHL (169). They express CD4 more often *(fig. 40)* than CD8 but can express either both together or neither. Residual or reactive B cells are present in variable amounts, often forming more or less atrophic follicles *(fig. 39)*. About 20 to 30% of T-cell NHL do not express the ß chain of the T-cell receptor (TCR) as shown by ßF1 antibody binding (170-172) *(fig. 41)*. This preliminary finding remains to be confirmed but could suggest different activation stages of tumour cells (173). In these cases, the δ chain of the TCR γδ is rarely expressed (174).

Some T-cell NHL, often associated with a nasopharyngeal involvement, have NK cell markers (175). T-cell NHL show a large range of mitotic rates as shown by Ki-67 anti-body expression (47) and, contrary to B-cell NHL, almost all T-cell NHL express the LFA-1 adhesion molecule (165,176).

Genotypic analysis

Demonstration of a unique TCR-Cß gene rearrangement is a reliable marker of clonality of T-cell NHL (34,158,177-179,181-184). This Cß gene rearrangement is often associated with a clonal rearrangement of γ and/or δ genes of the TCR γδ (185,186). This latter rearrangement may be used as a clonality marker in rare cases in which there is no Cß gene rearrangement. There also are exceptional cases of T-cell NHL with neither Cß gene nor Cγ gene rearrangement (187). Nevertheless, in most cases, molecular biology studies are not mandatory for the diagnosis of T-cell NHL if tumour cells have an abnormal T-cell phenotype, since it has been shown that there is a close relationship between such an abnormal phenotype and Cß gene rearrangement. On the other hand, normal T-cell phenotype is observed in the T-cell population of Hodgkin's disease and in reactive T-lymphoid hyperplasias (34).

Genomic study is however, useful for diagnosis (34,184,188):

- if the morphological and immunological patterns of the proliferation are heterogenous with an admixture of polyclonal B cells, CD4+ and CD8+ T cells, suggesting either a T-cell NHL or a non-malignant "dysimmune" disorder. Such patterns may be observed in angioimmunoblastic lymphadenopathy (AILD) (189-191) which is now considered to be a T-cell NHL. In "granulomatous" proliferations such as Liebow's lymphomatoid granulomatosis or polymorphic reticulosis, genomic studies have shown clonal rearrangements and these disorders are now considered to be angiocentric T-cell NHL (153,192,193);

- if the tumour cells do not express any pan-T antigen, especially CD3, or only express CD4 which can also be found on monocyte-macrophage cells (34,194); and

- if the malignant involvement is only partial, making morphological and immunological interpretations difficult(34). Genoty-pe studies allow the detection of a minority of 1 to 10% of clonal cells among all cells of the tissue sample (35).

Although the usefulness of genotype studies has been confirmed in these situations, two remarks must be made. First, the demonstration of a clonal proliferation does not *per se* allow us to ascertain its malignant nature. Other morphological and clinical data must also be taken into account. For instance, lymphomatoid papulosis is characterized by polymorphic skin lesions, a clonal Cß-TCR gene rearrangement but a slow and "benign" course (195). Secondly, both B- and T-cell receptor genes may be rearranged (34,196,197). Although such a finding is rare in post-thymic T-cell proliferations, phenotypic study results, showing that only one of these rearrangements is productive, must be used to confirm the cell origin.

5. Karyotype analyses in T-cell NHL most often do not show clonal chromosome abnormalities. In some cases, chromosome 14 may be the site of a translocation [t(11;14) or t(8;14)] or an inversion. The breakpoint is located close to TCR genes. In T cells with t(8;14), *c-myc* oncogene may be translocated close to TCRα genes (198,199).

If paraffin sections only are available, the T-cell phenotype can be recognized by anti-CD45(RO) (UCHL1) *(fig. 42a)* (200), ßF1 (170-172) and anti-CD3 (101) *(fig. 42b)*.

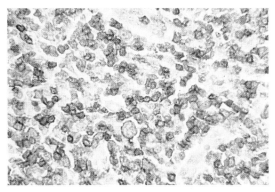

Fig. 42a

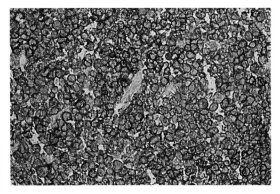

Fig. 42b

Fig. 42: **T-cell lymphoma**. *Immunoperoxidase staining on paraffin sections using monoclonal antibodies directed against CD45 RO (UCH-L1, fig. 42a) and CD3 (fig. 42b). Tumoral cells express CD45 RO and CD3.*

Low-grade T-cell lymphomas

Diffuse small T-cell NHL

A T-cell origin can be demonstrated in less than 5% of diffuse small-cell NHL. They have some clinical specificities such as extensive spleen enlargement, skin involvement and an unusually rapid course (201), but there are no sufficiently characteristic morphological differences between B- and T-small-cell NHL to allow their identification without the use of immunohistochemistry. On blood smears, 2 cell types have been described, one with an irregular nucleus and numerous protrusions ("knotty nuclear"), the other with multiple azurophilic granulations in the cytoplasm (202). In most cases, cells have a CD4+ helper/auxiliary phenotype (203).

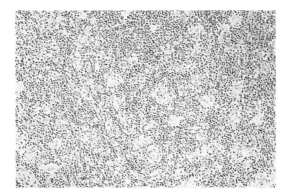

Fig. 43a

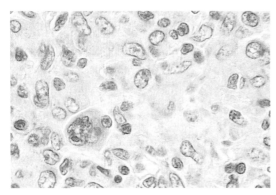

Fig. 43b

Fig. 43: **Lennert's lympho-epithelioid lymphoma.**
Morphological aspects at low (43a) and high magnification (43b). Pleomorphic T cells with irregular nuclei and presence of large cells resembling Reed-Sternberg cells.

Mycosis fungoides and Sézary syndrome will be described
in the chapter *"Cutaneous lymphomas".*
(pp. 207-225)

Lennert's lympho-epithelioid NHL

This lymphoma was first described by Lennert as a variant of Hodgkin's disease (12), but was rapidly considered to be a non-Hodgkin's T lymphoma with an unusually prominent epithelioid component (204,205). It is formed of numerous clusters of epithelioid cells admixed with a predominantly small lymphocyte proliferation with an irregular nucleus and some intermediate-size lymphoid cells and, in some cases, giant cells similar to Reed-Sternberg cells *(fig. 43)* (164,206). If these cells are numerous, a diagnosis of Hodgkin's disease has to

be ruled out. The pleomorphism and atypia of small lymphoid cells, their "abnormal" T-cell phenotype and a typical Cß clonal rearrangement point towards diagnosis of a T-cell NHL.

Several authors have suggested the T-cell origin of Lennert's lymphoma and it has been recently confirmed by phenotypic and genotypic studies. Malignant cells express a mature CD4+ T-cell phenotype (164,207) and have a clonal TCR gene rearrangement (164,207,208). Rare cases of Lennert's lymphoma with a B-cell phenotype have been described (209). Clonal chromosome-5 abnormalities have also been described (210). Patients with Lennert's lymphoma present with disseminated lymph-node involvement, often tonsil (164) and bone-marrow (209) involvement. Cutaneous involvement is rare (209). Because no prospective anatomo-clinical study has yet been done, the prognosis of Lennert's lymphoma remains unsettled. In a recently reported clinical study (209), patients with Lennert's lymphoma have a median survival period of 20 months. Their response to anthracycline-containing polychemotherapy regimens seems rather poor. Lennert's lymphoma may transform into T-cell NHL of a more aggressive histological type (207).

Angioimmunoblastic-like T-cell NHL

Angioimmunoblastic lymphadenopathy (AIL) was initially described by Frizzera (211) and by Lukes under the heading of "immunoblastic lymphadenopathy" (212). The morphological characteristics are *(fig. 44)*:

- disappearance of the normal lymph node architecture with some residual follicles;

- a polymorphic lymphoid proliferation comprising small lymphocytes, plasma cells, immunoblasts, mixed with eosinophils and histiocytes; epithelioid cells may be present (213); and

- a vascular proliferation predominantly involving post-capillary venules which have a turgescent endothelium.

Patients with AIL have disseminated lymph node, liver and spleen enlargement, fever,

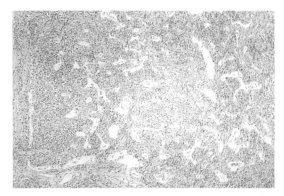

Fig. 44a

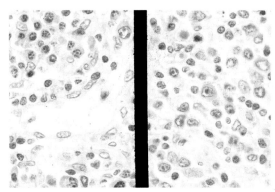

Fig. 44b

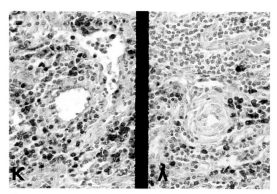

Fig. 44c

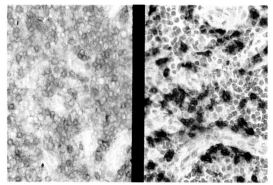

Fig. 44d

Fig. 44: **Angioimmunoblastic-like T-cell lymphoma.** Morphological aspects at low (44a) and high magnification (44b). Immunoperoxidase staining using polyclonal antibodies directed against kappa (44c, left) and lambda (44c, right) light-chain and monoclonal antibodies directed against CD4 (Leu 3, 44d left) and CD8 (Leu 2a, 44d right). B cells are polyclonal, expressing either kappa or lambda. Tumoral cells express CD4. Few reactive T cells express CD4 and CD8.

skin involvement, a polyclonal hypergammaglobulinaemia and a positive Coomb's test haemolytic anaemia.

Until recently, the nosology of AIL remained controversial (214). It has long been considered to be an initially non-malignant immune disorder. Despite a usually fatal course, several items of data now strongly suggest that most AIL cases are in fact T-cell NHL: (a) morphologically, clusters of large cells (164,190) or of intermediate-size lymphoid cells with a clear cytoplasm (158,164,215) may be seen; (b) immunohistochemical studies (158,191,216) have shown that T cells were predominant with a mixture of CD4+ and CD8+ T cells, although proliferating Ki- 67+ cells were mostly CD4+ T cells; (c) genotypic studies have revealed in most cases a clonal β or γ rearrangement (185,189,190,216), associated in some cases with a heavy chain gene rearrangement (191); and (d) clonal chromosome abnor-malities such as trisomy 3 or trisomy 5 have been found in some cases (217,218).

If morphological abnormalities suggestive of NHL are lacking, distinction from atypical T-cell hyperplasia, such as in those induced by drugs, may be difficult. In these cases, genotypic studies (158,190,191) or cytogenetic analysis (218) may be especially useful. In most cases, they suggest a malignant clonal proliferation. In rare cases, they are normal or suggest an oligoclonal disorder (218), sometimes fluctuating (219), and suggest a non-malignant immune disorder. These non-malignant immune-lymphoid disorders may nevertheless evolve towards an angioimmunoblastic-like malignant NHL (218,220). Whether these lymphoid disorders have to be treated from their presentation to prevent such an evolution remains unknown.

Between 10 and 25% of AILD cases transform into high-grade immunoblastic large-cell NHL (218,221). A selection of abnormal clones (222) and phenotypic changes may accompany such a transformation (220).

T-cell zone NHL

This subtype was initially described by Lennert (12) and Waldron (223) as a malignant NHL originating from T-cell zones and sparing B-cell follicles, at least at the initial stages of development (164) *(fig. 34)*. Its frequency is probably low. The proliferation consists of predominantly small lymphoid cells, with an irregular nucleus, mixed with rare cells of intermediate or large size. A diagnosis of malignancy may be difficult in cases with numerous hyperplastic reactive follicles. Atypical cells, an "abnormal" T-cell phenotype or a clonal Cß rearrangement may help in diagnosis. Although lymphoid cells include CD4+ and CD8+ T cells, most Ki-67+ proliferating cells are CD4+ (164). Most patients present with general symptoms. Pleural and/or pulmonary involvement seem unusually frequent (164,223).

Pleomorphic small T-cell NHL

Pleomorphic T-cell NHL form a heterogenous group of NHL with different histological patterns. In the updated Kiel classification (3), they include a low-grade small-cell NHL, and high-grade medium (98,100) and large-cell NHL (98). Whatever their size, tumour cells have an uneven and irregular nucleus surrounded by a clear cytoplasm.

Pleomorphic T-cell NHL may be observed in association with HTLV-1 (3). Pleomorphic T-cell NHL are post-thymic lymphomas (CD1-, CD2+, CD3+), usually CD4+ (99).

High-grade T-cell lymphomas

Pleomorphic medium and large T-cell NHL

These lymphomas are defined by a proliferation of medium and/or large cells, with irregular, sometimes convoluted or cerebriform, nuclei with abundant, clear, well-delineated cytoplasm (100).

Immunoblastic T-cell NHL

Immunoblastic NHL may have a B-cell or T-cell phenotype. B-cell immunoblastic NHL have been described above. Among immunoblastic NHL, the variants called clear-cell, polymorphic or with an epithelioid component often have a T-cell phenotype.

Their common feature is the prevalence of large cells with a clear, well-defined and abundant cytoplasm, a central nucleus containing a fine chromatin, and one or several small nucleoli. They are largely predominant in the clear-cell subtype *(fig. 45)*. In the polymorphic subtype, they are mixed with numerous small or intermediate-size cells. This latter subtype was created to include several T-cell NHL entities previously described by Japanese (99) and western groups, such as peripheral T-cell NHL, T-cell zone NHL, Pinkus multilobulated large-cell NHL, lymphoepithelioid NHL *(fig. 43)* (223,224). They differ from diffuse mixed NHL of the Japanese classification of NHL by the presence of multiple nuclear atypia of large cells resembling Reed-Sternberg cells and by considerable cell polymorphism (99).

Immunoblastic T-cell NHL have a post-thymic phenotype (CD1-, CD2+, CD3+) and are most often CD4+. Abnormal T-cell phenotypes are especially frequent in the

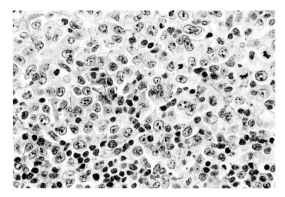

Fig. 45: **Immunoblastic T-cell lymphoma,** *clear-cell type.*

polymorphic subtype (100,120). Some rare immunoblastic large-cell NHL may express neither T- nor B-cell antigens. They may be true histiocytic lymphomas but there is at present no sensitive and specific marker for this subtype (225).

Lymphoblastic NHL

Lymphoblastic NHL originate from bone-marrow precursor cells. The cell characteristics are identical to those of acute lymphoblastic leukaemias. Their immunological characteristics are not identical: lymphoblastic NHL usually have a T-cell origin and their phenotype is more "mature" than that of acute lymphoblastic leukaemias (226,227).

Fig. 46: **Lymphoblastic lymphoma.** *Partial involvement of the paracortex, sparing lymphoid follicles.*

Clinical characteristics

Most lymphoblastic lymphomas occur in young males (sex-ratio of 2.5/1, median age of 30 yrs) (228). Most young patients present with a mediastinal tumour, often revealed by signs of compression and general symptoms (228-231). Bone-marrow involvement is found at presentation in 22 to 60% of cases (228,230,231). Liver and spleen enlargements are rare (232,233). In patients with blood involvement (11 to 40% of cases), there is no clinical, cytological or immunological criterion which allows distinction between lymphoblastic lymphomas and acute lymphoblastic leukaemias (228,230). Between 20 and 40% of patients have CNS involvement either at presentation or during the course of the disease (228-231).

Morphology

Lymph-node involvement is often partial in lymphoblastic lymphomas *(fig. 46)* (228). The proliferation has a diffuse architecture and consists of cells of intermediate size (15 to 20 µm). Their chromatin is fine, and nucleoli are absent or faint. The cytoplasm is rare and basophilic. Mitoses are numerous. Two cellular subtypes have been described: the convoluted type in which the nuclei of tumour cells are of varying size and shape, and, most often, a lobulated nucleus (fig.47). In the non-convoluted subtype, nuclei are regular, ovoid or round *(fig. 48).*

Immunological characteristics

Approximately 80% of lymphoblastic lymphomas have a T-cell phenotype (228,234). Tumour cells have either an early thymocyte phenotype CD1-, CD4-, CD8-, a common thymocyte phenotype CD1+, CD4+, CD8-, or a late thymocyte phenotype CD3+, CD4 or CD8+. In fact, diverse combinations of T-cell antigen expression are possible.

Other cases of lymphoblastic lymphomas either have a pre-B-cell phenotype with intracytoplasmic IgM or are called "common" since they express the common acute lymphoblastic leukaemia antigen CALLA CD10 *(fig. 49).* Most common lymphoblastic lymphomas have a "pre-pre-B" origin since they express some B-cell antigens

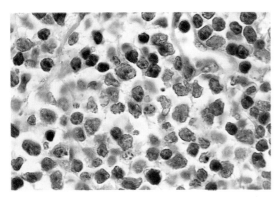

Fig. 47: **Lymphoblastic lymphoma,** convoluted type.

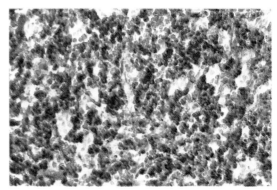

Fig. 49: **Lymphoblastic lymphoma.** Immunoperoxidase staining using monoclonal antibodies directed against CD10 (CALLA). Tumoral cells express CD10.

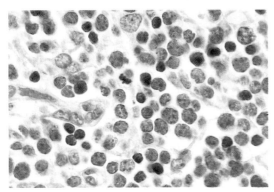

Fig. 48: **Lymphoblastic lymphoma,** non-convoluted type.

(most of them are CD19+ and 50% CD20+); they can be stimulated *in vitro* to produce immunoglobulins, and their immunoglobulin genes have rearranged (235). There is no relationship between the morphological aspects and the immunological phenotype: convoluted lymphoblastic lymphomas may have either a B-cell or a T-cell origin.

Angiocentric T-cell NHL

This group includes lymphomatoid granulomatosis (LG) as described by Lie-bow and polymorphic reticulosis (PR) or lethal midline granuloma, which have several morphological and evolutive characteristics in common (193) (*see pp. 231-239*). LG preferentially involves lungs and other extranodal organs (skin, kidneys, nasopharynx)

while PR affects the nasopharynx and palate. Lymph-node involvement can be seen and these angiocentric T lymphomas can present as pleomorphic peripheral T-cell NHL (236,238). Both disorders are characterized (fig.50) by an angiocentric and angiodestructive polymorphous proliferation, consisting of lymphocytes, plasma cells and histiocytes. The number of atypical and/or large cells varies from case to case. The venule and artery walls are progressively destroyed and this can lead to ischaemic necrosis. In several cases, evolution toward a monomorphous lymphoma has been described but LG and PR were initially considered as non-malignant granulomatous disorders. More recently, several immunohistochemical studies have shown the T-cell phenotype of the infiltrate, in most cases CD4+ and in some cases "abnormal" (192,193). Some genotypic studies have confirmed the clonal origin of T cells (192,193), a fact which justified the name of angiocentric T-cell NHL proposed by Jaffe.

Their cell characteristics and their prognosis are those of high-grade NHL (193). Their cure depends on obtaining complete remission by aggressive polychemotherapy (193).

There are important variations from case to case in the number of atypical lymphoid cells, and from lesion to lesion in the same patient. There is often a progressive increase in large cells, resulting in a large-cell NHL (192,193). There is a continuum of angiocentric lymphoid proliferations, from infiltrates containing very few atypical cells, which can be difficult to distinguish from Wegener's granulomatosis, to large-cell NHL. In the former cases, molecular biology is helpful if it shows a clonal rearrangement of T-receptor genes (192,193).

Anaplastic large-cell lymphoma (Ki-1+)

Anaplastic large-cell lymphomas (ALCL) have been recently recognized both on morphological criteria and on the expression of the Ki-1 (CD 30) antigen by tumour cells (239).

In 1982, Schwab et al. described a novel monoclonal antibody, Ki-1, prepared from a Hodgkin cell line (L 428) (240). The membrane-bound antigen - also called Ki-1 antigen or CD 30 - is a 120 kD glycoprotein, probably a phosphokinase (241,242). In the first studies, Ki-1 antibody appeared to react with Hodgkin and Reed-Sternberg cells in Hodgkin's disease and with a small population of large cells, preferentially located around B-cell follicles in reactive lymphoid tissue (243). Further, it was shown that Ki-1 antibody also binds to normal lymphoid cells activated *in vitro* by mitogens or allogenic cells (239,244), to virally transformed lymphocytes (239,244) and to macrophages derived *in vitro* from blood monocytes (245). Ki-1 antigen is also expressed by various permanent cell lines of lymphoid or histiocytic origin (239,244,245). Moreover, Ki-1 antigen is expressed by tumour cells in a subgroup of large-cell lymphomas with characteristic morphology, currently referred to as "Ki-1 lymphoma" (246,247).

Clinical studies

The frequency of Ki-1 lymphoma has not yet been assessed. It may represent 1 to 8% of all NHL (247, and French multicentre study of aggressive malignant lymphomas [GELA protocol]). In the first report on 45 cases, the median age was 41 years with 20% of the patients less than 20 years old (243). There were 29 males and 16

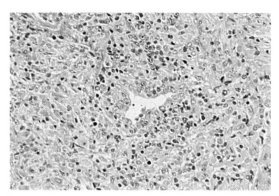

Fig. 50: **Angiocentric T-cell lymphoma.** *Angiocentric and angiodestructive polymorphous proliferation.*

females. In another series of patients with anaplastic large-cell lymphoma (most of them Ki-1-positive), 50% were less than 30 years old (246). Subsequently, several authors reported Ki-1 lymphomas in children (248,249).

There is no specific clinical presentation of Ki-1 lymphomas. Diagnosis was made on the basis of a lymph node biopsy in 89% of the cases reported by Stein et al. (243). Kadin et al. noticed that, in their paediatric population, peripheral lymphadenopathy and/or skin lesions were the most frequent clinical presentation (248,249). In fact, Ki-1 lymphoma may be encountered in any site and primary cutaneous anaplastic large-cell lymphoma has been described (250).

The prognosis of patients with Ki-1 lymphoma is controversial. In the updated Kiel classification for lymphomas (3), anaplastic large-cell lymphomas are included in the "high-grade" group. ALCL of the skin can be of good prognosis (250).

Pathological findings (239,246,251)

In the majority of cases the affected lymph nodes display a peculiar pattern of involvement. The neoplastic process partially infiltrates lymph-node tissue and is preferentially located in paracortical areas, sparing follicles *(fig. 51a)*. This infiltration is often associated with intrasinusoidal dissemination *(fig. 51b)*. Total destruction of the architecture can be observed.

The tumour cells *(fig. 52)* are large and pleomorphic. They have a large nucleus,

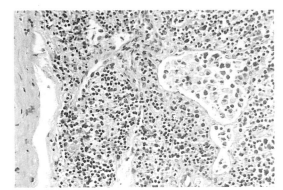

Fig. 51a

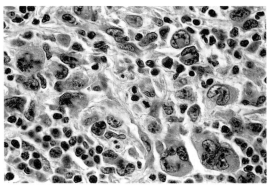

Fig. 52: **Anaplastic large-cell lymphoma.** *Pleomorphic lymphoid proliferation.*

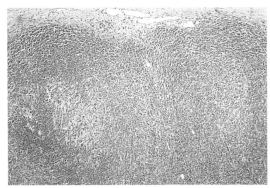

Fig. 51b

Fig. 51: **Anaplastic large-cell lymphoma** *or Ki-1 lymphoma: frequent tumoral infiltration of sinuses (51a) and paracortical involvement (51b).*

A histological subclassification of anaplastic large-cell lymphomas, based on cytological features, has recently been proposed (252).

These special histological features, associating preferential patterns of involvement (paracortical and sinusal infiltration) and pleomorphic large cells with possible erythrophagocytosis, explain why this tumour has raised important diagnostic difficulties. These ALCL were initially misdiagnosed and interpreted as malignant histiocytosis, metastatic carcinoma, or Hodgkin's disease of the lymphoid depletion type. Their lymphoid nature is now well-established using both immunohistochemical studies and genotypic analysis.

often irregular and multilobated, with one or more nucleoli, and clustered heterochromatin. Some cells are giant, multinucleated and may resemble Reed-Sternberg cells. The cytoplasm is large, sometimes vacuolated, and basophilic. Erythrophagocytosis in the tumour cells is a frequent and important feature *(fig. 53)*. Numerous mitoses and single-cell necrosis are common. However, in some cases, tumour cells are more monomorphous with round nuclei.

Stromal reaction is abundant, comprising numerous inflammatory cells associating small lymphocytes, plasma cells and eosinophils. Histiocytes are usually less frequent but can be very numerous. Fibrosis can be abundant with variable amounts of collagen fibres, both interstitial or in bands.

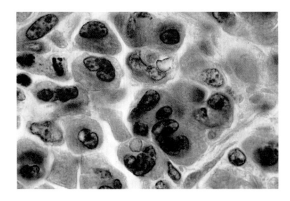

Fig. 53: **Anaplastic large-cell lymphoma.** *Pleomorphic tumoral cells and frequent erythrophagocytosis by tumoral cells.*

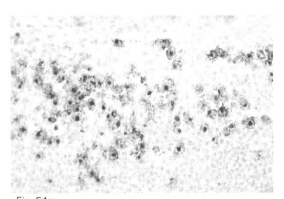

Fig. 54a:

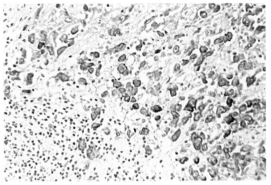

Fig. 54b

Fig. 54: **Anaplastic large-cell lymphoma**. Immunoperoxidase staining using monoclonal antibodies directed
against CD30. Ki-1 (fig. 54a, frozen section) a,d BerH2
(fig. 54b, paraffin section). Tumoral cells express CD30.

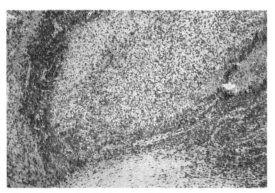

Fig. 55: **Anaplastic large-cell lymphoma**. Immunoperoxidase staining using monoclonal antibodies directed
against CD3 (Leu 4): tumoral cells are located in T zones
but do not express CD3.

Immunohistochemical studies (239, 246,
251) demonstrate a constant expression by
almost all tumour cells of the Ki-1 antigen
(CD 30) *(fig. 54)*. Most ALCLs commonly
express an abnormal T-cell phenotype (60%
to 80%) with no expression of one or more
pan-T antigens (such as CD 3) *(fig. 55)*.
The remaining cases express either B-cell-
related antigens (approximately 10%), both
B- and T-cell-related antigens, or are devoid
of B or T antigen ("null" phenotype).
Furthermore, most of them also express
activation-associated antigens such as CD
25 (Tac-p55 chain of the IL-2 receptor)
(fig. 56), Epithelial Membrane Antigen *(fig.
57)*, HLA-DR and transferrin receptor (CD
71). It has recently been hypothesised that
CD 25 expression may be involved in
tumour growth by a paracrine mechanism
considering the *in situ* production of IL-2 by
reactive T cells (253) *(fig. 58)*. Taken together,
these findings suggest that ALCL express-

ing the Ki-1 antigen are a neoplasm derived
from an activated lymphoid cell of either T
or B phenotype.

On paraffin sections, of diagnosis can be
performed using monoclonal antibodies
which bind to CD 45 antigen (leucocyte
common antigen) and CD 30 antigen (Ber-
H2) *(fig. 54b)* (254,255).

A translocation involving chromosome 5
(breakpoint of q35) and, in most cases,
chromosome 2 [t (2,5) (p23; q35)] has been
described as characteristic of Ki-1 lymphoma (256-261). This translocation had
been previously reported in several cases
considered as malignant histiocytosis (summarized in reference 259). These cases may

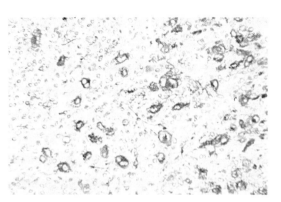

Fig. 56: **Anaplastic large-cell lymphoma**. Immunoperoxidase staining using monoclonal antibodies directed
against CD25: tumoral cells express the α chain of the
IL2 receptor.

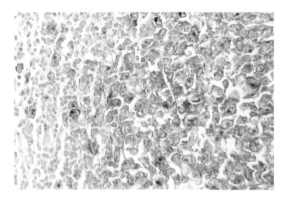

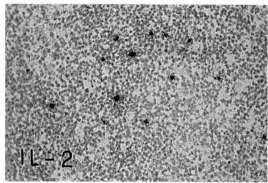

Fig. 57: **Anaplastic large-cell lymphoma**. *Immunoperoxidase staining on paraffin section using monoclonal antibodies directed against epithelial membrane antigen (EMA): tumoral cells express EMA.*

Fig. 58: **Anaplastic large-cell lymphoma**. *In situ hybridization using a specific IL2 RNA probe labelled with 35S: reactive T cells in close contact with tumour cells produce IL2 mRNA.*

be Ki-1 lymphomas. The breakpoint on chromosome 5 is located in the vicinity of c-fms proto-oncogene (5 q33 - q34) (260). Whether this oncogene is involved in Ki-1 lymphoma development remains to be seen.

Malignant histiocytosis was originally described as a neoplastic proliferation of cells of monocyte-macrophage origin (262). In fact, using immunohistochemistry and/or genotypic analysis, it has been shown that most - if not all - cases were of lymphoid origin. Several cases initially considered as malignant histiocytosis were in fact anaplastic large-cell lymphomas (246). It is now believed that if the histological characteristics suggest a diagnosis of malignant histiocytosis, it usually corresponds to either a malignant lymphoma or a virus-associated haemophagocytic syndrome (263).

TABLE I

Comparison of the Working Formulation for Clinical Usage with the Kiel Classification

Working Formulation		Kiel Classification
A.	Diffuse, small lymphocytic	Lymphocytic, CLL
B.	Follicular small cleaved cell	Centroblastic-centrocytic (small-cell) ± follicular ± diffuse
C.	Follicular mixed	
D.	Follicular large-cell	Centroblastic-centrocytic (large-cell), follicular ± diffuse
E.	Diffuse small cleaved cell	Centrocytic (small-cell)
F.	Diffuse mixed	Centroblastic-centrocytic diffuse Lymphoplasmacytic Lymphoplasmacytoid, polymorphic
G.	Diffuse large-cell	Centroblastic-centrocytic (large-cell), diffuse Centrocytic (large-cell) Centroblastic
H.	Large-cell, immunoblastic	Immunoblastic
I.	Lymphoblastic	Lymphoblastic
J.	Small non-cleaved cell	Lymphoblastic Burkitt-type or non-Burkitt-type

TABLE II

Correlation between histological and immunological phenotype

Histological type	Immunological phenotype	
	B	**T**
Small lymphocytic	95%	5%
Plasmacytoid	100%	
Follicular	100%	
Diffuse, small cleaved cell	100%	
Diffuse, mixed	40%	60%
Large-cell	90%	10%
Immunoblastic	60%	30%
Small non-cleaved cell:		
- Burkitt	100%	
- Non-Burkitt	85%	15%
Lymphoblastic	20%	80%

TABLE III

Differential diagnosis between lymphoid follicular hyperplasia and follicular lymphoma: morphological criteria

	Follicular hyperplasia	Follicular lymphoma
Architecture	**Preserved**	**Destroyed**
Follicles		
- size	variable	uniform
- shape	variable	often regular
- density	low	high
Germinal centers		
- mantle zone	visible	often absent
- polarization	usual	absent
- cytology	polymorphous	monomorphous
	numerous mitoses	few mitoses
	phagocytosis +++	no phagocytosis
Interfollicular areas		
- abundance	great	poor
- cytology	polymorphous	monomorphous when infiltrated
	with reactive cells	by tumour cells, or polymorphous
		with only reactive cells

TABLE IV

Differential diagnosis between lymphoid follicular hyperplasia and follicular lymphoma: immunohistochemical criteria

	Follicular hyperplasia	Follicular lymphoma
Follicles		
- follicular dendritic cell	regular network	often disrupted network
- extracellular binding with anti-Ig	present	absent
- mantle zone	polytypic μ+ δ+	often absent if present d+
- centre: B cell area	polytypic μ+ / δ-	monotypic m+ d+ sometimes g+
T cells	present	present (CD8 ↗ (?))
Interfollicular areas		
B cells	polytypic	sometimes monotypic
T cells	dispersed	around the periphery of follicles

TABLE V

Classification of extension in Burkitt's lymphoma (from Magrath)

Stade	Extension
A	Single extra-abdominal tumour
AR	Resected intra-abdominal tumour
B	Multiple extra-abdominal sites excluding bone narrow and CNS
C	Multiple and unresectable intra-abdominal tumours, with or without extra-abdominal tumour(s) excluding bone narrow and CNS
D	Bone narrow and/or CNS inoshemas

References

1. The non-Hodgkin's lymphoma pathologic classification project: National Cancer Institute sponsored study of classifications of non-Hodgkin's lymphomas.
   Summary and description of the Working Formulation for Clinical Usage.
   Cancer, 1982; 49: 2112-2135.

2. PORTLOCK CS
   Non-Hodgkin's lymphomas. Advances in diagnosis, staging, and management.
   Cancer, 1990; 65: 718-722.

3. STANSFELD AG, DIEBOLD J, KAPANCI Y et al.
   Updated Kiel classification for lymphomas.
   Lancet, 1988; 1: 292-293.

4. JAFFE ES, SHEVACH EM, FRANK MM, BERARD CW, GREEN I

Nodular lymphoma. Evidence for origin from follicular B lymphocytes.

N Engl J Med, 1974; 290: 813-819.

5. WARNKE RA, LEVY R

Immunopathology of follicular lymphomas. A model of B-lymphocyte homing.

N Engl J Med, 1974; 298: 481-486.

6. LUKES RJ, PARKER JW, TAYLOR CR, TINDLE BH, CRAMER AD, LINCOLN TL

Immunologic approach to non-Hodgkin's lymphomas and related leukemias. Analysis of the results of multiparameter studies of 425 cases.

Semin Hematol, 1978; 15: 322-351.

7. LUKES RJ, COLLINS RD

New approaches to the classification of the lymphomata.

Br J Cancer, 1975; 31 (suppl. 2): 1-28.

8. STRAUS DJ, FILIPPA DA, LIEBERMAN PH et al.

The non-Hodgkin's lymphomas. I. A retrospective clinical and pathologic analysis of 499 cases diagnosed between 1958 and 1969.

Cancer, 1983; 51: 101-113.

9. DABSKI K, BANKS PM, WINKELMANN RK

Clinicopathologic spectrum of cutaneous manifestations in systemic follicular lymphoma.

Cancer, 1989; 64: 1480-1485.

10. McCURLEY TL, GAY RE, GAY S et al.

The extracellular matrix in "sclerosing" follicular center cell lymphomas: an immunohistochemical and ultrastructural study.

Hum Pathol, 1988; 17: 930-937.

11 LENNERT K

Histopathologie des lymphomes malins non hodgkiniens.

Doin, Paris, 1981.

12. LENNERT K, MOHRI N, KAISERLING E et al.

Malignant lymphomas other than Hodgkin's disease.

In: Springer-Verlag, Berlin, Heidelberg, New York, 1978; p. 11.

13. METTER GG, NATHWANI BN, BURKE JS et al.

Morphological subclassification of follicular lymphoma: variability of diagnosis among hematopathologists, a collaborative study between the repository center and pathology panel for lymphoma clinical studies.

J Clin Oncol, 1985; 3: 25-34.

14. KAUFMAN AG, NATHWANI BN, PRESTON K

Subclassification of follicular lymphomas; computerized microscopy.

Hum Pathol, 1987; 18: 226-237.

15. MANN RB, BERARD CW

Criteria for the cytologic subclassification of follicular lymphomas: a proposed alternative method.

Hematol Oncol, 1983; 1: 187-192.

16. ELLISON DJ, NATHWANI BN, METTER GE et al.

Mitotic counts in follicular lymphomas.

Hum Pathol, 1987; 18: 502-509.

17. SCHULTZ HB, ERSBOLL J, HOUGAARD P

Prognostic significance of architectural patterns in non-Hodgkin's lymphomas.

Scand J Haematol, 1985; 35: 270-283.

18. EZDINLI EZ, COSTELLO W, LENHARD RE

Survival of nodular versus diffuse pattern in lymphocytic poorly differentiated lymphoma.

Cancer, 1978; 41: 1990-1996.

19. GLICK JH, McFADDEN E, COSTELLO W, EZDINLI EZ, BERARD CW, BENNETT JM

Nodular histiocytic lymphoma: factors influencing prognosis and implications for aggressive chemotherapy.

Cancer, 1982; 49: 840-845.

20. EZDINLI EZ, COSTELLO W, ICLI I et al.

Nodular mixed lymphocytic-histiocytic lymphoma (NM): response and survival.

Cancer, 1980; 45: 261-267.

21. WEST KP, POTTER LJ, HENDERSON SD, LAUDER I

A retrospective study of follicular lymphomas.

Histopathology, 1989; 14: 629-636.

22. NATHWANI BN, METTER GE, MILLER TP et al.

What should be the morphologic criteria for the subdivision of follicular lymphomas?

Blood, 1986; 68: 837-848.

23. HUBBARD SM, CHABNER BA, DE VITA VT et al.

Histologic progression in non-Hodgkin's lymphoma.

Blood, 1982; 59: 258-264.

24. QASI R, AISENBERG AC, LONG JC

The natural history of nodular lymphoma.

Cancer, 1976; 37: 1923-1927.

25. COIFFIER B, SEBBAN C, BERGER F et al.

Transformation histologique des syndromes lymphoprolifératifs de faible malignité. Etude clinique et évolutive de 32 cas.

Presse Méd 1985; 14: 1229-1236.

26. HARRIS NL, DATA RE

The distribution of neoplastic and normal B-lymphoid cells in nodular lymphomas: use of an immunoperoxidase technique on frozen sections.

Hum Pathol, 1982; 13: 610-617.

27. ANCELIN E, DELSOL G, MASON DY et al.

   In situ immunologic characterization of follicular lymphomas.

   Hematol Oncol, 1984; 2: 221-237.

28. SWERDLOW SH, MURRAY LJ, HABESHAW JA, STANSFELD AG

   B- and T-cell subsets in follicular centroblastic/centrocytic (cleaved follicular center cell) lymphoma: an immunohistologic analysis of 26 lymph nodes and three spleens.

   Hum Pathol, 1985; 16: 339-352.

29. STEIN H, GERDES J, MASON DY

   The normal and malignant germinal centre.

   Clin Haematol, 1982; 11: 531-559.

30. SCOAZEC JY, BERGER F, MAGAUD JP, BROCHIER J, COIFFIER B, BRYON PA

   The dendritic reticulum cell pattern in B cell lymphomas of the small cleaved, mixed- and large-cell types: an immunohistochemical study of 48 cases.

   Hum Pathol, 20: 124-131.

31. GLOGHINI A, COLOMBATTI A, BRESSAN G, CARBONE A

   Basement membrane components in lymphoid follicles: immunohistochemical demonstration and relationship to the follicular dendritic cell network.

   Hum Pathol, 1989; 20: 1001-1007.

32. RATECH H, LITWIN S

   Surface immunoglobulin light chain restriction in B-cell non-Hodgkin's malignant lymphomas.

   Am J Clin Pathol, 1989; 91: 583-586.

33. NGAN B, WARNKE A, CLEARY ML

   Variability of immunoglobulin expression in follicular lymphoma. An immunohistologic and molecular genetic study.

   Am J Pathol, 1989; 135: 1139-1144.

34. HENNI T, GAULARD P, DIVINE M et al.

   Comparison of genetic probe with immunophenotypic analysis in lymphoproliferative disorders: a study of 87 cases.

   Blood, 1988; 72: 1937-1944.

35. AISENBERG AC, WILKES BM, JACOBSON JO, HARRIS NL

   Immunoglobulin gene rearrangements in adult non-Hodgkin's lymphoma.

   N Engl J Med, 1987; 82: 738-744.

36. PAPADOPOULOS KP, BAGG A, BEZWODA WR, MENDELOW BV

   The routine diagnostic utility of immunoglobulin and T-cell receptor gene rearrangements in lymphoproliferative disorders.

   Am J Clin Pathol, 1989; 91: 633-638.

37. DVORETSKY P, WOOD GS, LEVY R, WARNKE RA

   T-lymphocyte subsets in follicular lymphomas compared with those in non-neoplastic lymph nodes and tonsils.

   Hum Pathol, 1982; 13: 618-625.

38. HARRIS NL, BHAN AK

   Distribution of T-cell subsets in follicular and diffuse lymphomas of B-cell type.

   Am J Pathol, 1983; 113: 172-180.

39. MILLER ML TUBBS RR, FISHLEDER AJ, SAVAGE RA, SEBEK BA, WEICK JK

   Immunoregulatory Leu-7+ and T8+ lymphocytes in B-cell follicular lymphomas.

   Hum Pathol, 1984; 15: 810-817.

40. STRICKLER JG, COPENHAUER CM, ROJAS VA, HORNING SJ, WARNKE RA

   Comparison of "host-cell infiltrates" in patients with follicular lymphoma with and without spontaneous regression.

   Am J Clin Pathol, 1988; 90: 257-261.

41. SWERDLOW SH, MURRAY LJ

   Natural killer cells (Leu-7+) cells in reactive lymphoid tissues and malignant lymphomas.

   Am J Clin Pathol, 1984; 81: 459-464.

42. GREIL R, GATTRINGER C, KNAPP W, HUBER H

   Growth fraction of tumour cells and infiltration density with natural killer-like (HNK 1+) cells in non-Hodgkin's lymphoma.

   Br J Haematol, 1986; 62: 293-300.

43. LAURENT G, AL SAATI T, OLIVE D et al.

   Expression of Tac antigen in B-cell neoplasms.

   Clin Exp Immunol, 1986; 65: 354-360.

44. SHEIBANI K, WINBERG CD, VAN DE VELDE S et al.

   Distribution of lymphocytes with interleukin-2 receptors (Tac antigens) in reactive lymphoproliferative processes, Hodgkin's disease, and non-Hodgkin's lymphoma. An immunohistologic study of 300 cases.

   Am J Pathol, 1987; 127: 27-38.

45. STRAUCHEN JA, BREAKSTONE BA

   IL-2 receptor expression in human lymphoid lesions. Immunohistochemical study of 166 cases.

   Am J Pathol, 1987; 126: 506-514.

46. PEUCHMAUR M, EMILIE D, CREVON MC, et al.

   IL-2 and interferon-gamma production in malignant follicular lymphomas.

   Am J Clin Pathol, 1991; 95: 55-62.

47. MEDEIROS LJ, STRICKLER JG, PICKER LJ et al.

   "Well-differentiated" lymphocytic neoplasms. Immunologic findings correlated with clinical presentation and morphologic features.

   Am J Pathol, 1987; 129: 523-535.

48. CHRISTENSON B, TRIBUKAIT B, LINDER I, ULLMAN B, BIBERFELD P

   Cell proliferation and DNA content in non-Hodgkin's lymphoma. Flow cytometry in relation to lymphoma classification.

   Cancer, 1986; 58: 1295-1302.

49. CIBULL ML, HERYET A, GATTER KC, MASON DY

The utility of Ki-67 immunostaining, nuclear organizer region counting, and morphology in the assessment of follicular lymphomas.

J Pathol, 1989; 158: 189-193.

50. NORTON AJ, ISAACSON PG

Lymphoma phenotyping in formalin-fixed and paraffin wax-embedded tissues. I. Range of antibodies and staining patterns.

Histopathology, 1989; 14: 437-446.

51. NORTON AJ, RIVAS C, ISAACSON G

A comparison between monoclonal antibody MT2 and immunoglobulin staining in the differential diagnosis of follicular lymphoid proliferations in routinely fixed wax-embedded biopsies.

Am J Pathol, 1989; 134: 63-70.

52. NGAN BY, CHEN-LEVY Z, WEISS LM et al.

Expression in non-Hodgkin's lymphoma of the bcl-2 protein associated with the t(14;18) chromosomal translocation.

N Engl J Med, 1988; 318: 1638-1646.

53. NATHWANI BN, WINBERG CD, DIAMOND LW, BEARMAN RM, KIM H

Morphologic criteria for the differentiation of follicular lymphoma from florid reactive follicular hyperplasia: a study of 80 cases.

Cancer, 1981; 48: 1794-1806.

54. CLEARY ML, SKLAR J

Nucleotide sequence of a t(14;18) chromosomal breakpoint in follicular lymphoma and demonstration of break-point cluster region near a transcriptionally active locus on chromosome 18.

Proc Natl Acad Sci USA, 1985; 82: 7439-7444.

55. WEISS LM, WARNKE RA, SKLAR J et al.

Molecular analysis of the t(14;18) chromosomal translocation in malignant lymphomas.

N Engl J Med, 1987; 317: 1185-1193.

56. YUNIS JJ, FRIZZERA G, OKEN MM et al.

Multiple recurrent genomic defects in follicular lymphoma: a possible model for cancer.

N Engl J Med, 1987; 316: 79-83.

57. WEISENBURGER DD, KIM H, RAPPAPORT H

Mantle-zone lymphoma. A follicular variant of intermediate lymphocytic lymphoma.

Cancer, 1982; 49: 1429-1438.

58. WEISENBURGER DD

Mantle-zone lymphoma. An immunohistologic study.

Cancer, 1984; 53: 1073-1080.

59. SAMOSZUK MK, EPSTEIN AL, SAID J, LUKES RJ, NATHWANI BN

Sensitivity and specificity of immunostaining in the diagnosis of mantle-zone lymphoma.

Am J Clin Pathol, 1986; 85: 557-563.

60. VAN DEN OORD JJ, DE WOLF-PEETERS C, PULFORD KAF, MASON DY, DESMET WJ

Mantle-zone lymphoma. Immuno and enzyme histochemical studies on the cell of origin.

Am J Surg Pathol, 1986; 10: 780-787.

61. POMPO DE OLIVEIRA MS, JAFFE ES, CATOVSKY D

Leukaemic phase of mantle zone (intermediate) lymphoma: its characterization in 11 cases.

J Clin Pathol, 1989; 42: 962-972.

62. ELLISON DJ, NATHWANI BN, CHO SY, MARTIN SE

Interfollicular small lymphocytic lymphoma: the diagnostic significance of pseudofollicles.

Hum Pathol, 1989; 20: 1108-1118.

63. KIM H, DORFMAN RF, RAPPAPORT H

Signet-ring cell lymphoma.

Am J Surg Pathol, 1978; 2: 557-563.

64. BENNETT MH

Sclerosis in non-Hodgkin's lymphomata.

Br J Cancer, 1975; 31 (supp. 1): 44-52.

65. ALBERTI A, NIEMAN RS

Lymphoplasmacytic lymphoma: a clinicopathologic study of a previously unrecognized composite variant.

Cancer, 1984; 53: 1103-1108.

66. LE TOURNEAU A, AUDOUIN J, CAPRON F, DIEBOLD J

Lymphomes malins folliculaires centroblastiques-centrocytiques associés à un lymphome malin lymphoplasmocytaire.

Ann Pathol, 1981; 1: 59-68.

67. PANGALIS GA, NATHWANI BN, RAPPAPORT H

Malignant lymphoma, well differentiated lymphocytic: its relationship with chronic lymphocytic leukemia and macroglobulinemia of Waldenström.

Cancer, 1977; 39: 999-1010.

68. DICK F, MACA R

The lymph node in chronic lymphocytic leukemia.

Cancer, 1978; 41: 283-292.

69. EVANS HL, BUTLER JJ, YOUNESS EL

Malignant lymphoma, small lymphocytic type.

Cancer, 1978; 41: 1440-1445.

70. LONG JC, AISENBERG AC

Richter's syndrome : a terminal complication of chronic lymphocytic leukemia with distinct clinicopathologic features.

Am J Clin Pathol, 1975; 63: 786-794.

71. HAROUSSEAU J, FLANDRIN G, BROUET JC, SELIGMANN M, BERNARD J

Malignant lymphoma supervening in chronic lymphocytic leukemia and related disorders.

Cancer, 1981; 48: 1302-1308.

72. NOWELL P, FINAN J, GLOVER D, GUERRY D

Cytogenetic evidence for the clonal nature of Richter's syndrome.

Blood, 1981; 58: 183-186.

73. VAN DONGEN JJM, HOOIJKAAS H, MICHIELS JJ et al.

Richter's syndrome with different immunoglobulin light chains and different heavy chain rearrangements.

Blood, 1984; 64: 571-575.

74. VAN DER REIJDEN HJ, VAN DER GAG R, PINKSTER J et al.

Chronic lymphocytic leukemia: immunologic markers and functional properties of the leukemic cells.

Cancer, 1982; 50: 2826-2833.

75. AISENBERG AC, WILKES BM

Monoclonal antibody studies in B-cell chronic lymphocytic leukemia and allied disorders.

Hematol Oncol, 1983; 1: 13-19.

76. STEIN H, LENNERT K, FELLER AC, MASON DY

Immunohistological analysis of human lymphoma. Correlation of histological and immunological categories.

Adv Cancer Res, 1984; 42: 67-147.

77. JOHNSTONE AP

Chronic lymphocytic leukaemia and its relationship to normal B lymphopoiesis.

Immunol Today, 1982; 3: 343-348.

78. TEFFERI A, LI CY, PHYLIKY RL

Correlation of clinical outcome with the degree of surface immunoglobulin (sIg) expression in B-cell chronic lymphocytic leukemia.

Am J Clin Pathol, 1989; 92: 82-85.

79. BURNS BF, WARNKE RA, DOGGETT RS, ROUSE RV

Expression of a T-cell antigen (Leu-1) by B-cell lymphomas.

Am J Pathol, 1983; 113: 165-171.

80. WORMSLEY SB, COLLINS ML, ROYSTON I

Comparative density of the human T-cell antigen T65 on normal peripheral blood cells and on chronic lymphocytic leukemia cells.

Blood, 1981; 57: 657-662.

81. CALIGARIS-CAPPIO F, GOBBI M, BOFILL M, JANOSSY G

Infrequent normal B lymphocytes express features of B-chronic lymphocytic leukemia.

J Exp Med, 1982; 155: 623,-628.

82. NADLER LM, ANDERSON KC, FISHER D, SLAUGHENHOUPT B, BOYD AW, SCHLOSSMAN SF

Immunologic classification of B-cell leukemias and lymphomas. UT M.D.

Anderson Clinical Conference on Cancer, 1984; 27: 225-239.

83. HARRIS NL, BHAN AK

B-cell neoplasms of the lymphocytic, lymphoplasmacytoid and plasma cell types: immunohistologic analysis and clinical correlation.

Hum Pathol, 1985; 16: 829-837.

84. VAN DER VALK P, JANSEN J, DAHA MR, MEIJER CJLM

Characterization of B-cell non-Hodgkin's lymphomas. A study using a panel of monoclonal and heterologous antibodies.

Virchows Arch (Pathol, Anat) 1983; 401: 289-305.

85. STEIN H, BONK A, TOLKSDORF G, LENNERT K, RODT H, GERDES J

Immunohistologic analysis of the organization of normal lymphoid tissue and non-Hodgkin's lymphomas.

J Histochem Cytochem 1980; 28: 746-760.

86. HABESHAW JA, BAILEY D, STANSFELD AG, GREAVES MF

The cellular content of non-Hodgkin's lymphomas: a comprehensive analysis using monoclonal antibodies and other surface marker techniques.

Br J Cancer, 1983; 47: 327-351.

87. NAIEM M, GERDES J, ABDULAZIZ Z, STEIN H, MASON DY

Production of a monoclonal antibody reactive with human dendritic reticulum cells and its use in the immunohistological analysis of lymphoid tissue.

J Clin Pathol, 1983; 36: 167-175.

88. COSSMAN J, NECKERS LM, HSU SM, LONGO D, JAFFE ES

Low-grade lymphomas: expression of developmentally regulated B-cell antigens.

Am J Pathol, 1984; 115: 117-124.

89. SWERDLOW SH, HABERSHAW JA, MURRAY LJ, DHALIWAL HS, LISTER TA, STANSFELD AG

Centrocytic lymphoma: a distinct clinicopathologic and immunologic entity. A multiparameter study of 18 cases at diagnosis and relapse.

Am J Pathol, 1983; 113: 181-197.

90. HARRIS NL, BHAN AK

Mantle zone lymphoma. A pattern produced by lymphomas of more than one cell type.

Am J Surg Pathol, 1985; 9: 872-881.

91 JENNETTE JC, REDDICK RL, SAUNDERS AW, WILKMAN AS

Diffuse T-cell lymphoma preceded by nodular lymphoma.

Am J Clin Pathol, 1982; 78: 242-248.

92. WEISENBURGER DD, NATHWANI BN, DIAMOND LW, WINDBERG CD, RAPPAPORT H

Malignant lymphoma, intermediate lymphocytic type: a clinicopathologic study of 42 cases.

Cancer, 1981; 48: 1415-1425.

93. WEISENBURGER DD, LINDER J, DALEY DJ, ARMITAGE JD
Intermediate lymphocytic lymphoma: an immuno-histologic study with comparison to other lymphocytic lymphomas.
Hum Pathol, 1987; 18: 787-795.

94. JAFFE ES, BOOKMAN MA, LONGO DL
Lymphocytic lymphoma of intermediate differentiation - mantle zone lymphoma: a distinct study of B-cell lymphoma.
Hum Pathol, 1987; 18: 877-890.

94a. LARDELLI P, BOOKMAN MA, SUNDEEN J, LONGO DL, JAFFE ES
Lymphocytic lymphoma of intermediate differentiation. Morphologic and immunophenotypic spectrum and clinical correlations.
Am J Surg Pathol, 1990; 14: 752-763.

95. STRICKLER JG, MEDEIROS LJ, COPENHAVER CM, WEISS LM, WARNKE RA
Intermediate lymphocytic lymphoma: an immunophenotypic study with comparison to small lymphocytic lymphoma and diffuse small cleaved cell lymphoma.
Hum Pathol, 1988; 19: 550-555.

96. NANBA K, JAFFE ES, BRAYLIN RC, OBAN EJ, BERARD CW
Alkaline-phosphatase-positive malignant lymphoma: a subtype of B-cell lymphomas.
Am J Clin Pathol, 1977; 68: 535-542.

97. SUCHI T, TAJMA K, NANBA K et al.
Some problems on the histopathological diagnosis of non-Hodgkin's malignant lymphoma: a proposal of a new type.
Acta Pathol, Jpn 1979; 29: 755-776.

98. WATANABE S
Pathology of peripheral T-cell lymphomas and leukemias.
Hematol Oncol, 1986; 4: 45.

99. SHIMOYAMA M, WATANABE S EDS
Symposium on T-cell malignancies.
Jpn J Clin Oncol, 1979; 9 (suppl. 1).

100. WEISS LM, CRABTREE GS, ROUSE RV ARNKE RA
Morphologic and immunologic characterization of 50 peripheral T-cell lymphomas.
Am J Pathol, 1985; 118: 316-324.

101. MASON DY, CORDELL J, BROWN M, PALLESEN G, RALFKIAER E, ROTHBARD J, CRUMPTON M, GATTER KC
Detection of T cells in paraffin wax-embedded tissue using antibodies against a peptide sequence from the CD3 antigen.
J Clin Pathol, 1989; 42: 1194-1200.

102. RAMSAY AD, SMITH WJ, ISAACSON PG
T-cell-rich B-cell lymphoma.
Am J Surg Pathol, 1988; 12: 433-439.

103. KATZIN WE, LINDEN MD, FISHLEDER AJ, TUBBS RR
Immunophenotypic and genotypic characterization of diffuse mixed non-Hodgkin's lymphomas.
Am J Pathol, 1989; 135: 615-621.

104. NG CS, CHAN JKC, HUI PK, LAU WH
Large B-cell lymphomas with a high content of reactive T cells.
Hum Pathol, 1989; 20: 1145-1154.

105. FOUCAR K, ARMITAGE JO, DICK FR
Malignant lymphoma, diffuse mixed small and large cell.
Cancer, 1983; 51: 2090-2099.

106. NATHWANI BN, METTER GE, GAMS RA et al.
Malignant lymphoma, mixed cell type, diffuse.
Blood, 1983; 62: 200-207.

107. ARMITAGE JO, DICK FR, PLATZ CE, CORDER MP, LEIMERT JT
Clinical usefulness and reproducibility of histologic subclassification of advanced diffuse histiocytic lymphoma.
Am J Med, 1979; 67: 929-934.

108. STRAUCHEN JA, YOUNG RC, DE VITA VT JR, ANDERSON T, FANTONE JC, BERARD CW
Clinical relevance of the histopathological subclassification of diffuse "histiocytic" lymphoma.
N Engl J Med, 1978; 299, 1382-1387.

109. COIFFIER B, BRYON PA, FRENCH M et al.
Intensive chemotherapy in aggressive lymphomas: updated results of LNH-80 protocol and prognostic factors affecting response and survival.
Blood, 1987; 70: 1394-1403.

110. COIFFIER B, LEPAGE E
Prognosis of aggressive lymphomas: a study of five prognostic models with patients included in the LNH-84 regimen.
Blood, 1989; 74: 558-564.

111. COIFFIER B, GISSELBRECHT C, HERBRECHT R, TILLY H, BOSLY A, BROUSSE N
LNH-84 regimen: a multicenter study of intensive chemotherapy in 737 patients with aggressive malignant lymphoma.
J Clin Oncol, 1989; 7: 1018-1026.

112. PINKUS GS, SAID JW, HARGREAVES H
Malignant lymphoma, T-cell type: a distinct morphologic variant with large multilobated nuclei, with a report of four cases.
Am J Clin Pathol, 1979; 72: 540-550.

113. HUI PK, FELLER AC, LENNERT K
High grade non-Hodgkin's lymphoma of B-cell type. I- Histopathology.
Histopathology, 1988; 12: 127-138.

114. WEISS RL, KJELDSBERG CR, COLBY TV, MARTY J

Multilobated B-cell lymphomas. A study of 7 cases.

Hematol Oncol, 1985; 3: 79-86.

115. ROSAS-URIBE A, RAPPAPORT H

Malignant lymphoma, histiocytic type with sclerosis (sclerosing reticulum cell sarcoma).

Cancer, 1972, 29: 946-953.

116. NEIMAN RS

Immunoblastic sarcoma.

Am J Surg Pathol, 1982; 6: 755-760.

117. SCHNEIDER DR, TAYLOR CR, PARKER JW, CRAMER AC, MEYER PR, LUKES RJ

Immunoblastic sarcoma of T- and B- cell types: morphologic description and comparison.

Hum Pathol, 1985; 16: 885-900.

118. WARNKE R, MILLER R, GROGAN T, PEDERSON M, DILLEY J, LEVY R

Immunologic phenotypes in 30 patients with diffuse large-cell lymphoma.

N Engl J Med, 1980; 303: 293-300.

119. DOGGETT RS, WOOD GS, HORNING S et al.

The immunologic characterization of 95 nodal and extranodal diffuse large-cell lymphomas in 89 patients.

Am J Pathol, 1984; 115: 245-252.

120. FREEDMAN AS, BOYD AW, ANDERSON KC et al.

Immunologic heterogeneity of diffuse large-cell lymphoma.

Blood, 1985; 65: 630-637.

121. JAFFE S, STRAUCHEN JA, BERARD CW

Predictibility of immunologic phenotype by morphologic criteria in diffuse aggressive non-Hodgkin's lymphomas.

Am J Clin Pathol, 1982; 77: 46-49.

122. MIRCHANDANI I, PALUTKE M, TABACZKA P, GOLDFARB S, EISENBERG L, PAK MSY

B-cell lymphomas morphologically resembling T-cell lymphomas.

Cancer, 1985; 56: 1578-1583.

123. SCHURMAN HJ, VAN BAARLEN J, HUPPES W et al.

Immunophenotyping of non-Hodgkin's lymphoma. Lack of correlation between immunophenotype and cell morphology.

Am J Pathol, 1987; 129: 140-152.

124. BOROWITZ MJ, BOUSVAROS A, BRYNES RK et al.

Monoclonal antibody phenotyping of B-cell non Hodgkin's lymphomas. The Southeastern Cancer Study Group experience.

Am J Clin Pathol, 1985; 121: 514-521.

125. ZIEGLER JL

Burkitt's lymphoma.

N Engl J Med, 1981; 305: 735-745.

126. MANN RB, JAFFE ES, BRAYLAN RC et al.

Non-endemic Burkitt's lymphoma. A B-cell tumor related to germinal centers.

N Engl J Med, 1976; 295: 685-691.

127. MURRAY LJ, HABESHAW JA, WIELS J, GREAVES MF

Expression of Burkitt lymphoma-associated antigen (defined by the monoclonal antibody 38.13) on both normal and malignant germinal-centre B cells.

Int J Cancer, 1985; 36: 561-565.

128. SHAM RL, PHATAK P, CARIGNAN J, JANAS J, OLSON JP

Progression of follicular large-cell lymphoma to Burkitt's lymphoma.

Cancer, 1989; 63: 700-702.

129. NKRUMAH FK, OLWENY CLM

Clinical features of Burkitt's lymphoma: the African experience.

In: Burkitt's lymphoma.

LENOIR G., O'CONNOR G., OLWENY C.L.M.

Eds. IARC Scientific Publications, Oxford Press, Oxford, 1985; p. 87-95.

130. OLWENY CLM, KATONGOLE-MBIDDE E, OTIM D, LWANGA SK, MAGRATH I, ZIEGLER JL

Long-term experience with Burkitt's lymphoma in Uganda.

Int J Cancer, 1980; 26: 261-266.

131. ZIEGLER JL, BLUMING AZ, MORROW RH, FASS L, CARBONE PP

Central nervous system involvement in Burkitt's lymphoma.

Blood, 1970, 36: 718-728.

132. ZIEGLER JL, BLUMING AZ, FASS L, MORROW RH

Relapse patterns in Burkitt's lymphoma.

Cancer Res, 1972, 32: 1267-1272.

133. ARSENEAU JC, CANELLOS GP, BANKS PM, BERARD CW, GRALNICK HR, DE VITA VT

American Burkitt's lymphoma: a clinicopathologic study of 30 cases. 1. Clinical factors relating to prolonged survival.

Am J Med, 1975; 58: 314-321.

134. PHILIP T

Burkitt's lymphoma in Europe.

In: Burkitt's lymphoma.

LENOIR G., O'CONNOR G., OLWENY C.L.M.

Eds. IARC Scientific Publications, Oxford Press, Oxford, 1985; p. 107-118.

135. MAGRATH IT, SARIBAN E

Clinical features of Burkitt's lymphoma in the USA.

In: Burkitt's lymphoma.

LENOIR G., O'CONNOR G., OLWENY C.L.M.

Eds. IARC Scientific Publications, Oxford Press, Oxford, 1985; p. 119-127.

136. SARIBAN E, EDWARDS B, JANUS C, MAGRATH I

Central nervous system involvement in American Burkitt's lymphoma.

J Clin Pathol, 1983; 1: 677-681.

137. COSSMAN J, JAFFE ES, FISHER RI

Immunologic phenotypes of diffuse, aggressive, non-Hodgkin's lymphomas. Correlation with clinical features.

Cancer, 1984; 54: 1310-1317.

138. CARBONE A, GLOGHINI A, PINTO A ATTADIA V, ZAGONEL V, VOLPE R

Monocytoid B-cell lymphoma with bone marrow and peripheral blood involvement at presentation.

Am J Clin Pathol, 1989; 92: 228-236.

139. SHEIBANI K, TRAWEEK T, BEN-EZRA J, et al.

Monocytoid B-cell lymphoma.

Am J Surg Pathol, 1989; 13: 902-904.

140. SHEIBANI K, SOHN CC, BURKE JJ et al.

Monocytoid B-cell lymphoma. A novel B-cell neoplasm.

Am J Pathol, 1986; 124: 310-317.

141. PIRIS MA, RIVAS C, MORENTE M et al.

Monocytoid B-cell lymphoma, a tumour related to the marginal zone.

Histopathology, 1988; 12: 383-390.

142. SHEIBANI K, BURKE JJ, SWARTZ WG et al.

Monocytoid B-cell lymphoma. Clinicopathologic study of 21 cases of a unique type of low-grade lymphoma.

Cancer, 1986; 62: 1531-1540.

143. BHAWAN J, WOLFF SM, UCCI AA, BHAN AK

Malignant lymphoma and malignant angioendotheliomatosis: one disease.

Cancer, 1985; 55: 570-576.

144. SHEIBANI K, BATTIFORA H, WINBERG CD, et al.

Further evidence that "malignant angioendotheliomatosis" is an angiotropic large-cell lymphoma.

N Engl J Med, 1986; 314: 943-948.

145. WICK MR, MILLS SE, SCHEITHAUER BW, COOPER PH, DAVITZ MA, PARKINSON K

Reassessment of malignant "angioendotheliomatosis". Evidence in favor of its reclassification as "intravascular lymphomatosis".

Am J Surg Pathol, 1986; 10: 112-123.

146. CARROLL TJ, SCHELPER R, GOEKEN JA, KEMP JD

Neoplastic angioendotheliomatosis: immunopathologic and morphologic evidence for intravascular malignant lymphomatosis.

Am J Clin Pathol, 1986; 85: 169-175.

147. DOMIZIO P, HALL PA, COTTER F, AMIEL S, TUCKER J, BESSER GM, LEVISON DA

Angiotropic large cell lymphoma (ALCL): morphological, immunohistochemical and genotypic studies with analysis of previous reports.

Hematol Oncol, 1989; 7: 195-206.

148. OTRAKJI CL, VOIGT W, AMADOR A, NADJI M, GREGORIOS JB

Malignant angioendotheliomatosis - a true lymphoma: a case of intravascular malignant lymphomatosis studied by Southern blot hybridization analysis.

Hum Pathol, 1988; 19: 475-478.

149. FERRY JA, HARRIS NL, PICKER LJ, WEINBERG DS, ROSALES RK, TAPIA J, RICHARDSON EP

Intravascular lymphomatosis (malignant angioendotheliomatosis). A B-cell neoplasm expressing surface homing receptors.

Modern Pathology, 1988; 1: 444-452.

150. D'AGATO V, SABLAY LB, KNOWLES DM, WALTER L

Angiotropic large cell lymphoma (intravascular malignant lymphomatosis) of the kidney: presentation as minimal change disease.

Hum Pathol, 1989; 20: 263-268.

151. YOUSEM SA, COLBY TV

Intravascular lymphomatosis presenting in the lung.

Cancer, 1990; 65: 349-353.

152. PIERARD GE, SOYEUR-BROUX M, FRIDMAN V, SADZOT B, DE LA BRASSINNE M, MOONEN G, BONIVER J

Lymphome angiotrope de type angioendothéliomatose proliférative systémique.

Ann Dermatol Venereol, 1988; 115: 333-336.

153. JAFFE ES

Pathologic and clinical spectrum of post-thymic T-cell malignancies.

Cancer Invest, 1984; 2: 413-435.

154. HORNING SJ, WEISS LM, CRABTREE GS, WARNKE RA

Clinical and phenotypic diversity of T-cell lymphomas.

Blood, 1986; 67: 1578-1587.

155. WEISENBURGER DD, LINDER J, ARMITTAGE JO

Peripheral T-cell lymphoma: a clinicopathologic study of 42 cases.

Hematol Oncol, 1987; 5: 175-189.

156. COIFFIER B, BERGER F, BRYON PA, MAGAUD JP

T-cell lymphomas: immunologic, histologic, clinical and therapeutic analysis of 63 cases.

J Clin Oncol, 1988; 6: 1584-1591.

157. KRAJEWSKI AS, MYSKOW MW, CACHIA PG et al.

T-cell lymphoma: morphology, immunophenotype and clinical features.

Histopathology, 1988; 13: 19-30.

158. TOBINAI K, MINATO K, OHTSU T et al.

Clinicopathologic, immunophenotypic and immunogenotypic analysis of immunoblastic lymphadenopathy-like T-cell lymphoma.

Blood, 1988; 72: 1000-1008.

159. WEISS JW, WINTER MW, PHYLIKY RL, BANKS PM

Peripheral T-cell lymphomas: histologic, immunohistologic and clinical characterization.

Mayo Clin Proc 1986; 61: 411-417.

160. GHERARDI R, GAULARD P, PROST C et al.

T-cell lymphoma revealed by a peripheral neuropathy. A report of two cases with an immunohistologic study on lymph node and nerve biopsies.

Cancer, 1986; 58: 2710-2720.

161. HANSON CA, BRUNNING RD, GAJL-PECZALSKA KJ et al.

Bone marrow manifestations of peripheral T-cell lymphoma. A study of 30 cases.

Am J Clin Pathol, 1986; 86: 449-456.

162. WHITE DM, SMITH AG, WHITEHOUSE JMA, SMITH JL

Peripheral T-cell lymphoma: value of bone marrow trephine immunophenotyping.

J Clin Pathol, 1989; 42: 403-408.

163. GAULARD P, ZAFRANI ES, MAVIER P et al.

Peripheral T-cell lymphoma presenting as predominant liver disease: a report of three cases.

Hepatology 1986; 6: 864-867.

164. SUCHI T, LENNERT K, TU LY et al.

Histopathology and immunohistochemistry of peripheral T-cell lymphomas: a proposal for their classification.

J Clin Pathol, 1987; 40: 995-1001.

165. PICKER LJ, WEISS LM, MEDEIROS LJ et al.

Immunophenotypic criteria for the diagnosis of non-Hodgkin's lymphoma.

Am J Med, 1987; 82: 738-746.

166. GROGAN TM, FIELDER K, RANGEL C et al.

Peripheral T-cell lymphoma: aggressive disease with heterogeneous immunotypes.

Am J Clin Pathol, 1985; 83: 279-288.

167. HOLLEMA H, POPPEMA S

T-lymphoblastic and peripheral T-cell lymphomas in the Northern part of the Netherlands.

Cancer, 1989; 64: 1620-1628.

168. PICKER LJ, WEISS LM, MEDEIROS LJ, WOOD GS, WARNKE RA

Immunophenotypic criteria for the diagnosis of non-Hodgkin's lymphoma.

Am J Pathol, 1987; 128: 181-201.

169. HASTRUP N, RALFKIAER E, PALLESEN G

Aberrant phenotypes in peripheral T-cell lymphomas.

J Clin Pathol, 1989; 42: 398-402.

170. PICKER LJ, BRENNER MB, WEISS LM et al.

Discordant expression of CD3 and T-cell receptor beta-chain antigens in T-lineage lymphomas.

Am J Pathol, 1987; 129: 434-441.

171. NG CS, CHAN JK, HUI PK et al.

Application of a T-cell receptor antibody beta F1 for immunophenotypic analysis of malignant lymphomas.

Am J Pathol, 1988; 132: 365-373.

172. KRAJEWSKI AS, MYSKOW MW, SALTER DM, CUNNINGHAM DS, RAMAGE EF

Diagnosis of T-cell lymphoma using beta F1, anti-T-cell receptor beta chain antibody.

Histopathology, 1989; 15: 239-247.

173. SU IJ, BALK SP, KADIN ME

Molecular basis for the aberrant expression of T-cell antigens in post-thymic T-cell malignancies.

Am J Pathol, 1988; 132: 192-201.

174. PICKER L, BRENNER M, MICHIE S, WARNKE R

Expression of T-cell receptor delta chains in benign and malignant T-lineage lymphoproliferations.

Am J Pathol, 1988; 132: 401-409.

175. NG CS, CHAN JK, LO ST

Expression of natural killer cell markers in non-Hodgkin's lymphomas.

Hum Pathol, 1987; 18: 1257-1263.

176. MEDEIROS LJ, WEISS LM, PICKER LJ, CLAYBERGER C, HORNING SJ, KRENSKY AM, WARNKE RA

Expression of LFA-1 in non-Hodgkin's lymphoma.

Cancer, 1989; 63: 255-259.

177. O'CONNOR NTJ, WEATHERALL DJ, FELLER AC et al.

Rearrangement of the T-cell receptor beta chain gene in the diagnosis of lymphoproliferative disorders.

Lancet 1985; 1: 1295-1299.

178. BERTNESS V, KIRSCH I, HOUIS G, JOHNSON B, BUNN PA JR

T-cell receptor gene rearrangements as clinical markers of human T-cell lymphomas.

N Engl J Med, 1985; 313: 534-540.

179. FLUG F, PELICCI PG, BONETTI F, DALLA-FAVERA R

T-cell receptor gene rearrangements as markers of lineage and clonality in T-cell neoplasms.

Proc Natl Acad Sci USA, 1985; 82: 7439-7445.

180. GRIESSER H, FELLER A, LENNERT K, MINDEN M, TAK W MAK

Rearrangement of the beta chain of T-cell antigen receptor and immunoglobulin genes in lymphoproliferative disorders.

J Clin Invest, 1986; 78: 1179-1188.

181. WILLIAMS ME, INNES DJ, BOROWITZ MJ et al.

Immunoglobulin and T-cell receptor gene rearrangements in human lymphoma and leukemia.

Blood, 1987; 69: 79-86.

182. O'CONNOR N1 J

Genotypic analysis of lymph node biopsies.

J Pathol, 1987; 151: 185-189.

183. KNOWLES DM

The human T-cell leukemias: clinical, cytomorphologic, immunophenotypic and genotypic characteristics.

Hum Pathol, 1986; 17: 14-19.

184. KNOWLES DM

Immunophenotypic and antigen receptor gene rearrangement analysis in T-cell neoplasia.

Am J Pathol, 1989; 134: 761-771

185. GRIESSER H, FELLER A, LENNERT K et al.

The structure of the T-cell gamma chain gene in lymphoproliferative disorders and lymphoma cell lines.

Blood, 1986; 68: 592-600.

186. TKACHUK D, GRIESSER H, TAKIHARA Y et al.

Rearrangement of T-cell δ locus in lymphoproliferative disorders.

Blood, 1988; 72: 353-359.

187. WEISS LM, PICKER LJ GROGAN TM et al.

Absence of clonal beta and gamma T-cell receptor gene rearrangements in a subset of peripheral T-cell lymphomas.

Am J Pathol, 1988; 130: 436-444.

188. O'CONNOR NT, GATTER KC, WAINSCOAT JS et al.

Practical value of genotypic analysis for diagnosing lymphoproliferative disorders.

J Clin Pathol, 1987; 40: 147-159.

189. O'CONNOR NTJ, CIRCK JA, WAINSCOAT JS, GATTER KC, STEIN H, FALINI B, MASON DY

Evidence for monoclonal T-lymphocyte proliferation in angioimmunoblastic lymphadenopathy.

J Clin Pathol, 1986; 39: 1229-1237.

190. WEISS LM, STRICKLER JG, DORFMANN RF, HORNING SJ, WARNKE RA, SKLAR J

Clonal T-cell populations in angioimmunoblastic lymphadenopathy and angioimmunoblastic lymphadenopathy-like lymphoma.

Am J Pathol, 1986; 122: 392-401.

191. FELLER A, GRIESSER H

Clonal gene rearrangement patterns correlate with immunophenotype and clinical parameters in patients with AILD.

Am J Pathol, 1988; 133: 549-560.

192. GAULARD P, HENNI T, MAROLLEAU JP et al.

Lethal midline granuloma (polymorphic reticulosis) and lymphomatoid granulomatosis: evidence for a monoclonal T-cell lymphoproliferative disorder.

Cancer, 1988; 62: 49-65.

193. LIPFORD EH, MARGOLICK JB, LONGO DL et al.

Angiocentric immunoproliferative lesions: a clinicopathologic spectrum of post-thymic T-cell proliferations.

Blood, 1988; 72: 1674-1680.

194. VAN HEERDE P, FELTKAMP CA, HART AAM, SOMERS R

Malignant histiocytosis and related tumors. A clinicopathologic study of 42 cases using cytological, histochemical and ultrastructural parameters.

Hematol Oncol, 1984; 2: 13-32.

195 WEISS LM, WOOD GS, TRELA M, WARNKE RA, SKLAR J

Clonal T-cell populations in lymphomatoid papulosis: evidence of a lymphoproliferative origin for a clinically benign disease.

N Engl J Med, 1986; 315: 475-479.

196 PELICCI PG, KNOWLES D, DALLA FAVERA G

Lymphoid tumors displaying rearrangements of both immunoglobulin and T-cell receptor genes.

J Exp Med, 1985; 162: 1015-1026.

197. SHEIBANI K, WU A, BEN-EZRA J et al.

Rearrangement of K-chain and T-cell receptor beta chain genes in malignant lymphomas of "T-cell" phenotype.

Am J Pathol, 1987; 129: 201-207.

198. DENNY CT, YOSHIKAI Y, MAK TW et al.

A chromosome 14 inversion is caused by site-specific recombination between immunoglobulin and T-cell receptor loci.

Nature, 1986; 320: 549-551.

199. LARSEN CJ, MATHIEU-MAHUL D, CAUBET JF et al.

    La translocation t(8;14) des leucémies et lymphomes T: un équivalent du modèle du lymphome de Burkitt.

    Med Sci, 1986; 2: 295-299.

200. CLARK JR, WILLIAMS ME, SWERDLOW SH

    Detection of B- and T-cells in paraffin-embedded tissue sections. Diagnostic utility of commercially obtained 4KB5 and UCHL-1.

    Am J Clin Pathol, 1990; 93: 58-69.

201. BROUET JC, FLANDRIN G SASPORTES AM, PREUD'HOMME JL, SELIGMANN M

    Chronic lymphocytic leukaemia of T-cell origin: immunological and clinical evaluation in eleven patients.

    Lancet, 1975; 2: 890-893.

202. COSTELLO C, CATOVSKY D, O'BRIEN M, MORILLA R, VARADI S

    Chronic T-cell leukaemias. I: Morphology, cytochemistry and ultrastructure.

    Leuk Res, 1980; 4: 463-476.

203. HUHN D, THIEL E, RODT H, SCHLIMOK G, THEML H, RIEBER P

    Subtypes of T-cell chronic lymphatic leukemia

    Cancer, 1983; 51: 1434-1447.

204 KIM H, NATHWANI BN, RAPPAPORT H

    So-called "Lennert's lymphoma". Is it a clinicopathologic entity?

    Cancer, 1980; 45: 1379-1399.

205. BEDETTI CD, OLLAPALLY E

    Malignant lymphoma with a high content of epithelioid histiocytes (so-called Lennert's lymphoma). Immunocytochemical and ultrastructural observations.

    Virchows Arch (Pathol Anat) 1983; 399: 255-264.

206. PATSOURIS E, NOEL H, LENNERT K

    Histological and immunohistological findings in lymphoepithelioid cell lymphoma (Lennert's lymphoma).

    Am J Surg Pathol, 1988; 12: 341-350.

207. FELLER AU, URIESSER GH, MAK TM et al.

    Lymphoepithelioid lymphoma (Lennert's lymphoma) is a monoclonal proliferation of helper inducer T-cells.

    Blood, 1986; 68: 663-670.

208. O'CONNOR NTJ, FELLER AC, WAINSCOAT JJ et al.

    T-cell origin of Lennert's lymphoma.

    Br J Haematol 1986; 64: 521-527.

209. SPIER CM, LIPPMAN SM, MILLER TP, GROGAN TM

    Lennert's lymphoma. A clinicopathologic study with emphasis on phenotype and its relationship to survival.

    Cancer, 1988; 61: 517-525.

210. GODDE-SALZ E, FELLER AC, LENNERT K

    Cytogenetic and immunohistochemical analysis of lympho-epithelioid cell lymphoma (Lennert's lymphoma): further substantiation of its T-cell nature.

    Leuk Res, 1985; 10: 313-321.

211. FRIZZERA G MORAN EM, RAPPAPORT H

    Angio-immunoblastic lymphadenopathy with dysproteinemia.

    Lancet 1974; 1: 1070-1073.

212. LUKES RJ, TINDLE BH

    Immunoblastic lymphadenopathy. A hyper immune entity resembling Hodgkin's disease.

    N Engl J Med, 1975; 292: 1-8.

213. PATSOURIS E, NOEL H, LENNERT K

    Angioimmunoblastic lymphadenopathy-type of T-cell lymphoma with a high content of epithelioid cells.

    Am J Surg Pathol, 1989; 13: 262-275.

214. WATANABE S, SATO Y, SHIMOYAMA M, MINATO K, SHIMOSATO Y

    Immunoblastic lymphadenopathy, angioimmunoblastic lymphadenopathy and IBL-like T-cell lymphoma. A spectrum of T-cell neoplasia.

    Cancer, 1986; 58: 2224-2233.

215. AOZASA K, OHSAWA M, FUJITA M et al.

    Angioimmunoblastic lymphadenopathy. Review of 44 patients with emphasis on prognostic behavior.

    Cancer, 1989; 63: 1625-1629.

216. NAMIKAWA R, SUCHI T, UEDA R et al.

    Phenotyping of proliferating lymphocytes in angioimmunoblastic lymphadenopathy and related lesions by the double immunoenzymatic staining technique.

    Am J Pathol, 1987; 127: 279-287.

217. GODDE-SALZ E, FELLER AC, LENNERT K

    Chromosomal abnormalities in lymphogranulomatosis X (LgrX)/ angioimmunoblastic lymphadenopathy (AILD).

    Leuk Res, 1987; 11: 181-191.

218. KANEKO Y, MASEKI N, SAKURAI M et al.

    Characteristic karyotypic pattern in T-cell lymphoproliferative disorders with reactive "angioimmunoblastic lymphoadenopathy with dysproteinemia type" features.

    Blood, 1988; 72: 413-420.

219. LIPFORD E, SMITH H, PITTALUGA S et al.

    Clonality of angioimmunoblastic lymphadenopathy and implications for its evolution to malignant lymphoma.

    J Clin Invest 1987; 79: 637-644.

220. WINSBERG CD, SHEIBANI K, KRANCE R, RAPPAPORT H

    Peripheral T-cell lymphoma: immunologic and cell-kinetic observations associated with morphological progression.

    Blood, 1985; 66: 980-990.

221. LIPPMAN SM, MILLER TP, SPIER CM et al.

The prognostic significance of the immunophenotype in diffuse large-cell lymphoma: a comparative study of T-cell and B-cell phenotype.

Blood, 1988; 72: 436-444.

222. NATHWANI BN, RAPPAPORT H, MORAN EM, PANGALIS GA, KIM H

Malignant lymphoma arising in angioimmunoblastic lymphadenopathy.

Cancer, 1978; 41: 578-606.

223. WALDRON JA, LEECH JH, GLICK AD, FLEXNER JM, COLLINS RD

Malignant lymphoma of peripheral T-lymphocyte origin: immunologic, pathologic and clinical features in six patients.

Cancer, 1977; 40: 1604-1617.

224. KADIN ME, BERARD CW, NANBA K, WAKASA H

Lymphoproliferative diseases in Japan and Western Countries: proceedings of the United States-Japan Seminar.

Hum Pathol, 1983; 14: 745-772.

225. ISAACSON PG

Histiocytic malignancy.

Histopathology, 1985; 9: 1007-1011.

226. COSSMAN J, CHUSED TM, FISHER RI, MAGRATH I, BOLLUM F, JAFFE ES

Diversity of immunological phenotypes of lymphoblastic lymphoma.

Cancer Res, 1983; 43: 4486-4490.

227. BERNARD A, BOUMSELL L, REINHERZ EL et al.

Cell surface characterization of malignant T cells from lymphoblastic lymphoma using monoclonal antibodies: evidence for phenotypic differences between malignant T cells from patients with acute lymphoblastic leukemia and lymphoblastic lymphoma.

Blood, 1981; 57: 1105-1110.

228. WEISS LM, BINDL JM, PICOZZI VJ, LINK MP, WARNKE RA

Lymphoblastic lymphoma: an immunophenotype study of 26 cases with comparison to T cell acute lymphoblastic leukemia.

Blood, 1986; 67: 474-478.

229. NATHWANI BN, DIAMOND LW, WINBERG CO et al.

Lymphoblastic lymphoma: a clinicopathologic study of 95 patients.

Cancer, 1981; 48: 2347-2357.

230. LEVINE AM, MEYER PR, LUKES RJ, FEINSTEIN DI

T cell convoluted/lymphoblastic undifferentiated lymphoma in adults.

In: U.T.M.D. Anderson Clinical Conference on Cancer. Vol. XXVII FORD R.J., p.327-332.

231. ROSEN PJ, FEINSTEIN DI, PATTENGALE PK et al.

Convoluted lymphocytic lymphoma in adults: a clinicopathologic entity.

Ann Intern Med, 1978; 89: 319-324.

232. STREULI R, KANEKO Y, VARIAKOJIS D et al.

Lymphoblastic lymphoma in adults.

Cancer, 1981; 47: 2510-2516.

233. SLATER DE, MERTELSMANN R, KOZINER B et al.

Lymphoblastic lymphoma in adults.

J Clin Oncol, 1986; 4: 57-67.

234. STEIN H, PETERSEN N, GAEDICKE G, LENNERT K, LANDBECK G

Lymphoblastic lymphoma of convoluted or acid phosphatase type: a tumor of T-precursor cells.

Int J Cancer, 1976; 17: 292-295.

235. AISENBERG AC, WILKES BM

The genotype and phenotype of T-cell and non-T, non-B acute lymphoblastic leukemia.

Blood, 1985; 66: 1215-1218.

236. DONNER LR, DOBIN S, HARRINGTON D, BASSION S, RAPPAPORT ES, PETERSON RF

Angiocentric immunoproliferative lesion (lymphomatoid granulomatosis). A cytogenetic, immunophenotypic, and genotypic study.

Cancer, 1990; 65: 249-254.

237. TROUSSARD X, GALATEAU F, GAULARD P et al.

Lymphomatoid granulomatosis in a patient with acute myeloblastic leukemia in remission.

Cancer, 1990; 65: 107-111.

238. CHOTT A, RAPPERSBERGER K, SCHLOSSAREK W, RADASZKIEWICZ T

Peripheral T-cell lymphoma presenting primarily as lethal midline granuloma.

Hum Pathol, 1988; 19: 1093-1101.

239. STEIN H, MASON DY, GERDES J et al.

The expression of the Hodgkin's disease-associated antigen Ki-1 in reactive and neoplastic lymphoid tissue: evidence that Reed-Sternberg cells and histiocytic malignancies are derived from activated lymphoid cells.

Blood, 1985; 66: 848-858.

240. SCHWAB U, STEIN H, GERDES J et al.

Production of a monoclonal antibody specific for Hodgkin and Sternberg-Reed cells of Hodgkin's disease and a subset of normal lymphoid cells.

Nature 1982; 299: 65-67.

241. FROSE P, LEMKE H, GERDES J, HAVSTEEN B, SCHWARTING R, HANSEN H, STEIN H

Biochemical characterization and biosynthesis of the Ki-1 antigen in Hodgkin-derived and virus-transformed human B- and T cell lines.

J Immunol 1987; 139: 2081-2087.

242. NAWROCKI JF, KIRSTEN ES, FISHER RI

Biochemical and structural properties of a Hodgkin's disease related membrane protein.

J Immunol, 1988; 141: 672-680.

243. STEIN H, GERDES J, SCHWAB U et al.

Identification of Hodgkin and Sternberg-Reed cells as a unique cell type derived from a newly-detected small-cell population.

Int J Cancer, 1982; 30: 445-459.

244. ANDREESEN R, OSTERHOLZ J, LOHR GW, BROSS KJ

A Hodgkin cell-specific antigen is expressed on a subset of auto- and alloactivated T (Helper) lymphoblasts.

Blood, 1984; 63: 1299-1302.

245. ANDREESEN R, BRUGGER W, LOHR GW, BROSS KJ

Human macrophages can express the Hodgkin's cell-associated antigen Ki-1 (CD30).

Am J Pathol, 1989; 134: 187-192.

246. DELSOL G, ALSAATI T, GATTER KC et al.

Coexpression of Epithelial Membrane Antigen (EMA), Ki-1 and Interleukin-2 receptor by anaplastic large cell lymphomas. Diagnostic value in so-called malignant histiocytosis.

Am J Pathol, 1988; 130: 59-70.

247. CARBONE A, GLOGHINI A, DE RE V, TAMARO P, BOIOCCHI M, VOLPE R

Histopathologic, immunophenotypic, and genotypic analysis of Ki-1 anaplastic large cell lymphomas that express histiocyte-associated antigens.

Cancer, 1990; 66: 2547-2556.

248. KADIN ME, SAKO D, BERLINER et al.

Chilhood Ki-1 lymphoma presenting with skin lesions and peripheral lymphadenopathy.

Blood, 1986; 68: 1042-1049.

249. SCHNITZER B, ROTH MS, HYDER DM, GINSBURG D

Ki-1 lymphomas in children.

Cancer, 1988; 61: 1213-1221.

250. KAUDEWITZ P, STEIN H, DALLENBACH F, ECKERT F, BIEBER K, BURG G, BRAUN-FALCO O

Primary and secondary cutaneous Ki-1+ (CD30) anaplastic large cell lymphomas.

Am J Pathol, 1989; 135: 359-367.

251. AGNARSSON BA, KADIN ME

Ki-1 positive large cell lymphoma. A morphologic and immunologic study of 19 cases.

Am J Surg Pathol, 1988; 12: 264-274.

252. CHAN JKC, NG CS, HUI PK, LEUNG TW, LO SF, LAU WH, Mc GUIRE LJ

Anaplastic large cell Ki-1 lymphoma. Delineation of 2 morphological types.

Histopathology, 1989; 15: 11-34.

253. PEUCHMAUR M, EMILIE D, CREVON MC, et al.

IL-2 m RNA expression in Tac-positive malignant lymphomas.

Am J Pathol, 1990; 136: 383-390.

254. HALL PA, D'ARDENNE AJ, STANSFELD AG

Paraffin section immunochemistry. II. Hodgkin's disease and large-cell anaplastic (Ki-1) lymphoma.

Histopathology, 1987; 13: 161-169.

255. SCHWARTING R, GERDES J, FALINI B, PILERI S, STEIN H

BER-H2: a new anti-Ki-1 (CD30) monoclonal antibody directed at a formol-resistant epitope.

Blood, 1989; 74: 1678-1689.

256. RIMOKH R, MAGAUD JP, BERGER R et al.

A translocation involving a specific breakpoint (q35) on chromosome 5 characteristic of anaplastic large-cell lymphoma ("Ki-1 lymphoma").

Br J Haematol 1989; 71: 31-36.

257. FICHER P, NACHEVA E, MASON DY et al.

A Ki-1 (CD30)-positive human cell line (Karpas 299) established from a high-grade non-Hodgkin's lymphoma showing a 2;5 translocation and rearrangement of the T-cell receptor -chain gene.

Blood, 1988; 72: 234-240.

258. KANEKO Y, FRIZZERA G, EDAMURA S et al.

A novel translocation, t (2;5) (p23 ; q35) in childhood phagocytic large T-cell lymphoma mimicking malignant histiocytosis.

Blood, 1989; 73: 806-813.

259. BENZ-LEMOINE E, BRIZARD A, HURET JL, et al.

Malignant histiocytosis: a specific t (2;5) (p23 ; q35).

Blood, 1988; 72: 1045-1047.

260. GROFFEN J, HEISTERKAMP N, SPURR N, DANA S, WASMUTH JJ, STEPHENSON JR

Chromosomal localization of the human c-fms oncogene.

Nucleic Acid Res, 1983; 11: 6331-6335.

261. BITTER MA, FRANKLIN WA, LARSON RA et al.

Morphology in Ki-1 (CD30)-positive non-Hodgkin's lymphoma is correlated with clinical feature and the presence of a unique chromosomal abnormality, t(2;5)(p23;q35).

Am J Surg Pathol, 1990; 14: 305-316.

262. WARNKE RA, KIM H, DORFMAN RF

Malignant histiocytosis (histiocytic medullary reticulosis). I. Clinicopathologic study of 29 cases.

Cancer, 1975; 35; 215-230.

263. RISDALL RJ, MC KENNA RW, NESBIT ME et al.

Virus-associated hemophagocytic syndrome. A benign histiocytic proliferation distinct from malignant histiocytosis.

Cancer, 1979; 44: 993-1002.

Childhood non-Hodgkin's lymphomas

C. PATTE, C. GISSELBRECHT

The non-Hodgkin's lymphomas (NHL) that typically occur in children differ from those common in adults in a number of important respects:

a - their architectural pattern is always different rather than nodular and their grade of malignancy is high;

b - their presentation is extranodal rather than nodal;

c - their dissemination is rapid and non-contiguous, with early involvement especially of bone marrow and the central nervous system.

Some 15 years ago, their prognosis was bad. Now, owing to a better understanding of the disease and to successive well-defined clinical trials with an optimal use of intensive treatment regimens, the cure rate has steadily increased and has become high.

In this chapter, only the specificities of childhood NHL will be detailed. Aspects shared with adult NHL will not be analyzed.

Burkitt-type lymphoblastic NHL [Kiel's classification (K)] (4,5) or small non-cleaved NHL [Working Formulation (WF)] (6) and non-Burkitt lymphoblastic NHL (K) or convoluted or non-convoluted lymphoblastic NHL (WF). Large-cell NHL or Ki-1+ anaplastic NHL occur more rarely and will not be detailed in this chapter.

Immunophenotypic studies have shown that Burkitt-type lymphomas belong to the B-cell lineage, whereas most lymphoblastic NHL are of T-cell lineage, with a small proportion having either a B-cell phenotype or a null phenotype similar to that of non-T non-B acute lymphoblastic leukaemias (7).

Any the usual t(8;14), t(2;8) or t(8;22) translocations are found in Burkitt's lymphoma (8) (*see pp. 41-47*). Cytogenetic anomalies are much less characteristic and frequent in T-cell lymphoblastic NHL. Chromosome 7 and/or chromosome 14 are most often involved.

Biological aspects

Childhood NHL always have a diffuse architecture (1-3). Diagnosis can therefore be established on the basis of a cell smear from a serous effusion or bone marrow.

Two histological types are by far the most frequent and show equal distribution:

Clinical aspects

NHL are rare before the age of 2 years. In 204 patients treated at the Institut Gustave-Roussy from 1974 to 1980, the median age was 7 years and the male predominance 3:1. The distribution of localizations found at presentation is reported in *Table I*. A nodal presentation was found in less than 10% of cases.

TABLE I

Breakdown of involved sites found at presentation in 204 children treated at the Institut Gustave-Roussy (1974-1980)

Abdomen	37%
Mediastinum	28%
Extracranial extranodal head-and-neck	17%
Nodal	9%
Miscellaneous	9%

Abdominal presentation

NHL with an abdominal presentation always have a B-cell phenotype. Most of them are Burkitt's type. They originate either from Peyer's patches or from mesenteric lymph nodes, usually in the ileocaecal region. They rapidly spread to contiguous organs, especially to the peritoneum with accompanying ascites. On rare occasions they may be revealed by an intussusception, but in most cases more often children present with an abdominal mass. Ultrasonography shows intraperitoneal tumours, often with ascites and involvement of other organs (liver, ovaries, pancreas, spleen, lombo-aortic lymph nodes). A laparotomy is required only in cases of emergency (perforation, intussusception) since, in most cases, diagnosis may be established on the basis of a cell smear from a serous effusion or by a transcutaneous needle biopsy.

Thoracic presentation

Except in rare cases, thoracic NHL in children originate from the thymus, are lymphoblastic and have a T-cell phenotype. Patients are at high risk of acute respiratory failure, either during mobilization and/or anaesthesia. The latter must be avoided whenever possible. Diagnosis is usually ascertained on the basis of cell smears from a pleural or pericardial effusion or bone-marrow aspiration or after a lymph-node aspiration or biopsy. Biopsy of the mediastinal tumour itself has rarely to be performed.

Other presentations

Of these, extracranial head-and-neck presentations are the most frequent, involving Waldeyer's ring or the maxillary bones (9). Any peripheral area may be involved in cases of nodal presentation. Other miscellaneous presentations are rarer and sometimes difficult to recognize and involve skin or subcutaneous tissue (10), breast, eyelids, orbit, thyroid, chest wall, bone(s) (11), kidney(s). With these sites immunophenotyping must be added to routine histology, since any immunophenotype may be found.

Pretreatment staging

In children, treatment must be initiated without any delay and staging procedures are limited.

Staging classifications

Because of the high frequency of extranodal involvement and of the mode of spreading, the Ann Arbor staging classification is not suitable. Several other classifications have been proposed. Murphy's classification is at present the one most routinely used *(Table II)* (1).

Staging procedure

Few staging procedures are mandatory: complete clinical examination, cavum and chest X-rays, abdomen ultrasonography, blood counts, bone-marrow aspiration in two separate areas, buffy-coat CSF examination. Other tests need to be performed less often: head-and-neck CT scan, bone gammography or radiography, CT scan or MR examination of the CNS in cases of neuromeningeal involvement.

Bone-marrow biopsy is not more sensitive than aspiration and is not useful.

TABLE II

**St Jude Children's Research Hospital (Murphy)
clinical staging system for childhood lymphomas (reference n°1)**

Stage	
I (8 %)*	A single extranodal tumour or a single anatomic nodal area, with the exclusion of mediastinum and abdomen
II (13 %)	A single extranodal tumour with regional node involvement or Two or more nodal areas on the same side of the diaphragm or Two extranodal tumours with or without regional node involvement on the same side of the diaphragm or A primary GI tract tumour, usually in the ileocaecal area, with or without involvement of associated mesenteric node only and completely surgically removed
III (48%)	Two extranodal tumours on opposite sides of the diaphragm or Two or more nodal areas above and below the diaphragm or All the primary intrathoracic tumours (mediastinal, pleural, thymic) or All extensive primary intra-abdominal disease or All paraspinal or epidural tumours
IV 31 %	Any of the above with initial CNS and or bone-marrow involvement

* Distribution of stages among 204 patients treated at the Institut Gustave-Roussy from 1974 to 1980

Abdomen ultrasonography is mandatory at staging and during follow-up. CT scan is rarely indicated at presentation: staging of the locoregional extension of a head-and-neck NHL, or of a stage I or stage II abdominal NHL, or to guide needle biopsy. It is more useful during follow-up, especially for careful assessment of the response in the mediastinum or in the abdomen.

The limit between NHL and leukaemia has been arbitrarily defined as a bone-marrow blast percentage of 25% but this is not correlated with differences in clinical or biological characteristics (12).

Besides staging, the general condition of the patient must be rapidly assessed. In some cases, because of certain sites or rapid tumour growth, emergency treatment may be necessary: acute respiratory failure from Waldeyer's ring or mediastinum involvement, surgical complication of an abdominal NHL, hypercalcaemia or renal failure. In this latter case, the mechanisms of kidney failure must be ascertained (ureteral compression, tumour infiltration of the kidneys, hyperuricaemia) and appropriate symptomatic treatment initiated (pyelostomy, urine alcalinization, urate oxidase) prior to chemotherapy.

Initial treatment with COP (Cyclophosphamide-Oncovin-Prednisone), as performed in recent studies of the Société Française d'Oncologie Pédiatrique (SFOP) (13,14), is a low-dose, non-haematotoxic regimen which allows the correction of acute complications before initiation of intensive chemotherapy and before the onset of bone-marrow aplasia.

Classification of NHL

Since the treatment procedures of all NHL in children depend on the immunological and histological characteristics, all cases must be classified into one of the two categories below.

B-cell NHL

– histology: Burkitt-type (small non-cleaved) or centroblastic type;
– immunohistology: monoclonal surface immunoglobulins or pan-B markers (CD19 to CD24);
– digestive tract involvement;
– translocation (8;14) or (2;8) or (8;22).

non-B cell NHL

– histology: lymphoblastic;
– immunohistology: T-cell proliferation (CD2, 3, 4, 5, 7, 8);
– immunocytochemistry: focal staining for alkaline phosphatase.
Non-T non-B NHL are included in this group except if they have a Burkitt-type histology or involve the digestive tract.

References

1. MURPHY SB
   Classification, staging and end-results of treatment of childhood non-Hodgkin's lymphomas: dissimilarities from lymphomas in adults.
   Semin Oncol, 1980; 7: 332-339.

2. PATTE C, GERARD-MARCHANT R, CAILLOU B, RODARY C, BAYLE C, HARTMANN O
   Les lymphomes malins non hodgkiniens de l'enfant. Aspects pratiques.
   Arch Fr Pediatr, 1981; 28: 359-367.

3. MURPHY SB, FAIRCLOUGH DL, HUTCHINSON RE, BERARD CW
   Non-Hodgkin's lymphomas in childhood: an analysis of the histology, staging, and response to treatment of 338 cases at a single institution.
   J Clin Oncol, 1989; 7: 186-193.

4. LENNERT K
   Lymphomas of high-grade malignancy.
   In Lennert K (Ed): Histopathology of non-Hodgkin's lymphomas. Berlin, Springer, 1981: pp. 72-102.

5. STANSFELD AG, DIEBOLD J, KAPANCI Y, KELENYI G, LENNERT K, MIODUSZEWSKA O, NOEL H, RILKE F, SUNDSTROM C, VAN UNNIK JAM, WRIGHT DH
   Updated Kiel classification for lymphomas.
   Lancet, 1988; 1: 293-294.

6. *National Cancer Institute sponsored study of classification of non-Hodgkin's lymphomas: summary and description of a working formulation for clinical usage.*
   Cancer, 1982; 49: 2112-2135.

7. BERNARD A, MURPHY SB, MELVIN S, BOWMAN WP, CAILLARD J, LEMERLE J, BOUMSELL L
   Non-T non-B lymphomas are rare in children and associated with cutaneous tumors.
   Blood, 1982; 59: 549-554.

8. LENOIR G, O'CONOR G, OLWENY CLM Eds
   Burkitt's lymphomas. A human cancer model.
   Lyon, IARC Scientific Publications n° 60, 1985.

9. BERGERON C, PATTE C, CAILLAUD JM, BERNARD A, BAYLE C, LUBOINSKI B, HARTMANN O, KALIFA C, FLAMANT F, LEMERLE J
   Aspects cliniques, anatomo-pathologiques et résultats thérapeutiques de 63 lymphomes malins non hodgkiniens ORL de l'enfant.
   Arch Fr Pediatr, 1989; 46: 583-587.

10. BERNARD A, BOUMSELL L, BAYLE C, RICHARD Y, COPPIN H, PENIT C, ROUGET P, LEMERLE J, DAUSSET J
    Subsets of malignant lymphomas in children related to the cell phenotype.
    Blood, 1979; 54: 1058-1068.

11. COPPES MJ, PATTE C, COUANET D, CAILLAUD JM, SALLOUM E, BRUGIERES L, HARTMANN O, KALIFA C, BERNARD A, LEMERLE J
    Chilhood malignant lymphoma of bone.
    Med Ped Oncol, 1991; 19: 22-27.

12. BERNARD A, BOUMSELL L, PATTE C, LEMERLE J
    Leukemia versus lymphoma in children. A worthless question?
    Med Ped Oncol, 1986; 14: 148-157.

13. PATTE C, PHILIP T, RODARY C, BERNARD A, ZUCKER JM, BERNARD JL, ROBERT A, RIALLAND X, BENZ-LEMOINE E, DEMEOCQ F, BAYLE C, LEMERLE J
    Improved survival rate in children with stage III and IV B-cell non-Hodgkin's lymphoma and leukemia using a multiagent chemotherapy: results of a study of 114 children from the French Pediatric Oncolocy Society.
    J Clin Oncol, 1986; 4: 1219-1229.

14. PATTE C, PHILIP T, RODARY C, ZUCKER JM, BEHRENDT H, GENTET JC, LAMAGNERE JP, OTTEN J, DUFILLOT D, PEIN F, CAILLOU B, LEMERLE J
    High survival rate in advanced stage B-cell lymphomas and leukemias without CNS involvement with a short intensive polychemotherapy. Results of a randomized trial from the French Pediatric Oncology Society (SFOP) on 216 children.
    J Clin Oncol, 1991; 9: 123-132.

Non-Hodgkin's lymphomas associated with human immunodeficiency virus (HIV) infection

P. SOLAL-CÉLIGNY, N. BROUSSE

Soon after the reporting of the first AIDS cases, several cases of NHL associated with opportunistic infections in patients at risk for AIDS were published in 1982 (1). Since 1985, patients with serological or viro-logical confirmation of HIV infection and high-grade NHL with a B-cell or a "null" phenotype have been included in the AIDS group (2). The pathogenesis of NHL associated with HIV infection remains unknown. The possible role of Epstein-Barr virus has been developed *on pp. 41-47.*

Epidemiology

NHL associated with HIV infection have some specificities (3-12). Initially, homosexuals were considered to be more often affected than other populations at risk (2-5). Currently, the incidence of NHL is similar in all populations at risk (6,10-12). The median age of patients varies from 30 to 39 years between series (3-12), lower among IV drug-users than among homosexuals (12). Mostly because of the increase in survival time in patients with HIV infection, the incidence of NHL in these patients is steadily increasing [10% (9) to 14.5% (13)]. For instance, in patients treated for at least 36 months with azidothymidine, the estimated probability of developing lymphoma was 46% (13).

NHL may occur at any stage of HIV infection:

- in some patients, it may reveal the viral infection and, for most authors, HIV-1 and HIV-2 serological testings must be performed in all patients with high-grade NHL (15 to 25% of cases);

- on the other hand, NHL may develop at the end stage of the disease, in patients with a previous history of multiple opportunistic infections and neoplastic disorders (40% of cases);

- occurrence of NHL is often preceded by a prodromal phase of lymphadenopathy syndrome (LAS) with disseminated lymph-node and sometimes spleen enlargement and serological and immunological manifestations of HIV infection (14,15) (25% of cases).

Lymphadenopathy syndrome

In patients with LAS, pathological examination of lymph nodes shows polyclonal B-cell follicular hyperplasia, often irregular, and paracortical hyperplasia (16-18) *(fig. 1).* The perifollicular lymphoid mantle-zone is thin, and may in certain cases contain a continuous solution which allows mantle-zone cells to penetrate into the germinal centre *(fig. 2).* Immunohistochemical studies show that germinal centres are made up of polytypic B cells and contain an increased number of T cells *(fig. 3),* which are mostly CD8+ *(fig. 4).* The network of dendritic reticulum cells is either preserved or partially disorganized *(fig. 5)* (20-27). This disorganization may promote the migration of cells from the mantle zone to the

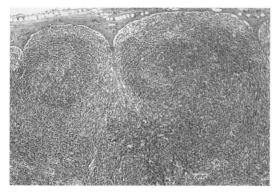

Fig. 1: **Lymphadenopathy syndrome.** Follicular and paracortical hyperplasia.

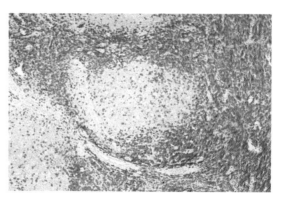

Fig.3a

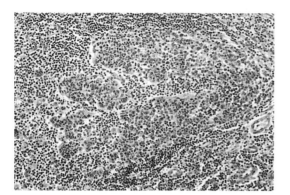

Fig. 2: **Lymphadenopathy syndrome.** Germinal centre with ill-defined limits and entry into the follicle of cells from the mantle zone.

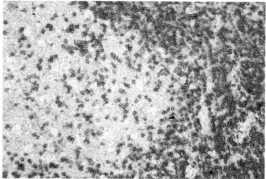

Fig. 3b

Fig. 3: **Lymphadenopathy syndrome.** Immunohistochemical study with an anti-T antibody (CD3). Increase in the total number of T cells (fig. 3a), especially in germinal centres (fig. 3b)

germinal centre *(fig. 6)* (26). When compared to normal lymph nodes, the numbers of T helper and T cytotoxic cells are reduced while the number of T suppressor cells is increased (27). There is a high rate of HIV replication in hyperplastic lymph nodes and a considerable immune reaction characterized by the production of cytokines such as γ IFN and IL-2. Gamma IFN is produced by CD8 cells which infiltrate the germinal centres. IL-2 and γ IFN may participate in the recruitment and activation of T cytotoxic cells specific for HIV (28). The follicular hyperplasia stage may be followed first by a stage of diffuse lymphoid hyperplasia, similar to angio-immunoblastic lymphadenopathy (23) then by a stage of lymphoid atrophy with fibrosis (20,22,24). These successive stages may precede the evolution towards AIDS (23,24). Using a monoclonal antibody specific for the core protein of the virus p18, immunohistochemical studies show the staining of lymphoid cells of the germinal centres and of large mono- or bi-

nucleated dendritic reticulum cells *(fig. 7)* (29). Using electronic microscopy, viral particles may be seen in the germinal centres, between the cytoplasmic extensions of dendritic reticulum cells (30).

In most paediatric cases, and some adult cases, LAS may be associated with a disseminated lymphoid hyperplasia of the lungs described as Lymphoid Interstitial Pneumonitis *(see pp. 231-239)*

Clinical and immunohistological features

NHL in HIV patients are characterized by a high incidence of extranodal involvement (80 to 90%), especially of the gastro-intestinal tract, the central nervous system, the

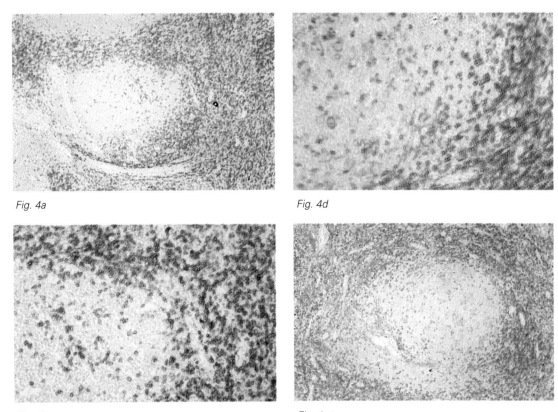

Fig. 4a

Fig. 4d

Fig. 4b

Fig. 4c

Fig. 4: **Lymphadenopathy syndrome.** Immunoperoxidase staining with antiCD8 and antiCD4 antibodies. Increase in suppressive CD8 T cells (fig. 4a) especially in germinal centres (fig. 4b) and decrease in CD4 T helper cells (figs 4c and 4d).

skin, the liver, the bone marrow and the muscles (*Table I*). Some previously almost unknown presentations have been reported: primary NHL of the rectum (8,31), the biliary tract (32), and the heart (33). In all patients with NHL and HIV infection, the extent of immune deficiency (blood level of CD4+ lymphocytes) and concomitant infections (viral hepatitis, cytomegalovirus, toxoplasma) must be sought.

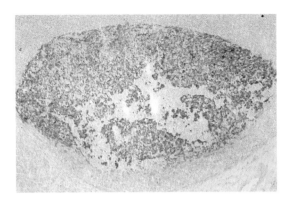

Fig. 5: **Lymphadenopathy syndrome.** Immunoperoxidase staining with an antibody directed dendritic reticulum cells (DCR 1). Disorganization of the germinal centre network.

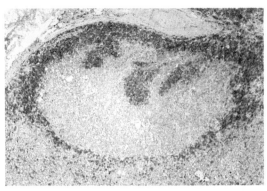

Fig. 6: **Lymphadenopathy syndrome.** Immunoperoxidase staining with an anti-IgD antibody. Thickening of the mantle zone with penetration of cells into the germinal centre.

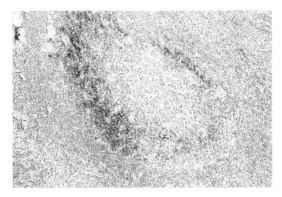

Fig. 7: **Lymphadenopathy syndrome.** *Immunoperoxidase staining with a monoclonal antibody directed against the p18 core protein of the virus (Dr. D. Klatzman). Staining of the lymphoid cells and of the reticulum dendritic cells of the germinal centre.*

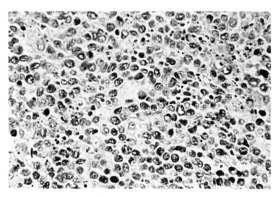

Fig. 9: **Lymph node.** *Small non-cleaved (Burkitt-type) NHL associated with HIV infection.*

The great majority of NHL in HIV patients are of high-grade malignancy. They are approximately equally distributed between diffuse large-cell (centroblastic) NHL (*fig. 8*) [24% in a combined series of 311 cases (10)], immunoblastic NHL (29%) and Burkitt's lymphonal or Burkitt-type NHL (36%) (*fig. 9*) (4-12). But in some cases, histological classification may be difficult. About 10% are low-grade follicular NHL. Diffuse large-cell lymphomas are often associated with severe immune deficiency and have a very poor prognosis. Burkitt's lymphoma often occurs earlier in the course of HIV infection and has a better response to chemotherapy (5,34).

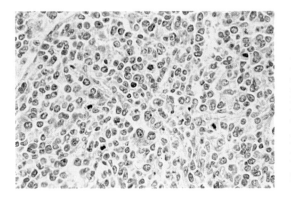

Fig. 8: **Lymph node.** *Diffuse large-cell (centroblastic) non-Hodgkin's lymphoma associated with HIV infection.*

Like most NHL occuring in patients with immune deficiency, the great majority of

TABLE I

Most frequently involved sites in NHL at diagnosis in patients with HIV infection

Reference	Number of pts	Frequency (%)					
		CNS	Liver	G.I. tract	Bone marrow	Lungs	Skin
Monfardini (12)	113	36	36	21	26	8	8
Ziegler (4)	88	43	9	17	34	9	16
Levine (11)	68	36	NP	26	25	9	NP
Knowles (7)	89	22	17	28	21	NP	NP
Lowenthal (8)	43	26	14	26	40	16	NP

them are of B-cell type. Burkitt-type NHL are CD10, CD20, CD22 and CD45 positive; large-cell NHL are usually CD10, CD19, CD20, CD22 and CD45 positive while immunoblastic NHL are CD10 and CD38 positive. A few cases of T-cell NHL in HIV patients have also been reported (35-37). As described *on pp. 41-47*, lymphoprolifera- tions in HIV patients often develop from an oligoclonal to monoclonal proliferation (38). A "relapse" of NHL in an HIV patient may - even if the histological type is identi- cal to the initial one - be due to the emer- gence of another malignant B-cell clone. In such cases, a treatment similar to that given initially may again be effective (39).

Treatment

In most series, the median survival of HIV patients with NHL is short, around 4 months (6-10). A poor response to chemotherapy, a high relapse rate and the fre- quent occurrence of opportunistic infections explain why the prognosis is so bad. The bone-marrow tolerance of aggressive che- motherapy is poor in these patients for several reasons: HIV directly infects mar- row precursors; the antiretroviral drug zidovudine is myelosuppressive; patients may have bone-marrow infection with micro- organisms such as *Mycobacterium avium intracellulare*. The prognosis of a given patient follows the usual prognosis parame- ters of NHL (dissemination, tumour burden, performance status, serum LDH, etc.) and on the underlying immune deficiency (previous opportunistic infections, blood level of CD4+ lymphocytes, etc.). The optimal treatment of NHL in HIV patients is still in debate. In patients with a severe immune deficiency or a concomitant opportunistic infection, only a symptomatic treatment can be proposed. Aggressive chemotherapy may only be proposed for patients with a good performance status, in whom NHL reveals the HIV infection, with no previous or concomitant opportunistic infection and a moderate immune deficiency (blood CD4+ lymphocyte count greater than 100/mm^3, i.e. CDC group II or III disease). A coope- rative group from France and Italy treated 60 patients fulfilling these criteria with a third-generation chemotherapy regimen

(LNH-84) and obtained a 72% complete remission rate with a median survival of 9 months (40). The toxicity of this regimen, myeloid in particular, was very high. Prophy- laxis of CNS involvement by radiotherapy and intrathecal chemotherapy must be per- formed concomitantly. Prophylaxis of *Pneu- mocystis carinii* pneumonia with aerosoli- zed pentamidine and concomitant anti-HIV treatment (azidothymidine) are probably useful. Other fair results of aggressive chemotherapy (MACOP-B) have been report- ed (41). However, other studies suggest that an aggressive treatment has deleterious effects on the survival of these patients (8,10,42). Haemopoietic growth factors (G- CSF, GM-CSF) are probably useful in associ- ation with chemotherapy in these patients. Prospective studies are in progress.

References

1. ZIEGLER JL, DREW WL, MINER RC et al.
   Outbreak of Burkitt's-like lymphoma in homosexual men.
   Lancet, 1982; 2: 631-633.

2. Center for Disease Control.
   Revision of the case definition of Acquired Immun- odeficiency Syndrome for national reporting.
   Ann Intern Med, 1985; 103: 402-403.

3. LEVINE AM, MEYER PR, BEGANOY MK et al.
   Development of B-cell lymphomas in homosexual men.
   Ann Intern Med, 1984; 100: 1007-1013.

4. ZIEGLER JL, BECKSTEAD JA, VOLBERDING PA et al.
   Non-Hodgkin's lymphoma in 90 homosexual men. Relation to generalized lymphadenopathy and the acquired immunodeficiency syndrome.
   N Engl J Med, 1984; 311: 564-570.

5. KALTER SP, RIGGS SA, CABANILLAS F et al.
   Aggressive non-Hodgkin's lymphomas in immuno- compromised homosexual males.
   Blood, 1985; 66: 655-659.

6. AHMED T, WORMSER GP, STAHL RE et al.
   Malignant lymphomas in a population at risk for acquired immune deficiency syndrome.
   Cancer, 1987; 60: 719-723.

7. KNOWLES DM, CHAMULAK GA, SUBAR M et al.

   Lymphoid neoplasia associated with AIDS. The New York Medical Center Experience with 105 patients (1981-1986).

   Ann Intern Med, 1988; 108: 744-753.

8. LOWENTHAL DA, STRAUS DJ, CAMPBELL SW et al.

   AIDS-related lymphoid neoplasia. The Memorial Hospital experience.

   Cancer, 1988; 61: 2325-2327.

9. KAPLAN LD, ABRAMS DE, FEIGAL E et al.

   AIDS-associated non-Hodgkin's lymphoma in San Francisco.

   JAMA, 1989; 261: 719-724.

10. KAPLAN LD

    AIDS-associated lymphoma.

    Clin Haematol, 1990; 3: 139-151.

11. LEVINE AM

    Malignant lymphoma associated with HIV infection.

    Semin. Oncol., 1990; 17: 104-112.

12. MONFARDINI S, VACCHER E, FOA R et al.

    AIDS-associated non-Hodgkin's lymphoma in Italy: intravenous drug users versus homosexual men.

    Ann Oncol, 1990; 1: 203-211.

13. PLUDA JM, YARCHOAN R, JAFFE ES et al.

    Development of non-Hodgkin lymphoma in a cohort of patients with severe human immunodeficiency virus (HIV) infection on long-term antiretroviral therapy.

    Ann Intern Med, 1990; 113; 276-282.

14. METROKA CE, CUNNINGHAM-RUNDLES S, POLLACK M et al.

    Generalized lymphadenopathy in homosexual men.

    Ann Intern Med, 1983; 99: 584-591.

15. MATHUR-WAGH V, SPIGLAND I, SACKS H et al.

    Longitudinal study of persistent generalized lymphadenopathy in homosexual men. Relation to acquired immuno-deficiency syndrome.

    Lancet, 1984; 1: 1033-1038.

16. DOMINGO J, CHIN NW

    Lymphadenopathy in a heterogeneous population at risk for the acquired immunodeficiency syndrome (AIDS). A morphologic study.

    Am J Clin Pathol., 1983; 80: 649-654.

17. GUARDA LA, BUTLER JJ, MARSELL P, HERSH ME, REUBEN J,NERVELL GR

    Lymphadenopathy in homosexual men. Morbid anatomy with clinical and immunological correlations.

    Am J Clin Pathol., 1983; 79: 559-568.

18. SAID JW, SHINTAKU IP, TEITELBAUM A, CHIEN K, SASSOON AF

    Distribution of T-cell phenotypic subsets and surface immunoglobulin-bearing lymphocytes in lymph nodes from male homosexuals with persistent generalized lymphadenopathy: an immunohistochemical and ultrastructural study.

    Hum Pathol, 1984; 15: 785-790.

19. BURNS BF, WOOD GS, DORFMAN RFL

    The varied histopathology of lymphadenopathy in the homosexual male.

    Am J Surg Pathol, 1985; 9: 287-297.

20. BARONI CD, PEZZELA F, STOPPACCIARO A et coll.

    Systemic lymphadenopathy (LAS) in intravenous drug abusers. Histology, immunohistochemistry and electron microscopy: pathogenic correlations.

    Histopathology, 1985; 9: 1275-1293.

21. JANOSSY G, PINCHING AJ, BOFILL M et al.

    An immunohistological approach to persistent lymphadenopathy and its relevance to AIDS.

    Clin Exp Immunol, 1985; 59: 257-266.

22. REICHERT CM, O'LEARTY TJ, LEVEUS DL, SIMRELL CR, MACHER AM

    Autopsy pathology in the acquired immune deficiency syndrome.

    Am J Path, 1983; 112: 357-382.

23. TURNER RR, MEYER PR, TAYLOR CR et al.

    Immunohistology of persistent generalized lymphadenopathy. Evidence for progressive lymph node abnormalities in some patients.

    Am J Clin Pathol, 1987; 88: 10-19.

24. IDACHIM HL, CRONIN W, ROY M, MAYA M

    Persistent lymphadenopathies in people at high risk for HIV infection. Clinicopathologic correlations and long-term follow-up in 79 cases.

    Am J Clin Pathol, 1990; 93: 208-218.

25. FERNANDEZ R, MOURADIAN J, METROKA C, DAVIS J

    The prognostic value of histopathology in persistent generalized lymphadenopathy in homosexual men.

    N Engl J Med, 1983; 309: 185-186.

26. WOOD GS, GARCIA CF, DORFMAN RF, WARNKE RA

    The immunohistology of follicle lysis in lymph-node biopsies from homosexual men.

    Blood, 1985; 66: 1092-1097.

27. WOOD GA, BURNS BF, DORFMAN RG, WARNKE RA

    In situ *quantitation of lymph node helper, suppressor and cytotoxic T-cell subsets in AIDS.*

    Blood, 1986; 67: 596-603.

28. EMILIE D, PEUCHMAUR M, CREVON MC, MAILLOT MC, BROUSSE N, DELFRAISSY JF, GALANAUD P

    Production of interleukins in HIV-1 replicating lymph nodes.

    J Clin Invest, 1990; 86: 148-159.

29. BARONI CD, PEZZELLA F, MIROLO M, RUCO LP, ROSSI GB
Immunohistochemical demonstration of p24 HTLV III major core protein in different cell types within lymph nodes from patients with lymphadenopathy syndrome (LAS).
Histopathology, 1986; 10: 5-13.

30. ARMSTRONG JA, HORNE R
Follicular dendritic cells and virus like particles in AIDS-related lympadenopathy.
Lancet, 1984; 2: 370-372.

31. BURKES RL, MEYER PR, GILL PS
Rectal lymphoma in homosexual men.
Arch Intern Med, 1986; 146: 913-915.

32. KAPLAN LD, KAHN J, JACOBSON M, BOTTLES K, CELLO J
Primary non-Hodgkin's lymphoma of extrahepatic bile ducts in Acquired Immunodeficiency Syndrome.
Ann Intern Med, 1989; 110: 161-162.

33. GUARNER J, BRYNES RK, CHAN WC, BIRDSONG G, HERTZLER G
Primary non-Hodgkin's lymphoma of the heart in two patients with the acquired immunodeficiency syndrome.
Arch Pathol Lab Med, 1987; 111: 254-256.

34. BOYLE MJ, SWANSON CE, TURNER JJ et al.
Definition of two distinct types of AIDS-associated non-Hodgkin lymphoma.
Br J Haematol, 1990; 76: 506-512.

35. NASR SA, BRYNES RK, GARRISON CP, CHAN WC
Peripheral T-cell lymphoma in a patient with acquired immune deficiency syndrome.
Cancer, 1988; 61: 947-951.

36. PRESANT CA, GALA K, WISEMAN C et al.
Human immunodeficiency virus-associated T-cell lymphoblastic lymphoma in AIDS.
Cancer, 1987; 60: 1459-1461.

37. STERNLIEB J, MINTZER D, KWA D, GLUCKMAN S
Peripheral T-cell lymphoma in a patient with the acquired immunodeficiency syndrome.
Am J Med, 1988; 85: 445.

38. LIPPMAN SM, VOLK JR, SPIER CM, GROGAN TM
Clonal ambiguity of human immunodeficiency virus-associated lymphomas. Similarity to post-transplant lymphomas.
Arch Pathol Lab Med, 1988; 112: 128-132.

39. BARRIGA F, WHANG-PENG J, LEE E et al.
Development of a second clonally discrete Burkitt's lymphoma in a human immunodeficiency virus-positive homosexual patient.
Blood, 1988; 72: 792-795.

40. GISSELBRECHT C, TIRELLI V, FARCET JP et al.
Non-Hodgkin's lymphomas associated with human immunodeficiency virus: treatment by LNH 84 regimen.
IVth International Conference on Malignant Lymphoma, Lugano, 1990: A60.

41. BERMUDEZ MA, GRANT KM, ROOVIEN R, MENDES F
Non-Hodgkin's lymphoma in a population with or at risk for acquired immunodeficiency syndrome: indications for intensive chemotherapy.
Am J Med, 1989; 86: 71-76.

42. GILL PA, LEVINE AM, FRAILO M et al.
AIDS-related malignant lymphoma: results of prospective treatment trials.
J Clin Oncol, 1987; 5: 1322-1328.

4.

EXTRA-NODAL NON-HODGKIN'S LYMPHOMAS

edited by

P. SOLAL-CÉLIGNY, N. BROUSSE

Malignant lymphomas of mucosa-associated lymphoid tissues (MALT)

N. BROUSSE, A. JARRY, N. CERF-BENSUSSAN

Introduction

Malignant lymphomas are tumoral prolifer ations of the lymphoid tissue, and are more frequently located in peripheral lymph nodes. But all organs, particularly those containing lymphoid tissue in normal subjects, can be the site of malignant lymphomas. Among these lymphoid organs, mucosae, normally containing lymphoid tissue called Mucosa-associated lymphoid tissue (MALT), are preferential targets for extranodal lymphomas.

Lymphomas of the MALT have been studied in particular by P. Isaacson (1,2), first in the gut (lymphomas of the GALT: "gut-associated lymphoid tissue") (3) and then in the lung (lymphomas of the BALT: "bronchus-associated lymphoid tissue") (4). The description of MALT lymphomas led to the study of

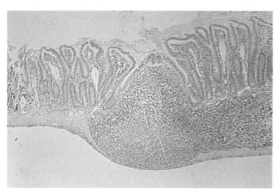

Fig. 1 : Overview of a Peyer's patch. The follicle-associated eptihelium (FAE) covers the dome region (D) and a lymphoid follicle (F).

lymphomas in other organs such as salivary glands (5), thyroid (6), or orbit (7).

In the MALT, B and T lymphocytes are present, and can generate B or T lymphomas of the MALT, of low- or high-grade malignancy. These lymphomas have been extensively studied in the gut. P. Isaacson has proposed a classification of these primary gut lymphomas, distinguishing between B and T lymphomas (8). Better knowledge of the normal MALT allows a better understanding of the origin of MALT lymphomas. For the description of the MALT, the gut has been selected in the present report.

Gut-associated lymphoid tissue (GALT) comprises lymphoid aggregates: Peyer's patches and mesenteric lymph nodes, as well as lymphoid cells scattered in the mucosa *(Fig. 1)* (9). Experimental studies in rodents have shown that lymphoid cells isolated in the mucosa, present both in the epithelium and in the lamina propria, are the effector cells of an intestinal immune response and that these cells are derived from precursors originating in Peyer's patches (10).

Lymphoid follicles and Peyer's patches

Lymphoid follicles, isolated or grouped in Peyer's patches, are present in the lower part of the mucosa and in the submucosa of the small intestine, colon, rectum, and appendix. Their structure allows the selective entry of antigens and the initiation of a gut immune response.

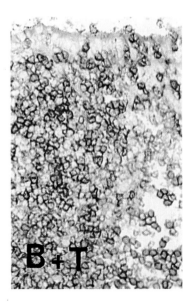

Fig. 2 : Follicle-associated epithelium and dome region. Double immunostaining with anti-Pan B CD22 conjugated to peroxidase an anti-Pan T CD3 conjugated to alkaline phosphatase, showing the distribution of B and T lymphoid populations in epithelium and dome region.

Peyer's patch consists of four distinct zones:

- The epithelium overlying lymphoid follicles is a specialized epithelium, whose structure is distinct from that of villous epithelium (11). This follicle-associated epithelium contains specialized epithelial cells termed M cells, interspersed between enterocytes, devoid of brush border and basal lamina, and possessing cytoplasmic processes enfolding CD4+ T lymphocytes, B lymphocytes *(Fig. 2)*, IgM+ plasma cells, and macrophages (11). Electron-microscopic have shown showed that M cells selectively endocytose and transport numerous intraluminal antigens (bacteria, viruses, etc.). These antigens are transported from the surface of Peyer's patches to the underlying dome and then to the lymphoid follicles, where the intestinal immune response is initiated (12).

- The dome, located immediately beneath the follicle-associated epithelium, contains a mixture of B lymphocytes (termed "cen-

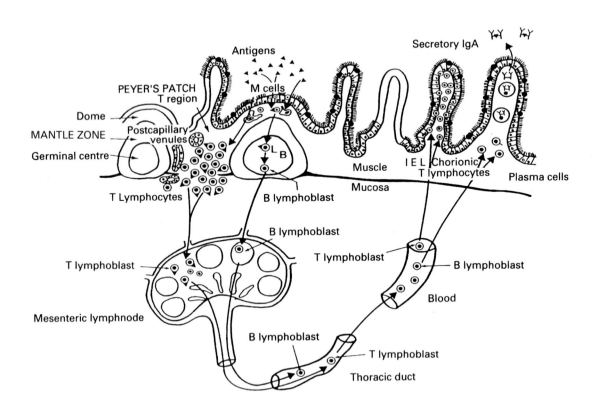

Fig. 3 : Haemolymphatic cycle of T lymphocytes and IgA plasma cells in gut.

trocyte-like cells" by Isaacson (3)), IgM+ plasma cells, predominantly CD4+ T lymphocytes *(Fig. 2)*, and macrophages (13).

- The lymphoid follicles, under the dome, constitute the B-cell proliferation site. When activated by antigenic stimulation, lymphoid follicles consist of a germinal centre surrounded by a mantle of small IgM+ IgD+ B lymphocytes. The germinal centres of Peyer's patches are rich in dividing blast cells bearing surface IgM and IgA, contrary to peripheral lymph node germinal centres, which express only surface IgM (14). The germinal centres of MALT lymphoid follicles also contain T lymphocytes, mostly CD4+, and cells of the histiomonocytic lineage (follicular dendritic reticulum cells).

- The T-cell zone or thymodependent zone, the proliferation site for T lymphocytes, is located between lymphoid follicles. It consists of T lymphocytes, mostly CD4+, macrophages, and numerous post-capillary high endothelial venules (HEV) which permit the migration of T lymphocytes from blood into Peyer's patches (11).

Experimental studies in rodents have shown that Peyer's patches contain the immature precursors of plasma cells (B blasts pre-differentiated towards IgA synthesis) and of T lymphocytes (T blasts) present in the intestinal mucosa. These progenitors follow a haemolymphatic cycle (10) *(Fig. 3)*, through which they mature and at the end of which they home back to the intestinal mucosa, where they differentiate into mature IgA-secreting plasma cells or into mature T lymphocytes which colonize either the epithelium or the lamina propria. This cycle is suggested but not proven in humans. Mechanisms regulating lymphocyte traffic in and through the intestine are not well-known. They could result from an interaction between lymphocyte receptors and homing receptors present on the endothelial cells of mucosa vessels (15-18). Peripheral lymphocytes express two types of surface receptors, one allowing binding to lymph-node HEV, the other binding to Peyer's-patch HEV. Lymph-node and Peyer's-patch HEV express different endothelial receptors. Presumably, the precursors of mucosal lymphocytes, after being

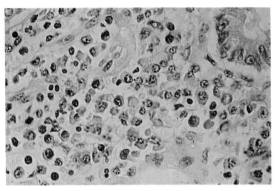

Fig. 4 : Normal human mucosa of the small intestine. Lamina propria contains lymphocytes, plasma cells and macrophages.

primed in Peyer's patches, may lose their receptors for lymph-node HEV, keeping only their receptors for Peyer's patches and lamina propria endothelial cells, and thus being able to home back to intestinal mucosa. Peyer's-patch lymphocytes can also migrate into other mucosae (bronchus, salivary glands, uterus and mammary gland during lactation). MALT originates from the spreading and exchange of immunological information between the various mucosae.

Immune cells scattered in the normal intestinal mucosa

These immune cells can be studied in humans either *in situ* on tissue sections with immunohistochemical methods using specific antibodies, or *in vitro* after isolating them from the mucosa, which permits the study of their functional properties.

Lymphocytes

The intestine, like every lymphoid organ, contains B lymphocytes which initiate humoral responses leading to immunoglobulin synthesis, and T lymphocytes responsible for cellular immunity.

a) **B lymphocytes** are present in the lamina propria. They are different from the B lym-

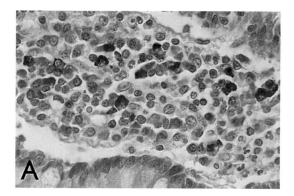

Fig. 5 : Phenotype of lamina propria plasma cells. Indirect immunoperoxidase technique (PAP) on paraffin sections with an anti-IgA antibody. IgA+plasma cells are predominant.

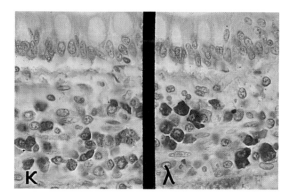

Fig. 6 : Plasma cells are polytypic : they synthesize either kappa or lambda light chain. Indirect immunoperoxidase technique (PAP) on paraffin sections with anti-kappa (6a) and anti-lambda (6b) monoclonal antibodies.

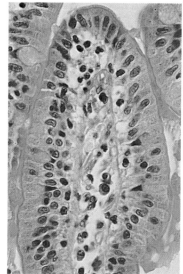

Fig. 7 : Intestinal villi : epithelium, overlying lamina propria, contains lymphocytes differing from their lamina propria counterparts.

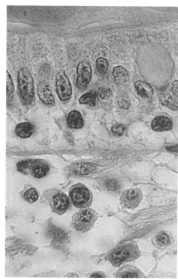

Fig. 8 : Intraepithelial lymphocytes (IEL). Intestinal epithelium contains numerous IEL, located against the basal lamina, between epithelial cells.

phocytes of other lymphoid organs. They are mostly plasma cells *(Fig. 4)*, which secrete IgA (75%) *(Fig. 5)*, but also IgM (20%) and IgG (5%). These plasma cells are polytypic, secreting twice as many kappa light chains as lambda light chains *(Fig. 6)*. Intestinal IgA are dimeric and contain 50% IgA1 and 50% IgA2, contrary to serum IgA, which are monomeric and mostly of the IgA1 subclass. The dimeric structure of intestinal IgA allows their binding to a membrane receptor: the secretory component, synthesized by epithelial cells. These IgA-secretory component complexes, termed secretory IgA, are transported to the apical pole of enterocytes and released into the gut lumen, in which they exert their protective functions towards epithelium (elimination of pathogenic microorganisms, inhibition of the absorption of food antigens, etc.) (19).

b) T lymphocytes (CD3+) are present both in the lamina propria and in the epithelium *(Figs 7 and 8)*. They acquire in the thymus a receptor for antigens called T-cell receptor (TCR), which allows antigen recognition. There are two different types of TCR:

1) the TCRαβ, composed of an alpha chain and a beta chain, is present on the majority

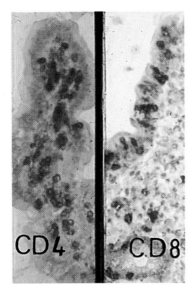

Fig. 9 : Phenotype of normal human intestinal mucosa T lymphocytes. Indirect immunoperoxidase technique on frozen tissue sections with anti-CD4 (9a) and anti-CD8 (9b) monoclonal antibodies : lamina propria lymphocytes are predominantly CD4+ (helper phenotype), whereas most of the IEL are CD8+ (cytotoxic /suppresor phenotype).

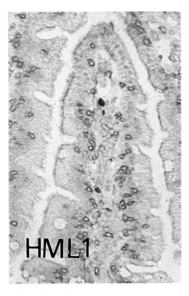

Fig. 10 : Phenotype of normal human intestinal mucosa T lymphocytes. Indirect immunoperoxidase technique on frozen tissue sections with HML1 monoclonal antibody. All IEL are stained with HML1.

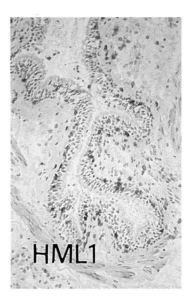

Fig. 11 : Phenotype of epithelial T lymphocytes of the human normal bronchus. Indirect immunoperoxidase technique on frozen tissue sections with HML1 monoclonal antibody. IEL of the bronchus epithelium are labelled with HML1.

of mature T lymphocytes; and 2) the TCRγδ, composed of a γ chain and a δ chain, was recently found on immature thymocytes and on a very small number of peripheral-blood T lymphocytes.

Most of the lamina propria T lymphocytes, like those of blood and peripheral lymphoid organs, express CD4 (helper phenotype) (60%) *(Fig. 9)* and TCR αβ. Lymphocytes associated with intestinal epithelium, termed intraepithelial lymphocytes (IEL), are almost exclusively T lymphocytes and differ from lamina propria T lymphocytes in several phenotypical features: 1) the majority of IEL (60 to 80%) express CD8 (cytotoxic/suppressor phenotype) *(Fig. 9)* and TCRαβ; 2) Thirteen per cent (2 to 30%) of IEL express TCRγδ, incontrast with blood and lamina propria T lymphocytes (5%). These TCRγδ + IEL are mostly CD4- CD8-. The function of this subset is unknown, but recent experiments in mice showed that TCRγδ + IEL are able to differentiate, owing to the inductive property of intestinal epithelium (20); and 3) a minor subset is specific to intestinal epithelium (10%); it does not express any mature T-cell markers, but it bears CD7, an antigen present on immature T cells. These CD3- CD7+ cells bear neither TCRαβ nor TCRγδ (21).

All these IEL subsets express the membrane antigen defined by monoclonal antibody HML1 *(Fig. 10)* (23). This antigen is absent on resting T lymphocytes in blood and peripheral lymphoid organs, but expressed on activated blood T lymphocytes, mostly CD8+. The possible function of this antigen present on IEL is unknown; however, its presence seems to be strongly correlated with the ability of lymphocytes to bind to epithelia, since this antigen is observed on lymphocytes associated with normal epithelia (bronchus *(Fig. 11)*, mammary gland...), as well as with inflammatory (skin) or tumoral epithelia (22, 23).

The study of immune deficiencies in humans (congenital deficiencies of cellular immunity and AIDS) clearly shows the crucial role of intestinal T lymphocytes in mucosal defence. However, the workings of T lymphocytes have not been totally elucidated. They may act either by secreting soluble factors called lymphokines which favour the local production of immunoglobulins, or by exerting a cytotoxic activity. *In vitro* studies of isolated cells suggest that intestinal mucosa contains a fair amount of cytotoxic T cells, whose targets remain to be defined (virus-infected or tumoral epithelial cells? microorganisms?).

Other types of immune cells

Lamina propria also contains macrophages, mast cells and eosinophils.

Macrophages, numerous in the axis of intestinal villi, bear class II molecules of the major histocompatibility complex (HLA-DR) which enable them to present antigens to neighbouring T lymphocytes.

Mucosa **mast cells** have long been insufficiently known, owing to researchers' failure to visualize them in formalin-fixed samples. Mast cells, which are few in number in normal subjects, increase in a variety of pathological processes including allergies and parasitic infections, when they can enter intestinal epithelium. They differ from connective-tissue and skin mast cells since they possess different granulations and above all

because their proliferation and maturation depend on interleukin 3 (IL3), a soluble factor secreted by activated T lymphocytes, as is stated in studies on mice (24).

A detailed characterization of intestinal immune cells allows a better understanding of MALT-malignant lymphomas, especially of low-grade malignancy, which are described in all organs containing MALT and which have been wrongly called "pseudolymphomas". Immunohistochemical findings have proved the monotypic proliferation of these so-called "pseudolymphomas" (25); DNA analyses have confirmed the clonality of these tumours (26). B lymphomas of low-grade malignancy arising in the stomach may derive from B lymphocytes of the marginal zone or dome zone covering lymphoid follicles, or from B lymphocytes of the follicle-associated epithelium. Indeed, IgM+ B lymphocytes are present in both these zones, and nowhere else in the intestine. Paradoxically, in normal subjects, gastric lymphoid tissue is rare and does not contain well-defined lymphoid follicles. How normal gastric mucosa develops isolated lymphoid hyperplasia and then lymphoma is unknown. Conversely, lymphoid tissue is abundant in the small intestine, where primitive lymphomas of low-grade malignancy are rare, apart from Mediterranean lymphomas, in particular the alpha-chain disease in which morphological lesions similar to those of gastric lymphomas have been described.

MALT lymphomas of low-grade malignancy have common morphological characteristics, whatever their location along the digestive tract:

- a monoclonal proliferation of small B lymphocytes, which are "centrocyte-like" cells;

- lymphoepithelial lesions, resulting from the tendency of "centrocyte-like" cells to invade mucosal epithelium;

- a frequent polytypic follicular lymphoid hyperplasia, subsequently invaded by "centrocyte-like" cells, and thus becoming monotypic;

- plasma-cell differentiation of tumour cells, in about a third of cases; and

- a frequent invasion of other MALT.

"Centrocyte-like" tumour cells might develop from parafollicular B lymphocytes.

In the stomach, lymphoepithelial lesions are pathognomonic features of MALT malignant lymphomas. In other sites, these lymphoepithelial lesions can be found in non-tumoral proliferations, for example in Hashimoto's thyroiditis or in sialadenitis (where they are named lymphomyoepithelial lesions). Immunohistochemical studies have allowed demonstration of the polytypic or monotypic nature of B lymphoid cells invading mucosal epithelium and have helped to rectify or ascertain the diagnosis of malignant lymphoma.

In allowing precise determination of a lymphoid infiltrate, immunohistochemistry is, at present, the best criterion when making a differential diagnosis distinguishing between lymphoid hyperplasia and malignant lymphoma.

Present results thus suggest continuity between "pseudotumoral" lymphoid hyperplasias and lymphomas of low-grade malignancy, as well as between low-grade and high-grade malignancy lymphomas.

Primitive malignant lymphomas of the MALT display important features which differ from those of lymph node lymphomas: MALT lymphomas of low-grade malignancy are localized in their initial site for a long time, in contrast with nodal B lymphomas of low-grade malignancy, which are often disseminated when the diagnosis is made. When MALT lymphomas are invasive, they preferentially invade other MALT organs. This could result from the lymphocyte traffic called "homing" (27). MALT lymphomas of high-grade malignancy are rarely disseminated. Surgical resection remains an important factor in treatment.

References

1. ISAACSON PG, WRIGHT DH
   Malignant lymphoma of mucosa-associated lymphoid tissue. A distinctive type of B-cell lymphoma.
   Cancer, 1983; 52: 1410-1416.

2. ISAACSON PG
   Lymphomas of mucosa-associated lymphoid tissue (MALT).
   Histopathology, 1990; 16: 617-619.

3. ISAACSON PG, SPENCER J
   Malignant lymphoma of mucosa-associated lymphoid tissue.
   Histopathology, 1987; 11: 445-462.

4. ADDIS BJ, HYJEK E, ISSACSON PG
   Primary pulmonary lymphoma: a reappraisal of its histogenesis and its relationship to pseudolymphoma and lymphoid interstitial pneumonia.
   Histopathology, 1988; 13: 1-12.

5. HYJEK E, SMITH WJ, ISAACSON PG
   Primary B-cell lymphoma of salivary glands and its relationship to myoepithelial sialadenitis.
   Hum Pathol, 1988; 19: 766-776.

6. HYJEK E, ISAACSON PG
   Primary B-cell lymphoma of the thyroid and its relationship to Hashimoto's thyroiditis.
   Hum Pathol, 1988; 19: 1315-1326.

7. MEDEIROS LJ, HARRIS NL
   Lymphoid infiltrates of the orbit and conjunctiva.
   Am J Surg Pathol, 1989; 13: 459-471.

8. ISAACSON PG, SPENCER J, WRIGHT DH
   Classifying primary gut lymphomas.
   The Lancet, 1988; ii: 1148-1149.

9. JARRY A, CERF-BENSUSSAN N, FLEJOU JF, BROUSSE N
   Le système lymphoïde du tube digestif chez l'homme.
   Ann Pathol, 1988; 8: 265-275.

10. GUY-GRAND D, GRISCELLI C, VASSALLI P
    The mouse-gut T lymphocyte, a novel type of T cell. Nature, origin, and traffic in mice in normal and graft-versus-host conditions
    J Exp Med, 1978; 148: 1661-1677.

11. ROBASZKIEWICZ M, JARRY A, BROUSSE N, POTET F
    Cellule M et épithélium associé aux follicules lymphoïdes du tube digestif.
    Gastroentérol Clin Biol, 1989; 13: 473-478.

12. WOLF JL, BYE WA
    The membraneous epithelial (M) cell and the mucosal immune system.
    Ann Rev Med, 1984; 35: 95-112.

13. SPENCER J, FINN T, PULFORD KAF, MASON DY, ISAACSON PG

    The human gut contains a novel population of B lymphocytes which resemble marginal zone cells.

    Clin Exp Immunol, 1985; 62: 607-612.

14. SPENCER J, FINN T, ISAACSON PG

    Human Peyer's patches: an immunohistochemical study.

    Gut, 1986; 27: 405-410.

15. STOOLMAN LM

    Adhesion molecules controlling lymphocyte migration.

    Cell, 1989; 56: 907-910.

16. STREETER PR, BERG EL, ROUSE BTN, BARGATZE RF, BUTCHER EC

    A tissue-specific endothelial cell molecule involved in lymphocyte homing.

    Nature, 1988; 331: 41-47.

17. JALKANEN S, NASH GS, DE LOS TOYOS J, MACDERMOTT RP, BUTCHER EC

    Human lamina propria lymphocytes bear homing receptors and bind selectively to mucosal lymphoid high endothelium.

    Eur J Immunol, 1989; 19: 63-68.

18. SCHMITZ M, NUNEZ D, BUTCHER EC

    Selective recognition of mucosal high endothelium by gut intraepithelial lymphocytes.

    Gastroenterology, 1988; 94: 576-581.

19. KAGNOFF MF

    Immunology of the digestive system.

    In: Physiology of the gastrointestinal tract. Ed. L.R. Johnson.

    Raven Press NY, 1987; 1699-1727.

20. GUY-GRAND D, CERF-BENSUSSAN N, MALISSEN B, MALLASSIS-SERIS M, BRIOTTET C, VASSALLI P

    Two gut intraepithelial CD8+ lymphocyte populations with different T cell receptors: a role for the gut epithelium in T cell differentiation.

    J Exp Med, 1991; 173: 471-481.

21. JARRY A, CERF-BENSUSSAN N, BROUSSE N, SELZ F, GUY-GRAND D

    Subsets of CD3+ (TcR αβ or γδ) and CD3- lymphocytes isolated from normal human gut epithelium display phenotypical features different from their counterparts in peripheral blood.

    Eur J Immunol, 1990; 20: 1097-1103.

22. CERF-BENSUSSAN N, JARRY A, BROUSSE N, LISOWSKA-GROSPIERRE B, GUY-GRAND D, GRISCELLI C

    A monoclonal antibody (HML-1) defining a novel membrane molecule present on human intestinal lymphocytes.

    Eur J Immunol, 1987; 17: 1279-1285.

23. JARRY A, CERF-BENSUSSAN N, BROUSSE N, GUY-GRAND D, MUZEAU F, POTET F

    The same peculiar subset of HML1+ lymphocytes present within normal intestinal epithelium is associated with tumoral epithelium of gastrointestinal carcinomas.

    Gut, 1988; 29: 1632-1638.

24. GUY-GRAND D, DY M , LUFFAU G, VASSALLI P

    Gut mucosal mast cells. Origin, traffic and differentiation.

    J Exp Med, 1984; 160: 12-28.

25. MYHRE MJ, ISAACSON PG

    Primary B-cell gastric lymphoma - A reassessment of its histogenesis.

    J Pathol, 1987; 152: 1-11.

26. SPENCER J, DISS TC, ISAACSON PG

    Primary B-cell gastric lymphoma. A genotypic analysis.

    Am J Pathol, 1989; 135: 557-564.

27. PALS ST, HORST E, SCHEPER RJ, MEIJER CJLM

    Mechanisms of human lymphocyte migration and their role in the pathogenesis of disease.

    Immunol Reviews, 1989; 108: 111-133.

Primary gastrointestinal non-Hodgkin's lymphomas

A. FOURMESTRAUX-RUSKONE, J.-C. RAMBAUD

The digestive tract is frequently involved late in the course of previously diagnosed malignant lymphomas, but primary presentations in this site are much rarer, even if the restrictive definition of primary digestive-tract lymphoma is extended to include all patients with predominant gut lesions without previously diagnosed involvement of peripheral lymph nodes, or who presented initially with symptoms caused by gastrointestinal involvement (1-3). Lymphomas of the western type have to be clearly separated from those of the Mediterranean type (4).

Western-type lymphomas are characterized by focal lesions in the gut with large residual non-lymphomatous areas.

Mediterranean-type non-Hodgkin's lymphomas (NHL) are characterized by an extensive infiltration of the whole or most of the small intestine (and sometimes stomach and colon). They include Immunoproliferative Small Intestinal Disease (IPSID), mainly alpha-chain disease, and nodular and diffuse small cleaved lymphomas often associated with benign follicular lymphoid hyperplasia (5,6).

Lymphomas of the Western type

Epidemiology: premalignant conditions

The reported frequency of gastrointestinal NHL is only 4.5 to 8.7% of all NHL (3).

However, the gastrointestinal tract is the most frequent site of primary extranodal lymphomas (36%). Primary gastrointestinal lymphomas (PGIL) account for 3% of malignant tumours of the stomach, less than 1% of those of the colon and rectum but 12.5% to 18% of those of the small bowel (4,7). Most patients are in the fifth or sixth decade of life and there is a male preponderance (sex-ratio 2:1). Most childhood tumours are Burkitt's or Burkitt-like lymphomas of predominantly ileocaecal location and usually occur in males.

Contrary to former claims, it does not seem that the PGIL of the Western type is more frequent in under-developed countries than in the industrialized world. However, it affects younger patients (6,8).

The aetiology of PGIL has not yet been determined. Adult coeliac disease and the similar small intestinal lesions of dermatitis herpetiformis may be complicated by small bowel lymphomas. A prevalence of 7% of this complication in British patients with adult coeliac disease has been reported, but recent data suggest a much lower frequency (9,11). Usually, NHL complicating adult coeliac disease are located in the small bowel, especially the jejunum (83%), rarely in the stomach (3%) and exceptionally in the colon (1.5%) . Treatment by gluten-free diet seems to decrease the risk (10,11). Interestingly, the mucosal lesions of adult coeliac disease may be in complete remission at the time of diagnosis of NHL whereas, in other cases, lymphoma can be found involved concomitantly with villous atrophy. Primary gut lymphoma can also complicate ulcerative colitis, Crohn's disease and nonspecific jejunoileitis (3,8,12). Extensive small intestinal follicular lymphoid hyperplasia can be associated with or complicated by lymphoma in the absence of immunoglobulin deficiency (3) but not when this pathological entity is associated with common variable hypogamma globulinaemia or selective IgA deficiency.

Other types of immunodeficiency syndromes may be complicated by PGIL: chromosome-related immunodeficiency the with increased IgM, the Wiskott-Aldrich syndrome. The gut is frequently involved in patients with NHL and the acquired immunodeficiency syndrome (17% small bowel and 3.4% rectum), with the majority of them having disseminated lesions (13). Such tumours may also be seen in patients previously treated with radiotherapy, chemotherapy or immunosuppressive therapy (12).

Pathology

Gross features and spread

Non-Hodgkin's PGIL of the Western type are characterized by focal or multifocal (20%) tumours in one or several sections of the gastrointestinal tract. In all series the stomach was the most frequently involved site, 37% to 77% of PGIL (mean=53%), compared with 9% to 55% (mean=29%) and 5% to 20% (mean=11%) of cases in the small bowel and colon respectively (1,2,3,7,12,19). Ileocaecal involvement represents 10% to 20% of cases (mean= 11%), with most cases being reported in children. Appendix involvement is rare and oesophageal involvement is exceptional (1,2,3,7,12,19).

In the small bowel, the frequency of the disease increases from the pylorus to the ileocaecal valve. In the colon, the caecum is more frequently involved, often together with the ileum; rectal tumours are rare.

In the stomach, several patterns may be observed (3,16,21). Large ulcerated lesions completely infiltrating the gastric wall, often multiple, are the most frequent pattern. The depth and size of the ulceration(s) are variable. Large superficial ulcers, especially when they are multiple, may suggest a diagnosis of lymphoma. However, peptic ulcer-like lesions, or more often, erosions with abnormal erythematous intervening mucosa are not rare. Infiltration of the gastric wall often results in giant mucosal folds, which may be associated with the previously described involvement patterns. A nodular or multinodular aspect may be observed.

In the small bowel, different gross patterns have been described (3,22). Large polypoid masses are mostly located in the distal ileum and are often responsible for intussusception. Aneurysmal tumours are pathognomonic of lymphoma, whereas deep ulcerations with raised margins simulate an adenocarcinoma: both are frequently complicated by perforation (20). Annular infiltrations of variable length, sometimes associated with small protruding nodules in the lumen, lead to intestinal obstruction. Composite gross patterns may be observed and multiple lesions in the small bowel are highly suggestive of lymphoma (3).

In the colon, the most frequent appearance of lymphoma is a large, unifocal, circumferential infiltrating and ulcerated mass (22). It is mainly located in the caecum, and it often extends to the terminal ileum. Multiple small polypoid tumours spreading to the whole length of the colon and simulating colonic polyposis may be observed.

Infiltration into surrounding structures is reported to occur in 41% of cases (22). However, it has been claimed that even large tumours can be more easily cleaved from adjacent organs than carcinomas. In our experience, large lesions are often difficult to remove surgically.

Lymphatic spread occurs frequently, and the draining lymph-node groups are involved early in the course of the disease. Thoracic and peripheral lymph nodes are rarely involved. Remote spread to liver, spleen, Waldeyer's ring, bone marrow, meningeal tissues and central nervous system appears more frequent in recent series of carefully staged patients.

The mode of dissemination of PGIL may be different from that of primary nodal or spleen NHL. Indeed, gut-associated lymphoid cells form a distinct compartment with a specific traffic and this could explain the frequency of multiple lesions in the gut and of the association of Waldeyer's ring and gastrointestinal sites (23).

Clinical features

Whatever the site of the lymphoma, three main presenting features can be distinguished (1,3,12,14,22): a) a vague symptomatology, non-specific to gastrointestinal lesion; b) symptomatology suggesting gastrointes-

tinal involvement; c) a surgical complication revealing the lymphoma, often preceded by a period of non-specific symptoms.

The frequency of presenting symptoms and signs in several large series is given in *Table I*. The most common presenting complaint of a patient with PGIL is abdominal pain. The location and character of the pain is dependent upon the site of involvement. Epigastric pain frequently reveals gastric lymphomas. Small bowel and ileocaecal tumours often have a surgical presentation, but it is usually difficult to distinguish in reported series between acute and chronic obstruction and intussusception. However, in the unselected series of small intestinal lymphoma patients reported by Green et al. (20), 60% of patients were first seen with surgical emergencies including 40% with

TABLE I

Presenting symptoms and signs in primary gastrointestinal lymphomas
(Survey of the literature)

	Stomach %	Small bowel %	I. caecum %	Colon-rectum %
Symptoms, %				
Abdominal pain a	54-90	28-79	79-100	50-83
Nausea/vomiting	19-60	17-55	14-38	0-25
Diarrhoea	0-4	3-33	21-38	5-50
Constipation	8-10	8-27	17	0-100
Bleeding	9-32	7-37	14-29	30-62
Anorexia	15-32	11-54	7-23	12-17
Malaise/fatigue	21-31	11-50	-	16-17
Signs, %				
Fever	-	44	+ b	-
Weight loss	18-90	11-94	21-31	12-50
Abdominal or rectal mass	14-30	21-78	29	25-100
Intestinal obstruction	-	16-45	29	11-30
Intussusception	-	0-12	53	0
Peritonitis	4	3-16	0	0

a Including surgical emergencies
b + = Frequent.
Only extreme values are reported because of the lack of homogeneity of different series
(Ref.: 1,2,8,18,40).

peritonitis and 20% with acute obstruction. A period of malaise, fatigue and vague pain often precedes these complications. Weight loss is often said to be mild and the contrast between a short-term clinical history (mean of 6 months) with minimal emaciation and the finding of an abdominal mass is highly suggestive of a lymphoma, but rare. Gastrointestinal bleeding is common in patients with colon or rectal involvement. It is malabsorption syndrome is unusual and is almost always due to coeliac disease associated with the lymphoma and, more rarely, with the spread of tumoral lesions or with the presence of blind loop syndrome.

Diagnosis

Routine biochemical, haematological and immuno-logical investigations are of little help. Anaemia is frequent, but often mild. An increased serum lactate dehydrogenase level indicates rapid growth and/or necrosis of the tumour. As already stressed, malabsorption syndrome (or a protein-losing enteropathy) is rare. There is usually no serum monoclonal immunoglobulin (3,8).

Radiological and endoscopic findings reflect the gross appearance of the lesion. Radiological investigations concern mainly the small intestine (3,24,25): "aneurysmal" dilatation with frequent fissure formation, multiple or extensive abnormalities, and extrinsic compression are highly suggestive of lymphoma (1/3 of cases). However, it is often difficult to distinguish small intestinal lymphoma from other malignant lesions or from a benign tumour or Crohn's disease. Moreover, small bowel X-rays may often miss the lesions.

Endoscopic investigations are not only essential for gastroduodenal and proximal jejunum lesions but also for rectocolic and distal ileal sites. Endoscopy is, of course, combined with multiple-target biopsies and the possibility of macrobiopsy may improve the diagnosis.

The only precise information available concerning the sensitivity of endoscopy and biopsy is for small series of gastric lymphomas. Sensitivity of gastric fribroscopy was 61% for Nelson and Lanza (26) and 62% for Mainget et al. (27), rising to respectively, 90 (27), 92 (28), and 93% (29) with biopsies. However, histological typing of lymphoma on endoscopic biopsies needs qualified pathologists. In 1993, Brousse et al. reported accurate diagnosis of 59% rising to 85% in the case of renewed examination of the histological samples after post-operative confirmation of the lymphoma (30). These data do not take into account the recent progress of immunohistochemistry, which allows precise typing of the cellular infiltrate. Diagnosis specificity of endoscopy with biopsies has not yet been assessed.

Sonography and computed tomography may be of value for the diagnosis of an abdominal mass, but are especially useful for staging and follow-up of the patients (31-33). Guided micro-biopsy and cytological puncture may enhance their diagnostic usefulness. Gastric endoscopic ultrasonography seems a valuable tool in the diagnosis and management of gastric lymphomas. A characteristic endoscopic ultrasonography pattern has been described (thickening of the second, the second and third layers, or a diffuse, transmural thickening of the entire wall), which was confirmed at surgery (34,35). The stage of the tumour was also accurately predicted. It seems possible that in the future endoscopic ultrasonography could play an important role in the detection, the staging, and the treatment planning of gastric lymphomas. Finally, in a very few cases laparotomy may be the only way to confirm a diagnosis of lymphoma (37).

Course

Most deaths from PGIL occur within the first or second year after diagnosis (14,36). Patients without recurrence after a 5-year follow-up are likely to be cured (3,20).

Several prognostic factors have been shown to influence the course of PGIL. The influence of histological type is difficult to assess since in old series the classifications used are obsolete. According to their definition, low-grade lymphomas have a slow course, whereas patients with high-grade tumours have a short survival period. Treament has modified this scheme: whereas a growing proportion of high-grade lymphomas is cured, the long-term survival of low- grade lymphomas has not been markedly improved by chemotherapy. They eventually progress to high-grade lesions. In all series the initial extent of the disease is a significant determinant of PGIL outcome (3,19,38-41). According to the Ann Arbor staging system modified by Musshoff (*Table II*), localized lymphomas (stage IE-II1E) have a significantly better prognosis than disseminated disease (stage II2E, IIIE, IV). Other anatomical parameters are also of importance: large tumours which often invade adjacent tissues and thus cannot be resected surgically point to a poor survival. Age and severe malnutrition often preclude any curative treatment. Some iatrogenic complications specific to PGIL also influence the outcome (3,37). The influence of the above factors on prognosis cannot be dissociated from the therapeutic methods employed. Chemotherapy adapted to the type and stage of the lymphoma has usually been used, invalidating the prognostic value of these parameters.

Therapeutic particularities of PGIL

If chemotherapy (adapted to the histological grade) is the main therapeutic arm in high-grade PGIL as in nodal lymphomas (3,8,19,38,42-44), its place in the treatment of low-grade tumours is much less certain. There is also no current general agreement on the role of locoregional treatment, i.e. surgery or radiotherapy.

Before the introduction of chemotherapy and radiotherapy into the treatment of PGIL, surgery alone was reported to be curative in some "localized" cases. In recent retrospective (42,43,45,46) and prospective studies (19,38,47,48) the influence of tumoral resection on the outcome is clearly suggested. However, it may be suggested that unresectability of the tumour is merely evidence of the poor prognosis of large bulky lesions. There is current agreement that adjuvant chemotherapy is necessary after surgery in high-grade PGIL, with the possible exception of small tumours at stage I. In low-grade tumours, chemotherapy may be unnecessary after a complete surgical resection. The place of abdominal radiotherapy is very ill-defined. It is recommended by some authors instead of surgical resection, but others report a high incidence

TABLE II

Modified Ann Arbor Staging Classification for Digestive Tract non-Hodgkin's Lymphomas.

I_E	Involvement of one or more localized sites of the digestive tract without any lymph-node involvement.
II_E	Involvement of one or more localized sites of the digestive tract and regional lymph nodes without any extra-abdominal lymphomatous involvement. Modification proposed by Musshoff : Stage IIE divided into cases with involvement of regional lymph nodes (II_{1E}) and involvement of regional but non-contiguous lymph nodes (II_{2E}).
III_E	Involvement of lymph-node regions on both sides of the diaphragm with localized involvement of the digestive tract.
IV	Diffuse or disseminated involvement of one or more extralymphatic organs or tissues, with or without associated lymph-node involvement.

of complications related to radiotherapy. In our opinion, this treatment has limited indications, such as localized residual or recurrent lesions or if too large a surgical resection would be necessary in low-grade lymphomas. So far, the superiority of one of these therapeutic schemes over the other has not been demonstrated. Before assessing their therapeutic efficacy by controlled studies, they should be evaluated separately according to clearly identified prognostic factors (37).

Alpha-chain disease, immunoproliferative small intestinal disease and Mediterranean lymphomas

Alpha-chain disease

Alpha-chain disease (alpha-CD) is one of the group of immunoproliferative small intestinal disease, which, by definition, includes all small intestinal lymphoid proliferations with the same pathology as that of alpha-CD, whatever their immunoglobulin product (49).

Epidemiology and aetiopathogenesis

The digestive tract form of alpha-CD mostly affects subjects 15 to 40 years old, without sex predominance. The majority of registered patients originated from the Mediterranean area or from the Middle East, but numerous cases have been reported in subjects from Eastern Europe, the Indian subcontinent, the Far East, Central and South America and sub-Saharan Africa (52). The only common denominators of these patients of various racial and ethnic origin were poor socio-economic status and hygiene.

These particular epidemiological features, together with the complete remissions achieved by antibiotic treatment alone, strongly suggest that sustained intestinal antigenic stimulation, operative since early infancy (in keeping with the young age of most patients), could play a major role in the pathogenesis of the disease (50,51).

According to this hypothesis, it is remarkable that the putative antigenic stimulation leads in nearly all cases to alpha-CD rather than to myeloma. The alpha-CD clone could have a selective advantage for proliferation because of the lack of idiotypic determinants on the surface of the cells, allowing them to elude the normal immunoregulatory process (53).

The postulated environmental antigenic stimulus might be associated with an underlying immunodeficiency (51). This could be a defect which makes the host more susceptible to infection with oncogenic organisms, or a basic defect of the feedback mechanisms controlling the cellular proliferative response to stimulation. Immunodeficiency could be due to malnutrition, especially in early infancy, as suggested by Dutz et al. (54) or to unknown genetic factors.

Pathology

Small-bowel lesions extend to the whole length of the organ or sometimes spare the distal ileum (55,56). When histological lesions are grade A or B, the small intestine has a normal gross external appearance, but there is thickening of the mucosal folds.

At grade C, the small intestinal wall appears diffusely thickened with occasional circumscribed gross tumours frequently located in the jejunum; ulcerations and internal fistulae may also be observed.

Alpha-chain disease lesions can spread to the stomach and the colon and rectum. In a few cases, the disease was limited to one or two of these organs, mainly the stomach, or to the thyroid, and spared the small intestine. One case of generalized lymph-node involvement sparing all mucosae has been recently reported (57). Dissemination of the disease to retroperitoneal, mediastinal, and peripheral lymph nodes, to Waldeyer's ring, to bone marrow, liver and spleen may be observed.

Clinical features

Clinical history and presentation of the intestinal form of alpha-CD are well known (50,52). In short, most patients present either with a malabsorption syndrome and a protein-losing enteropathy, or (especially in underprivileged countries, in which a more delayed diagnosis is frequent), with symptoms, signs or complications of intra-abdominal tumours, usually but not always preceded by chronic diarrhoea.

As alpha-CD intestinal lesions nearly always affect the duodenum and the jejunum, fibre-optic endoscopy with biopsies, using a long-end viewing instrument, is a promising tool for its diagnosis. The Tufrali Group in Tunisia evaluated its usefulness as the first procedure in the investigation of patients suspected clinically of suffering from small intestinal Mediterranean lymphoma (58).

Five primary endoscopic patterns were defined, occurring either alone or in various combinations. The "infiltrated" pattern was the most sensitive (0.80) and specific (0.96) finding, with predictive positive and negative values reaching 0.88 and 0.93; it was followed by the nodular pattern (sensitivity 0.6, specificity 0.84). Other patterns had a low sensitivity and/or specificity. However, the endoscopic appearance of proximal small intestine could not differentiate alpha-CD from non-IPSID ESIL (Extensive Small Intestine Lymphoma), as defined later, whereas endoscopic biopsies with immunohistochemical study of Ig chains in the cytoplasm of infiltrating cells was able to ascertain the diagnosis of alpha-CD in 92% of cases, with no false-positive cases (58).

Immunological diagnosis

In most patients, the alpha-CD protein is present in the serum, but its concentration is low or very low in more than 50% of cases (51). Several methods may be used to ascertain the presence in biological fluids of incomplete alpha chains not linked to light chains. Immunoelectrophoresis combined with immunoselection, using for the latter strong anti-κ and anti-λ antisera to precipi-

tate residual normal IgA proteins, is the most sensitive and 100% specific *(Fig. 1)* (59). It is worth noting that in all cases so far studied the alpha-CD protein belonged to the α-1 sub-class, whereas the percentage of IgA2-cells among IgA-synthesizing plasma cells in the normal intestine is higher than in spleen or peripheral lymph nodes (51,52). Alpha-CD protein is sometimes found in intestinal (60) or gastric (61) juice, being absent from serum.

The synthesis of α-CD protein by the proliferating cells has been demonstrated by immunohistochemical and/or immunocytochemical molecular biology (62,63) methods and by biosynthesis studies *in vitro* (60,61). The latest, as well as membrane-bound Ig studies, have shown that immunoblastic cells of stage C of the disease did synthesize the α-CD protein (51). Moreover, these techniques and molecular biology studies allowed the diagnosis of two "non-secretory" forms of the disease in which the abnormal protein was absent from serum, urine and jejunal juice (59,66).

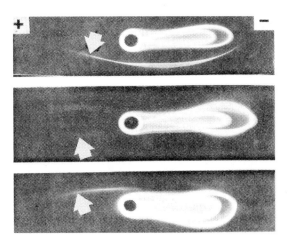

Fig 1: Immunoselection plate of the serum of 3 patients with α-CD. The serum samples have been electrophoresed in agar containing anti-κ and anti-λ antibodies. The troughs contain anti-α antiserum. The precipitin lines given by the freely mobile α-CD proteins are shown by an arrow. (reproduced with permission from Doe et al. Clin Exp Immunol, 1979; 36: 189-197)

Until recently, the monoclonal character of the α-CD proliferation was doubtful. However, the observation in a few cases of κ-chains and no λ-chains bound to cell membrane together with α-chains (64,67) suggested that α-CD was in fact a monoclonal proliferation.

This has been confirmed by recent cytogenetic and molecular biology studies in typical cases of α-CD (62,63,68). In three of four cases, cytogenetic studies on an intestinal tumour or on metastatic mesenteric lymph nodes showed clonal chromosomal abnormalities (69), involving in two cases band 14 q32 of chromosome 14.

Molecular biology studies of the two previous cases with chromosome 14 rearrangement showed three rearranged α bands (62,63). The α-chain mRNA was short (1.2 kb) as compared to that of a normal control (2.0 kb). The cloned α-CD protein cDNA contained about 300 nucleotides 5' at the beginning of the hinge region sequences. These nucleotide sequences differed in the two cases, and, in one of them, did not resemble any previously described sequence.

The α-CD productive genes were modified, as compared to a normal $\alpha 1$ rearranged gene, by the presence of two major deletions, one of the V_H region, and the other of the S α-C_{HI} region. In one of the two cases, two insertions were found.

The establishment of the sequence of these productive α-CD protein [lacking V_H] genes resulted in the production of an abnormal α 1 mRNA lacking V_H, and C_{HI} sequences. Finally, it is worth noting that, although most alpha-CD cellular proliferations do not express light chains, in the two cases mentioned above, a short κ-mRNA (0.9 kb) were found (67). Interestingly, a short κ-chain mRNA has been observed in three other cases of α-CD, in which no synthesis of κ-chains could be detected (67). A possible simultaneous defect of heavy and light chain genes in α (and γ) heavy chain diseases would raise the possibility of a coordinated mechanism related to the oncogenic event leading to these diseases.

These data from molecular biology indicate that genomic abnormalitites are at least partly responsible for the production of alpha-CD proteins and that these proteins are monoclonal from the so-called "benign" phase of the disease. Indeed, in one case mentioned above (66), the same α-gene clonal rearrangement was present from the first stage A of the disease until the final immunoblastic stage C.

Course and treatment

The spontaneous course of α-CD may be relentless or, more frequently, interrupted by periods of clinical improvement often induced by a blind course of antibiotics. Death may occur at any stage because of complications (infections, hypoglycaemia, surgical emergencies) or of cachexia due to malabsorption and tumour growth (6).

Treatment may avoid this fatal outcome. Its modalities depend upon precise knowledge of the extent and histological stage of the disease. Owing to the frequent asynchronism of the histological lesions from one site to another, sampling at a single site is inadequate and laparotomy must be performed. Complete remission should always be ascertained by multilevel gastric, small and large intestinal biopsies studied by immunohistochemical techniques including doublelabelling of κ and λ light chains. A second laparotomy may be necessary in a few cases for accurate evaluation.

Our present therapeutic guidelines are as follows (6). Patients with stage A lesions limited to the gut and to mesenteric lymph nodes should be treated first by oral antibiotics, including metronidazole, which also eradicates frequent infestation by *Giardia lamblia*. Any other parasite should also be eradicated. 39% of 28 patients achieved complete clinical, histological and immunological remission with antibiotic therapy alone, including a case treated without tetracycline. Antibiotics usually have a dramatic effect on the malabsorption syndrome, whether or not a true remission of the disease is obtained.

At stages B and C, antiparasitic and antibiotic treatments are also useful, as they may improve the malabsorption syndrome. Stage C patients with disseminated immunoblastic lesions of the small intestine require an intensive chemotherapy regimen, as far as is allowed by their nutritional state. When a focal tumour is found, its surgical resection followed by combination chemotherapy including an anthracycline may induce a complete and prolonged remission.

Patients with stage-B lesions or with stage-A lesions showing no marked improvement after a 6-month course of antibiotic treatment or a complete remission within 12 months should be given combination chemotherapy. Some of these patients progress to stage-C lesions and die, whereas others apparently remain at stage A and asymptomatic for long periods of time on tetracyclin treatment. The overall complete remission rate in all Tunisian patients was 52% (64.3% for stages B and C), with a survival rate of 67% at 3 years (6). Relapses, sometimes after a long disease-free interval, may occur after treatment at any stage of the disease. As most patients are young, those with disseminated stage-C lesions showing a good response after four cycles of conventional or salvage chemotherapy may be submitted to intensive chemotherapy with autologous bone-marrow transplantation (6).

Supportive therapy by intravenous infusion of water, electrolytes, calcium and magnesium salts, blood or albumin and, in some cases, enteral or total parenteral nutrition, is often necessary before laparotomy and during the early phase of the treatment.

Immunoproliferative small intestinal disease (IPSID) distinct from alpha-chain disease

In a few patients with the typical clinical and pathological features of α-CD, either another monoclonal Ig or polyclonal IgA was secreted (70). Thus, in two cases of IPSID, a complete monoclonal IgA was produced and in a third gamma heavy-chain disease protein was secreted by the cellular proliferation. In the majority of patients (6), the massive small intestinal plasma-cell infiltrate was polyclonal. Among these latter patients, some had very high plasma levels of polymeric IgA. In two such patients in whom detailed immunological studies were performed (71,72), the serum IgA was mostly polymeric, contained J chain and in one case (72) bound to human secretory component (SC) in vitro, and was actively transported in rat bile. Immunohistochemical (71) or jejunal perfusion (73) studies strongly suggested that the availability of SC, which is of epithelial cell origin, and is not regulated by IgA disposal, was the rate-limiting step for the transport of polymeric IgA into the intestinal lumen.

Finally, in some IPSID patients from the Third World, the prominent cell type was mature lymphocyte and non-α-CD protein was found in the serum (74). No cell-marker studies were available in these patients; however, they were performed in two French subjects with similar lesions (74). In one case a polyclonal B-lymphocyte population was found, while in the other a small B-cell component with light-chain restriction was associated with a homogeneous but not necessarily monoclonal population of mature CD8+ cells. No evolution towards an overt lymphoma was observed in any of these patients.

Mediterranean lymphomas

Mediterranean lymphomas were described a few years before α-CD. In spite of repeated attempts to clarify their relationships, confusing reports are still published on this topic. Since the first publications on α-CD, the similarity of epidemiology and clinical pattern with those of the Mediterranean lymphoma as previously described in Israel was stressed, and we have suggested that most of these lymphomas could be unrecognized cases of α-CD (53,75). Thus, we (53) and the WHO (49) have proposed that the term of Mediterranean lymphoma should be restricted to small intestinal lymphomas whose pathology is identical to that of α-CD at any of its histological stages, irrespective of the type of Ig synthesized by the proliferating cells. The two entities were unified by the WHO under the acronym of IPSID.

As outlined above, most patients with IPSID, according to the WHO definition, had secreting and sometimes non-secreting forms of α-CD. On the other hand, is it accurate to classify all cases previously described as Mediterranean lymphoma as IPSID?

In 1982, we reported the study of four young patients born in countries where IPSID is observed and with a clinical history and presentation completely identical to those of this syndrome (73). However, the pathological lesions, consisting of extensive follicular (or nodular) lymphoid hyperplasia of the small intestine associated in one case with multicentric follicular centre-cell (or centrocytic-like) lymphoma or, in some places, higher grade lymphoma, were quite different from those of α-CD, and immunological studies were unable to disclose α-CD protein synthesis or primary Ig deficiency (72). A review of the literature revealed that the few previously described cases of this entity, which must not be confused with multiple lymphomatous polyposis of the gut, had been mainly observed in the same epidemiological context as IPSID.

Thus, one of the goals of the Tufrali Group in Tunisia was to re-evaluate prospectively in this developing Mediterranean country the underlying diseases which would have been previously classified together under the term Mediterranean lymphomas. All patients referred to the Group with suspected intestinal lymphoma from 1981 to 1985 were thoroughly investigated. Among the 55 patients included in the study, 39% had IPSID and α-CD protein synthesis was demonstrated in all of them; 46% showed an extensive cellular proliferation infiltrating either all or the proximal half of the small intestinal mucosa and submucosa, and consisting of follicular lymphoid structures of benign appearance surrounded and more or less destroyed by a malignant lymphoid proliferation of centrocyte-like cells (76). Gross tumour foci, usually of higher malignancy than the diffuse lesions, were found in association with the latter proliferation in nearly half the cases (77). A provisional denomination of non-IPSID ESIL (and not "IPSID without alpha-chain disease"), can be given to these lymphoid proliferations. Finally, 15% of the patients had a Western type, i.e. localized, small intestinal lymphoma, associated in three cases with coeliac disease.

Although IPSID and non-IPSID extensive small intestinal lymphomas have clearly distinctive features in most cases, the findings in a few cases of α-CD associated with follicular lymphoid hyperplasia and centrocytie-like lymphoma suggest the possibility of a transition between the two entities (76).

References

1. LEWIN KJ. RANCHOD H, DORFMAN RF.
   Lymphomas of the gastrointestinal tract. A study of 177 cases presenting with gastrointestinal disease.
   Cancer, 1978; 42: 693 - 707

2. HERRMANN R, PANAHON AM, BARCOS MP, WALSH D, STUTZMAN L.
   Gastrointestinal involvement in non Hodgkin's lymphoma.
   Cancer, 1980; 46: 215 - 222

3. RAMBAUD JC, RUSKONE A.
   Small intestinal lymphomas
   Surv Dig Dis, 1985; 3: 95-113

4. RAMBAUD JC, RUSKONE A.
   Small intestinal lymphomas and alpha-chain disease.
   Clin Gastroenterol, 1983; 12: 743-766

5. RAMBAUD JC, JIAN R, GALLIAN A, SELIGMAN M.
   Maladie des chaînes alpha.
   Presse Med, 1985; 14: 1551 - 1556

6. RAMBAUD JC, HALPHEN M.
   Immunoproliferative small intestinal disease (IPSID) : relationships with alpha-chain disease and "Mediterranean" lymphomas.
   Gastroenterol Int, 1989; 2: 33-41

7. RUSKONE-FOURMESTRAUX A.
   Localisations digestives primitives des lymphomes malins non hodgkiniens de type occidental. Pronostic et traitement.
   Thèse Médecine, Paris, 1986

8. RAMBAUD JC, RUSKONE A, LE LOUARGANT M.
   Localisations digestives des hémopathies malignes.
   In Zittoun R. éd., Encyclopédie des cancers, Paris, Flammarion Médecine Siences, 1987; 423-451

9. SALMERON M, MODIGLIANI R.
   Lymphome malin et maladie coeliaque de l'adulte.
   Gastroenterol Clin Biol, 198; 8: 248-252

10. SPENCER JO, MACDONALD TT, DISSE TC, WALKER-SMITH JA, CICLITIRA PJ, ISAACSON PG.

Changes in intra-epithelial lymphocyte subpopultations in celiac disease and enteropathy associated T cell lymphoma (malignant histiocytosis of the intestine).

Gut, 1989; 30: 339-346

11. LOGAN RF, RIFKIND EA, TURNER ID, FERGUSON A

Mortality in celiac disease.

Gastroenterology, 1989; 97: 265-271

12. SKUDDER PA, SCHWARTZ SI

Primary lymphoma of the gastrointestinal tract.

Surg Gyn Obst, 1985; 160: 5-8

13. ZIEGLER JL, BECKSTEAS JA, VOLBERDING AP et al

Non-Hodgkin's lymphoma in 90 homosexual men.

N Engl J Med, 1984; 311: 565-570

14. BLACKELEDGE G, BUSH H, DODGE OG, CROWTHER D

A study of gastro-intestinal lymphoma.

Clin Oncol, 1979; 5 : 209-219

15. BLACKSHAW AJ

Non-Hodgkin's lymphomas of the gut.

Clin Gastroenterol, 1980; suppl. I: 213-240

16. BROOKS J, ENTERLINE HT

Primary gastric lymphoma. A clinicopathologic study of 58 cases with long term follow-up and literature review.

Cancer, 1983; 51: 701-711

17. FREEMAN C, BERG JW, CUTLER SJ

Occurrence and prognosis of extranodal lymphomas.

Cancer, 1972; 29: 252-260

18. LOEHR JN, MUJAHED Z, ZAHN FD, GRAY GR, THORBJARNARSON B

Primary lymphoma of the gastrointestinal tract : a review of 100 cases.

Am Surg, 1969; 170: 232-238

19. RUSKONE-FOURMESTRAUX and Groupe d'étude des lymphomes malins digestifs de l'adulte. Fondation Française de Cancérologie digestive

Résultats préliminaires.

Gastroenterol Clin Biol, 1989; 13 (2 bis): 6

20. GREEN JA, DAWSON AA, JONES PF, BRUNT PW

The presentation of gastrointestinal lymphoma : a study of a population.

Br J Surg, 1979; 66: 798-801

21. MING SC

Tumors of the oesophagus and stomach.

In : Atlas of tumor pathology, fasc 7. Washington DC US Armed Forces Institute of Pathology 1973

22. WOOD DA

Tumors of the intestine.

In : Atlas of tumor pathology, section VI fasc 22 Washington DC US Armed Forces Institute of Pathology 1967

23. ARNAUD-BATTANDIER F

Le système lymphoïde intestinal ; conceptions actuelles.

Gastroentérol Clin Biol, 1984; 8: 632-640

24. CUPP RE, HODGSON JR, DOCKERTY MB, ADSON MA

Primary lymphoma in the small intestine : problems of roentgenologic diagnosis.

Radiology, 1969; 92: 1355-1362

25. MARSHAK RH, LINDNER AE, MAKLANSKY D

Lymphoreticular disorders of the gastrointestinal tract : roentgenographic features.

Gastrointest Radiol, 1979; 4: 103-120

26. NELSON RS, LANZA FL

The endoscopic diagnosis of gastric lymphoma; gross characteristics and histology.

Gastrointestinal Endoscopy, 1974; 21; 66-68

27. MAINGUET P, DUMONT A, GRUSELLE P, MAOT J

Efficacité diagnostique des biopsies endoscopiques dans les lymphomes gastriques.

Acta Endosc, 1979; 9: 111-117

28. VOINCHET O, YOSHII Y, PROLLA J, KIRSNER JB

Rôle de l'endoscopie dans le diagnostic des tumeurs intramurales de l'estomac.

Arch Fr Mal App Dig, 1975; 62: 385-392

29. SPINELLI, LOGALLO C, PIZZETTI P :

Endoscopic diagnosis of gastric lymphoma.

Endoscopy, 1980; 12: 211-214

30. BROUSSE N, FOLDES C, BARGE J, MOLAS G, POTET F

Intérêt des biopsies endoscopiques dans le diagnostic des lymphomes malins primitifs de l'estomac : études de 29 cas.

Gastroenterol Clin Biol, 1983; 7: 145-149

31. FAKHYR JR, BERK RN

The "target " pattern : characteristic sonographic features of stomach and bowel abnormalities.

Am J Roentgenol, 1981; 137: 969-972

32. NEUMANN CH, ROBET NF, ROSENTHAL D, CANELLOS G

Clinical value of ultrasonography for the management of non-Hodgkin lymphoma patients as compared with abdominal computed tomography

J Comp Ass Tomogr, 1983; 7: 666-669

33. MEGIBOY AJ, BALTHAZARE EJ, NAIDICH DP, BOSNIAK MA

Computed tomography of gastrointestinal lymphoma.

Am J Roentgenol, 1983; 141: 541-547

34. TIO TL, HARTOT TAGER FCA, TYTGAT GN

    Endoscopic ultrasonography in detection and staging of gastric non-Hodgkin's lymphoma. Comparison with gastroscopy, barium meal, and computerized tomography scan.

    Scand J Gastroenterol, 1986; 123 suppl: 52-58

35. CALETTI GC, LORENA Z, BOLONDI L, GUIZZARDI G, BROCCHI E, BARBARA L

    Impact of endoscopic ultrasonography on diagnosis and treatment of primary gastric lymphoma.

    Surgery, 1988; 103: 315-320

36. CONTREARY K, NANCE FC, BECKER WF

    Primary lymphoma of the gastrointestinal tract.

    Ann Surg, 1980; 191: 593-598

37. RAMBAUD JC, NAJMAN A

    Les lymphomes malins primitifs du tube digestif de l'adulte ont des traits particuliers. La laparotomie garde une place pour le diagnostic et le traitement.

    Gastroenterol Clin Biol, 1984; 8: 432-435

38. HERRERA A, SOLAL-CELIGNY Ph, GAULARD P et al

    Lymphomes primitifs du tube digestif. Résultats thérapeutiques dans une série de 35 cas.

    Gastroenterol Clin Biol, 1984; 8: 407-413

39. FILIPPA DA, DE COSSE JJ, LIEBERMAN P, BRETSKY SS, WEINGRAD DN

    Primary lymphomas of the gastrointestinal tract. Analysis of prognosis factors with emphasis on histological type.

    Am J Surg Pathol, 1983; 7: 363-372

40. DAWSON IMP, CORNES JS, MORSON B

    Primary malignant lymphoid tumours of the intestinal tract. Report of 37 cases with a study of factors influencing prognosis.

    Br J Surg, 1961; 49: 80-89

41. FU YS, PERKIN K

    Lymphosarcoma of the small intestine. A clinicopathologic study.

    Cancer, 1972; 29: 654-659

42. RICHARDS MA, GREGORY WM, HALL PA, et al.

    Management of localized non-Hodgkin's lymphoma : the experience at St Bartholomew's Hospital 1972-1985.

    Hematol Oncol, 1989; 7: 1-18

43. BELLESI G, ALTERINI R, MESSORI A et al.

    Combined surgery and chemotherapy for the treatment of primary gastrointestinal intermediate or high-grade non-Hodgkin's lymphomas.

    Br J Cancer, 1989; 60: 244-248

44. RODER JD, FINK U, BABIC R, GOSSNER N, SIEWERT JR

    Primary extranodal non-Hodgkin's lymphomas of the stomach. Value of surgery within the scope of a multimodality treatment concept.

    Chirurg, 1989; 60: 157-162

45. ROSEN HR, HEINZ R, MARCZELL AP, HANAK H

    Lymphoma of the gastrointestinal tract.

    Chirurg, 1988; 59: 244-247

46. MENTZER ST, OSTEEN RT, PAPAAS TN, ROSENTHAL DS, CANELLOS GP, WILSON RE

    Surgical therapy of localized abdominal non-Hodgkin's lymphomas.

    Surgery, 1988; 103: 609-614

47. STEWARD WP, HARRIS M, WAGSTAFF J. et al

    A prospective study of the treatment of high grade histology non-Hodgkin's lymphoma involving the gastrointestinal tract.

    Eur J Cancer Clin Oncol, 1985; 21: 1195-1200

48. SHERIDAN WP, MEDLEY G, BRODIE GN

    Non-Hodgkin's lymphoma of the stomach : a prospective pilot study of surgery plus chemotherapy in early and advanced disease.

    J Clin Oncol, 1985; 3: 495-500

49. World Health Organization Memorandum

    Alpha-chain disease and related lymphoma.

    Bull WHO, 1976; 54: 615-624

50. RAMBAUD JC, SELIGMANN M

    Alpha-chain disease.

    Clin Gastroenteral, 1976; 5: 314-358

51. SELIGMANN M, RAMBAUD JC

    Alpha-chain disease : a possible model for the pathogenesis of human lymphomas.

    In : Good RA, Day SB, eds Comprehensive Immunology, vol IV : The immunology of lymphoreticular neoplasms. New York and London : Plenum Med Book Company, 1978; 425-547

52. RAMBAUD JC

    Maladie des chaînes alpha et lymphome méditerranéen.

    In : Zittoun R, ed. Hémopathies malignes. Paris, Flammarion Médecine-Science, 1986; 554-568

53. RAMBAUD J, MATUCHANSKY C

    Alpha-chain disease. Pathogenesis and relation to Mediterranean lymphoma.

    Lancet, 1973; 1: 1430-1432

54. DUTZ W, ASVADI S, SADRI S, KOHOUT E

    Intestinal lymphoma and sprue : a systematic approach.

    Gut, 1971; 12: 804-810

55. GALIAN A, LECESTE MJ, SCOTTO J, BOGNEL C, MATUCHANSKY C, RAMBAUD JC

    Pathological study of alpha-chain disease with special emphasis on evolution.

    Cancer, 1977; 39: 2081-2101

56. GALIAN A, LE CHARPENTIER Y, RAMBAUD JC

    La maladie des chaînes lourdes alpha.

    In : Nezelof C, ed. Nouvelles acquisitions en pathologie. Paris: Hermann, 1983; 73-112

57. TAKAMASHI K, NAITO M, MATSUOKA Y, TAKATSUKI K

A new form of alpha disease with generalized lymph node involvement.

Path Res Pract, 1988; 183: 717-723

58. HALPHEN M, NAJJART T, JAAFOURA H, CAMMOUN M, Group TUFRALI

Diagnostic value of upper intestinal fiber endoscopy in primary small intestinal lymphoma.

Cancer, 1986; 58: 2140-2145

59. DOE WF, DANON F, SELIGMANN M

Immunodiagnosis of alpha-chain disease.

Clin Exp Immunol, 1979; 36: 189-197

60. RAMBAUD JC, GALIAN A, DANON F, et al

Alpha-chain disease without qualitative serum IgA abnormality. Report of two cases, including a "non-secretory" form.

Cancer, 1983; 51: 683-686

61. COULBOIS J, GALLIAN P, GALLIAN A, COUTEAUX B, DANON F, RAMBAUD JC

Gastric form of alpha-chain disease.

Gut, 1986; 27: 719-725

62. TSARIS A, BENTAROULET M, PILET P et al.

The productive gene for alpha-heavy chain disease protein MA1 is highly modified by insertion deletion.

J Immunol, 1989; 143: 3821-3827

63. BENTABOULL TH, MIHAESCO C, GENDRON MC, BROUET JC, TSARIS A

Genomic aberrations in a case of alpha-chain disease leading to the generation of composite exons from the JH region.

Eur J Immunol, 1989; 19: 2093-2098

64. PREUD'HOMME JL, BROUET JC, SELIGMANN M

Cellular immunoglobulins in human α and δ-chain diseases.

Clin Exp Immunol, 1979; 37: 283-291

65. SELIGMANN M, MIHAESCO E, HUREZ D, MIHAESCO C, PREUD'HOMME JL, RAMBAUD JC :

Immunochemical studies in four cases of alpha chain disease.

J Clin Invest, 1969; 48: 2374-2388

66. MATUCHANSKY C, COGNE M, LEMAIRE M, et al

Maladie des chaînes alpha (MC a) non secrétante de l'intestin : démonstration par l'étude des acides nucléiques.

Gastroenterol Clin Biol, 1988; 12: A 123

67. SMITH WJ, PRICE SK, ISAACSON PG

Immunoglobulin gene rearrangement in immunoproliferative small intestinal disease (IPSID)

J Clin Pathol, 1987; 40: 1291-1297

68. PILLET R, BERGER R, BERNHEIM A, BROUET JC, TSAPIS A.

Molecular analysis of a t (9; 14) (p 11; q 32) translocation occurring in the case of alpha-chain disease

Oncogene, 1989; 4: 653-657

69. BERGER R, BERNHEIM A, TSAPIS A, BROUET JC, SELIGMANN M

Cytogenetic studies in four cases of alpha-chain disease.

Cancer Genet Cytogenet, 1986; 22: 219-223

70. SELIGMANN M, MIHAESCO E, PREUD'HOMME JL, DANON F, BROUET JC

Heavy-chain diseases: current findings and concepts.

Immunol Rev, 1979; 48: 145-167

71. BAKLIEN K, FAUSA O, BRANDTZAEG P, FROLAND S, GJONE E

Malabsorption, villous atrophy, and excessive serum IgA in a patient with unusual intestinal immunocyte infiltration.

Scand J Gastroenterol 1977; 12: 421-432

72. COLOMBEL JF, RAMBAUD JC, VAERMAN JP et al

Massive plasma cell infiltration of the digestive tract. Secretory component as the rate-limiting factor of immunoglobulin secretion in external fluids.

Gastroenterology, 1988; 95: 1106-1113

73. RAMBAUD JC, de SAINT-LOUVENT P, MARTI M et al

Diffuse follicular lymphoid hyperplasia of the small intestine without primary immunoglobulin deficiency.

Am J Med, 1982; 73: 125-132

74. MATUCHANSKY C, TOUCHARD G, BABIN P, LEMAIRE M, COGNE M, PREUD'HOMME JL

Diffuse small intestinal lymphoid infiltration in non-immuno deficient adults from Western Europe.

Gastroenterology, 1988; 95: 470-477

75. SELIGMANN M, RAMBAUD JC

IgA abnormalities in abdominal lymphoma (α–chain disease)

Isr J Med Sci, 1969; 5: 151-157

76. ISAACSON PG, DOGAN A, PRICE SK, SPENCER J

Immunoproliferative small intestinal disease. An immunohistochemical study.

Am J Surg Pathol, 1989; 13: 1023-1033

77. CAMMOUN C, JAAFOURA H, TABBANE F, MOURALI N, HALPHEN M, TUFRALI G

Immunoproliferative small intestinal disease without alpha-chain disease : pathological study.

Gastroenterology, 1989; 96: 750-763

Pathology of gastrointestinal non-Hodgkin's lymphomas

N. BROUSSE, A. GALIAN

Gastrointestinal NHL comprise 2 groups: (1) primary gastrointestinal NHL in which patients present with digestive symptoms and have no previously known superficial lymph-node involvement; (2) secondary gastrointestinal involvement with the same pathological pattern as the primary site. Only primary gastrointestinal NHL will be detailed. They

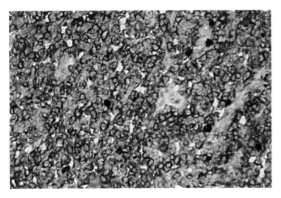

Fig. 1a

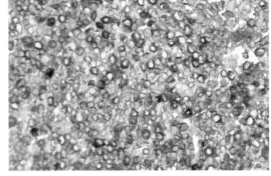

Fig. 1c

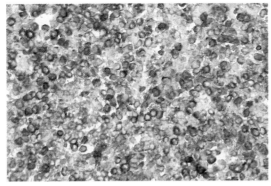

Fig. 1b

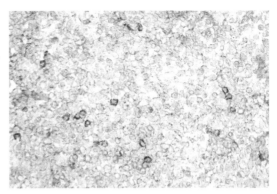

Fig. 1d

Fig. 1: Primary large non-cleaved cell non-Hodgkin's lymphoma of the stomach. Phenotype of tumour cells. Immunoperoxidase technique using anti-pan B CD22 (1a), anti-IgM (1b), anti-kappa (1c) and anti-lambda (1d) monoclonal antibodies. Tumour cells have a B IgM κ phenotype.

TABLE I

Categories of primary gastrointestinal lymphomas
(from P.G. Isaacson (8))

B-cell

1) Low-grade B-cell lymphoma of MALT

2) High-grade B-cell lymphoma of MALT, with or without evidence of a low-grade component

3) Mediterranean lymphoma (immunoproliferative small intestinal disease), low-grade, mixed, or high-grade

4) Malignant centrocytic lymphoma (lymphomatous polyposis)

5) Burkitt-like lymphoma

6) Other types of low- or high-grade lymphoma corresponding to peripheral lymph-node equivalents

T-cell

1) Enteropathy-associated T-cell lymphoma (EATCL)

2) Other types unassociated with enteropathy

---

are usually separated into primary "Western" type and "Mediterranean" type B-cell NHL and T-cell NHL.

All primary digestive NHL originate from the Gut-Associated Lymphoid Tissue (GALT), also called MALT (Mucosa-Associated Lymphoid Tissue) (1), and include B- and T- cell NHL with low- or high-grade malignancy. They include primary NHL of the gastro-intestinal tract and primary NHL of mesenteric lymph-nodes. Classifications of nodal NHL can be used for primary digestive NHL but the distribution between histological types is different (2-4). Among primary gastrointestinal NHL, aggressive histological types are more frequent. Diffuse large-cell and immunoblastic NHL represent 70 to 80% of primary digestive NHL while low-grade NHL represent 20 to 30%. Follicular NHL, such as Burkitt's lymphoma or lymphoblastic NHL, are rarely observed (less than 10%). Conversely, primary mesenteric lymph-node NHL have the same histological patterns as nodal NHL.

Immunohistochemical studies have allowed specification of the phenotype of primary NHL of the gastrointestinal tract. In a recent study of 25 cases (5), 84% were B-cell NHL, with most expressing IgM (*fig. 1*), 8% were T-cell NHL and 8% were of an undetermined phenotype.

Improved knowledge of the normal functions the B and T lymphoid cells of the gastrointestinal mucosa (6,7) and in the clinical, histological, immunological and progressive features of primary digestive NHL has led P. Isaacson to propose a classification (8) (*Table I*).

Gastrointestinal lymphomas of B-cell type

Most often, primary gastrointestinal NHL have a B-cell phenotype, and synthesize κ light chains rather than λ light chains. The

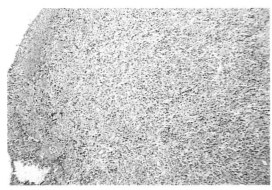

Fig. 2a

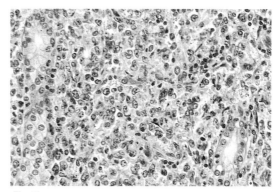

Fig. 3a

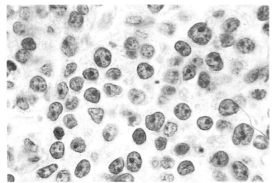

Fig. 2b

Fig. 2: Gastric involvement in a large non-cleaved cell NHL. Low magnification (2a). High magnification (2b).

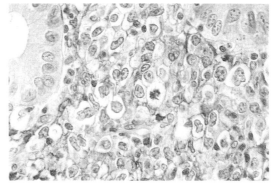

Fig. 3b

IgA phenotype is more frequent in Mediterranean NHL while the IgM phenotype predominates among Western-type NHL. Clinical and pathological data differentiate Western-type NHL from Mediterranean-type NHL.

Gastrointestinal NHL of the Western-type

Diagnostic problems are related to the characteristics of the lymphoid cell proliferation. The malignancy of small-cell proliferations must be confirmed, while large-cell NHL must be distinguished from carcinoma.

Large B-cell NHL (centroblastic or immunoblastic) are the most frequent primary B-cell NHL. In most cases diagnosis is

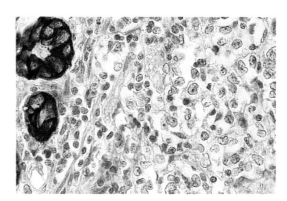

Fig. 3c

Fig. 3: Undifferentiated malignant tumour of the stomach. Pathological pattern of the proliferation (3a). Positive staining of tumour cells with an anti-pan-leukocyte mAb (3b). Negative staining of tumour cells with an anti-cytokeratin mAb while normal epithelial glandular cells express the corresponding antigen (3c). Thus, the immunohistochemical study confirms the lymphoid origin of this tumour.

easily ascertained, even on endoscopic biopsy specimens. The malignant proliferation destroys the mucosa, forming large ulcerations and consists of a diffuse and dense close infiltrate of large cells, with a basophilic cytoplasm and a round and uncleaved nucleus of the centroblastic type (*fig. 2*) or of the immuno-blastic type. Mitoses are numerous. There are often necrotic areas.

When the histological study suggests a diagnosis of "undifferentiated" malignant proliferation, immunohistochemical studies on paraffin-embedded tissues allow easy confirmation of the diagnosis of large-cell NHL. Several monoclonal antibodies (mAB) must be used: one mAb directed against the commom leucocyte antigen (CD45) expressed by lymphoid cells, and one anticytokeratin mAb (KL1) which binds to normal and malignant epithelial cells, even if undifferentiated (*fig. 3*). Using these techniques, it appeared that undifferentiated gastrointestinal carcinomas were very rare. Other mAb can be used to detect epitopes which have not been destroyed by routinely used fixative (9,10) (formalin) and which specify the lymphoid cell pheno-type: most B-cell NHL express CDw75 (LN1), CD74 (LN2) and CD20 (L26). They do not express CD45R0 (UCHL-1), which is expressed on normal and malignant T cells.

Small B-cell NHL must be distinguished from **localized lymphoid hyperplasias:** most (50 to 60%) of these lymphoid hyperplasias are observed in the **stomach:** they are often associated with other disorders: peptic ulcer, chronic gastritis due to *Helicobacter pylori* or follicular gastritis (11-13). In such disorders, lymphoid hyperplasia is an associated immune reaction to the gastric lesion.

In the **rectum**, lymphoid hyperplasia may be observed in several conditions. The most frequent are observed in children, and lymphoid hyperplasia forms "polyps" or "lymphoid polyps" made of lymphoid follicles with large germinal centres. Lymphoid hyperplasia may also be found in ulcerative rectitis, in follicular lymphoid proctitis (16) or in "blind" rectums. All of these disorders have distinctive pathological and immunohistochemical specificities. But in all of them there are large lymphoid follicles with polytypic germinal centres.

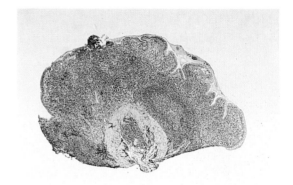

Fig. 4: Gastric endoscopic biopsy. Low-grade malignant NHL of the stomach. Dense infiltration of the mucosa associated with a lymphoid follicle.

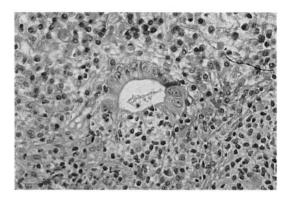

Fig. 5: Gastric endoscopic biopsy. Lymphoepithelial lesion in a low-grade malignant NHL. While plasma cells are found in the superficial part of the lamina propria, deeper zone contains centrocyte-like cells which invade the glandular epithelium.

Like "benign" lymphoid hyperplasias, most primary digestive NHL are located in the stomach. As previously mentioned, small lymphoid cell infiltrations of the stomach suggest either a non-malignant hyperplasia, or a small-cell NHL. In the stomach, 20 to 30% of primary NHL are low-grade small-cell NHL. Most of these cases have been previously classified as non-malignant "pseudolymphomas". Recently, the studies of P. Isaacson and co-workers have led to these entities being considered as primary gastric NHL arising from B lymphocytes of GALT (17). Immunohistochemical and molecular studies have confirmed the monoclonality of the B-cell infiltrate. Pathological characteristics have been extensively described and are found in almost all cases: they include a small-cell infiltrate of the

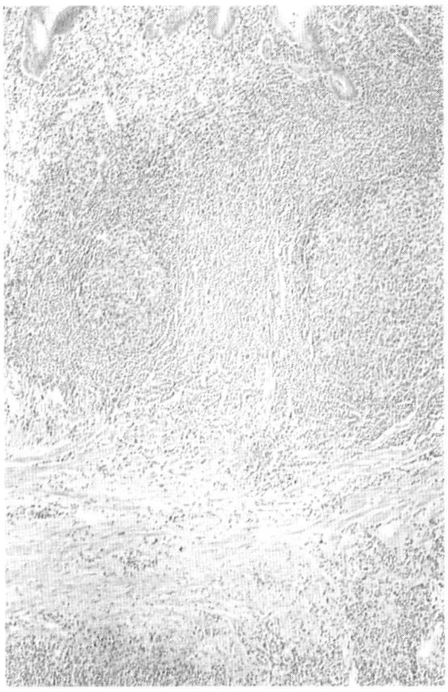

Fig. 6: Follicular hyperplasia in a low-grade malignant NHL of the stomach. Lymphoid follicles usually have a large germinal centre.

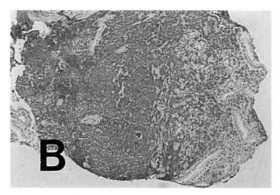

Fig. 7a

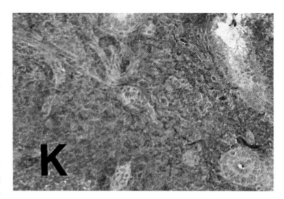

Fig. 7b

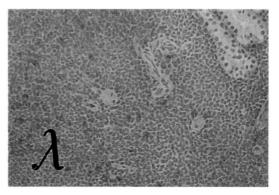

Fig. 7c

Fig. 7: Endoscopic biopsy of the stomach. Low-grade malignant NHL. Phenotype of tumour cells using an immunoperoxidase technique on frozen sections with anti-pan B (CD22) (7a), anti-κ (7b) and anti-λ (7c) mAbs. Tumour cells have a B κ phenotype.

mucosa, lymphoepithelial lesions and follicular hyperplasia. The mucosa contains a close cellular infiltrate (fig. 4), often polymorphous and formed of small lymphocytes, plasma cells, and eosinophil granulocytes, especially in the superficial area of the mucosa. The lymphoid infiltrate is made up of small- or medium-sized cells, with an indented or a cleaved nucleus and a large and clear cytoplasm. These cells have been designated "centrocyte-like" cells (fig. 5) by P. Isaacson.

Plasma cells of the superficial mucosa are most often polytypic (fig. 5). In 30% of cases, they are monotypic and have the same phenotype as the lymphoid infiltrate, demonstrating a plasmocytic differentiation of the malignant B-cell proliferation. Lymphoepithelial lesions are constantly found and are a unique characteristic of this NHL type (fig. 5). They are formed by an infiltration of the glandular epithelium by clusters of centrocyte-like cells. Lymphoepithelial lesions must be distinguished from normal intra-epithelial T lymphocytes, which are isolated and located above the basal membrane. The follicles, located under the centrocyte-like cell proliferation, are hyperplastic with large germinal centres (fig. 6). They are polytypic and non-malignant. They may

be progressively infiltrated and destroyed by the malignant lymphoid cells.

Immunohistochemical studies have confirmed the monotypy of the lymphoid infiltration. Tumour cells express IgM or IgA. They are CD22+ and CD35+ (*fig. 7*). They do not express IgD, CD23 and CD5 antigens. This phenotype is identical to that of normal lymphoid B cells located in the "dome" of the follicles and/or of the normal lymphoid B cells located in the epithelium covering the follicles of Peyer's patches.

Molecular studies have confirmed the clonality of the B-cell proliferation. All these results explain why the name "pseudolymphoma" should no longer be used (18). Recent cytogenetic studies have sought evidence of the bcl-2 gene associated with a t(14;18) translocation in primary digestive NHL. They did not find such a rearrangement in the 21 cases studied, but demonstrated it in 6 of 8 follicular lymph-node NHL. These results suggest that primary digestive NHL of low-grade malignancy do not have a centrofollicular origin (19).

Primary low-grade gastric NHL have a slow course and remain localized in the stomach for a long time. In locally involved lymphnodes, the initial topography is particular, around the follicles. In some cases of smallcell NHL, clusters of large lymphoid cells have been described. In these cases, immunohistochemical studies show the same light-chain isotype of the large-cell component as in the small-cell proliferation, suggesting that large-cell NHL arise from small-cell NHL (20).

In conclusion, not all small-cell lymphoid hyperplasias of the digestive tract are malignant NHL: follicular lymphoid hyperplasia may be found around peptic ulcers; in the ulcerative areas, the cell infiltrate is polymorphous and glands may be destroyed. In such cases, the glands are infiltrated by polymorphonuclears but not by lymphocytes. A diagnosis of NHL must rely on the demonstration of true lymphoepithelial lesions. It is not usually urgent to distinguish between a benign lymphoid hyperplasia and a malignant small-cell NHL lymphoma of low grade malignancy. In some cases, complementary studies are required: multiple sections to demonstrate lymphoepithelial lesions, new endoscopic biopsies and endo-

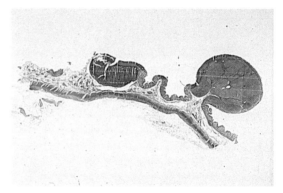

Fig. 8: Lymphomatous polyposis of the small intestine. Multiple polyps at low magnification.

scopic search for multiple lesions. In most cases, a diagnosis of small-cell malignant NHL of the stomach can be ascertained from endoscopic biopsies (*fig. 4*).

Digestive multiple lymphomatous polyposis is a rare (less than 10%) variant type of primary digestive NHL. The clinical and pathological features are typical (21,22). The lesions are disseminated in the gastrointestinal tract. Colonic involvement is almost constant, associated or not with small intestinal involvement. Gastric involvement is frequent. Endoscopy suggests a diagnosis of multiple digestive polyposis and the pathological studies confirm the lymphoid nature of these polyps (*fig. 8*) (23). Typical pathological and immunological features include a monomorphous proliferation of small lymphoid cells, with cleaved nuclei and scanty cytoplasm. They gather to form nodules (*fig. 9*). There is no lymphoepithelial lesion; lymphomatous polyposis is a low-grade malignant NHL, arising from the B cells of the mantle-zone of follicles. Like normal cells of the mantle zone, they express IgM, IgD (*fig. 10*) and CD35 (C3b). Tumour cells also express CD5 (*fig. 10*), normally found on circulating T cells and a minority of normal B cells ("autoreactive" B cells). They do not express CD10 (CALLA). Bone marrow and/or blood, spleen, liver, and peripheral lymph-nodes are frequently involved during the course of multiple lymphomatous polyposis. This entity has not been treated separately in the Working For-

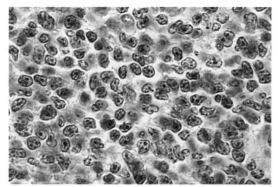

Fig. 9: Lymphomatous polyposis. Polyps are made of a monomorphous proliferation of small cleaved lymphoid cells.

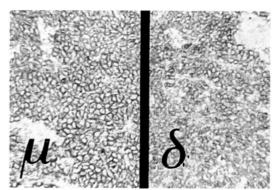

Fig. 10a

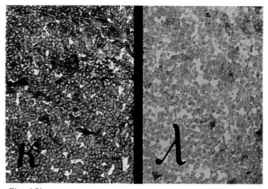

Fig. 10b

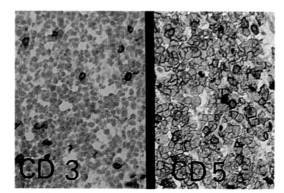

Fig. 10c

Fig. 10: Lymphomatous polyposis. Phenotype of tumour cells using an immunoperoxidase technique on frozen sections with anti-IgM and anti-IgD (10a), anti-κ and anti-λ (10b), anti-CD3 and anti-CD5 (10c) mAbs. Tumour cells have a B, IgM and IgD, κ, CD5+ phenotype.

mulation or in the updated Kiel classification. It has been distinguished in Isaacson's classification (8).

Digestive multiple lymphomatous polyposis must be distinguished from diffuse nodular lymphoid hyperplasia, which has been described in children and adults, associated or not associated with an immune deficiency (24). Diffuse nodular lymphoid hyperplasia is characterized by the development of multiple nodules in the small intestine and/or the colon. These nodules consist of a polyclonal follicular lymphoid hyperplasia, with well-defined germinal centres. Rare associations of diffuse small intestinal nodular lymphoid hyperplasia and malignant lymphoma, most often of high grade, have been described (25,26).

Mediterranean lymphomas, alpha-chain disease and immunoproliferative small-intestinal disease (IPSID)

The relationships between Mediterranean lymphomas, alpha-chain disease and IPSID are confused. As initially described, Mediterranean NHL form an extensive and continuous malignant lymphoid proliferation of the small intestine without any remaining normal mucosa. Alpha-chain disease belongs to the Mediterranean NHL entity. IPSID are disseminated lymphoid proliferations of the small intestine including malignant ones, such as Mediterranean NHL and alpha-chain disease, and non-

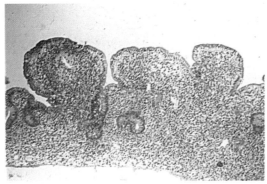

Fig. 11a

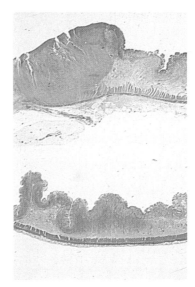

Fig. 12a

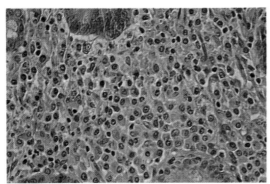

Fig. 11b

Fig. 11: Stage A alpha-chain disease. Jejunum biopsy. A dense infiltration of the lamina propria (11a) with "normal-looking" plasma-cells (11b) may be observed.

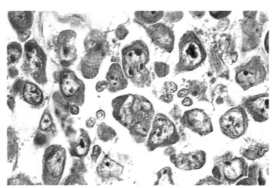

Fig. 12b

Fig. 12: Stage C alpha-chain disease. Multiple tumours infiltrating the jejunum wall (12a). Tumours are formed by an immunoblastic NHL with plasma-cell differentiation (12b).

malignant ones, such as benign lymphoplasmacytic infiltrations of the small intestine.

Pathological characteristics of alpha-chain disease have been described by Galian and co-workers (27,28). In the small intestine, the whole mucosa is involved. Gastric and colonic mucosa may also be involved. Pathological lesions are stratified into 3 stages. In stage A lesions, the cell infiltration is non-invasive, usually limited to the lamina propria and consists of plasma cells of normal appearance (fig. 11). In some cases, lymphocytes are predominant. An immunoblastic NHL with plasma-cell differentiation is typical of stage C lesions (fig. 12). It forms large ulcerating tumours or long thickenings of the small intestine wall. Stage B lesions are an intermediate state between stages A and C: the infiltration involves the submucosa; plasma cells have

significant cytological abnormalities and immunoblasts may be present in the deepest part of the infiltration, sometimes forming clusters. With time, pathological lesions may progress from stage A to stage B and then to stage C. These different stages may also be simultaneously observed in the same digestive segment or in different segments.

Mesenteric lymph-nodes are usually involved except in stage A patients. As in the small intestine, 3 pathological stages

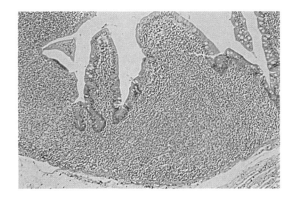

Fig. 13a

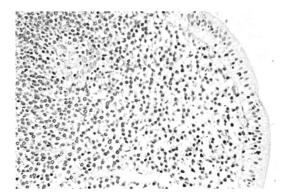

Fig. 13b

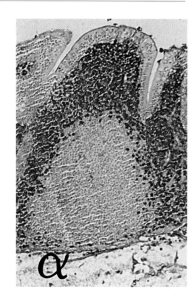

Fig. 13c

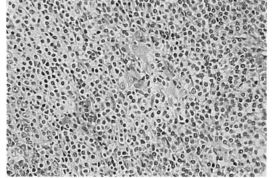

Fig. 13d

Fig. 13: Alpha-chain disease. Follicular lymphoid hyperplasia in the deepest zones of the mucosa (13a). In the superfical parts of the mucosa, the infiltration is made of plasma cells (13b) synthetizing alpha chain (13c). In the intermediate zone, centrocyte-like cells form lymphoepithelial lesions (13d).

have been described, according to infiltration, cell-type and architectural destruction.

Immunohistochemical studies are most useful to establish the diagnosis, especially in non-secreting variants and in the course of the disease if α heavy-chain proteins can no longer be detected in the serum or in the digestive juice while the lymphoproliferation remains detectable in the intestine wall. They disclose α heavy chains in the cytoplasm of tumour cells without any light chain.

In the first studies of MALT lymphomas, Isaacson suggested that α-chain disease had a centrofollicular origin (29). But, more recent studies have demonstrated some similarities between Western type and Mediterranean primary digestive NHL. For instance, in some cases of α-chain disease, appear-

ance is peculiar (fig. 13): a plasma-cell infiltration synthesizing α chains may be seen in the most superficial parts of the lamina propria, associated with a centrocyte-like cell infiltration in the mid zone, and a follicular hyperplasia in the deepest zones. The polyclonal follicles are progressively broken up by the malignant centrocyte-like cell proliferation. The infil-tration of the intestinal crypts, frequently described even in patients with stage A alpha-chain disease, is very similar to the lymphoepithelial lesions of

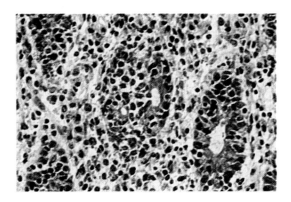

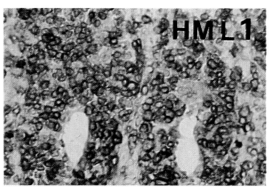

Fig. 14: T-cell NHL of the small intestine associated with coeliac disease. Infiltration of the glandular crypts by tumour cells (Photography by Pr. PG Isaacson).

Fig. 15: T-cell NHL of the small intestine associated with coeliac disease. Phenotype of tumour cells on frozen sections using anti-HML1 MoAb. Tumour cells infiltrating the lamina propria and the epithelium of the crypts express HML1 antigen.

Western-type primary digestive NHL. In alpha-chain disease, centrocyte-like cells contain the same alpha-chain as plasma-cells and have the same clonal origin (30). Although they have different pathological patterns, Mediterranean and Western-type primary digestive NHL probably arise from the same cells of the GALT. They both contain lymphoepithelial lesions and may have a plasmacytic differentiation, constant in alpha-chain disease, and frequent in MALT-derived Western-type NHL.

Gastrointestinal lymphomas of T-cell type

Primary intestinal T-cell NHL have been extensively described and distinguished in Isaacson's classification (8). They are rare, accounting for less than 5% of primary gastrointestinal NHL. Most of them are located in the small intestine. The first primary T-cell NHL were observed in patients with coeliac disease and initally considered as malignant histiocytosis of the small intestine on pathological (azurophilic granules considered as lysosomes) and histochemical criteria (positive stainings for acid phosphatase, non-specific esterase, α1-antitrypsin, lysozyme and chymotrypsin) (31,32). Recently, immunological and molecular studies (33) have confirmed the

T-cell origin of primary digestive NHL associated with coeliac disease. At pathological examination, an infiltration of the epithelium of intestinal glands, which is unusual in primary digestive NHL, has been described (fig. 14). Tumour cells have a peculiar immunological phenotype: they are CD7+ CD3± CD5- CD4- CD8-. They also express an antigen recognized by HML1 mAb (34) (fig. 15), which binds to normal intraepithelial digestive lymphocytes (35). All these results suggest that T-cell NHL associated with coeliac disease originate from intraepithelial lymphocytes. Other phenotypes such as CD4+ and CD8+ have also been described. This primary NHL is now termed "Enteropathy-Associated T-Cell Lymphoma" because of its association with villous atrophy and hyperplasia of mucosal crypts in non-tumoral zones. Enteropathy-associated T-cell lymphomas have a high grade of malignancy. They are pleomorphic with a mixture of large cells, intermediate-size cells, immunoblasts, some showing features of phagocytosis, and eosinophil leucocytes. The epithelium of atrophic but non-tumoral zones may nevertheless contain a few scattered tumour cells. The significance of the villous atrophy remains unknown: whether it is primary, preceding the development of the NHL, or secondary to the T-cell proliferation. In most cases, coeliac disease is discovered simultaneously with the NHL, but in some cases the coeliac desease may precede the dicovery of the NHL. Some patients with adult onset of coeliac disease may have low-grade lymphoma from the onset of their illness (36).

Shepherd (37) has described a T-cell NHL of the small intestine associated with an intense eosinophilic reaction. The tumours are often multiple, sometimes necrotic or ulcerated, and may be revealed by an intestinal perforation. The infiltrate consists of scattered large cells, sometimes multinucleated, and similar to Reed-Sternberg cells. The eosinophilic reaction may be induced by the release by tumoral T cells of eosinophil chemotactic factor (ECF), or interleukins such as IL5 (eosinophilic differentiation factor). Other rare and isolated cases of primary digestive T-cell NHL have been described: immunoblastic CD8+ NHL with azurophilic granules in the cytoplasm of tumour cells (38), or low-grade T-cell NHL (39).

References

1. ISAACSON PG, SPENCER J
   Malignant lymphoma of mucosa-associated lymphoid tissue.
   Histopathology, 1987; 11: 445-462.

2. BROUSSE N, FOLDES C, BARGE J, MOLAS G, POTET F
   Intérêt des biopsies endoscopiques dans le diognostic des lymphomes malins primitifs de l'estomac : étude de 29 cas.
   Gastroenterol Clin Biol, 1983; 7: 145-149.

3. MOORE I, WRIGHT DH
   Primary gastric lymphoma: a tumour of mucosa-associated lymphoid tissue. A histological and immunohistochemical study of 36 cases.
   Histopathology, 1984; 8: 1025-1039.

4. BROOKS JJ, ENTERLINE HT
   Primary gastric lymphoma. A clinicopathologic study of 58 cases with long-term follow-up and literature review.
   Cancer, 1983; 51: 701-711.

5. GROBY WW, WEISS LM, WARNKE RA, MAGIDSON JG, HU E, LEWIN KJ
   Gastrointestinal lymphomas. Immunohistochemical studies on the cell of origin.
   Am J Surg Pathol, 1985; 9: 328-337.

6. JARRY A, CERF-BENSUSSAN N, FLEJOU JF, BROUSSE N
   Le système lymphoïde du tube digestif chez l'homme.
   Ann Pathol, 1988; 8: 265-275.

7. BRANDTZAEG P, HALSTENSEN TS, KETT K et al.
   Immunobiology and immunopathology of human gut mucosa; humoral immunity and intraepithelial lymphocytes.
   Gastroenterology, 1989; 97: 1562-1584.

8. ISAACSON PG, SPENCER J, WRIGHT DH
   Classifying primary gut lymphomas.
   Lancet, 1988; ii: 1148-1149.

9. NORTON AJ, ISAACSON PG
   Lymphoma phenotyping in formalin-fixed and paraffin wax-embedded tissues: I. Range of antibodies and staining patterns.
   Histopathology, 1989; 14: 437-446.

10. NORTON AJ, ISAACSON PG
    Lymphoma phenotyping in formalin-fixed and paraffin wax-embedded tissues: II. Profiles of reactivity in the various tumour types.
    Histopathology, 1989; 14: 557-579.

11. ZAZI JI, SINNIAH R, JAFFREY NA et al.
    Cellular and humoral immune responses in Campylobacter pylori-*associated chronic gastritis.*
    J Pathol, 1989; 159: 231-237.

12. ODES HS, KRAWIEC J, YANAI-INBAR I, BAR-ZIV J.
    Benign lymphoid hyperplasia of the stomach. Report in a young girl and review of the literature.
    Pediatr Radiol, 1981; 10: 244-246.

13. STOLTE M, EIDT S
    Lymphoid follicles in antral mucosa: immune response to campylobacter pylori ?
    J Clin Pathol, 1989; 42: 1269-1271.

14. MOLAS G, POTET F, NOGIG P
    Hyperplasie lymphoïde focale (pseudo-lymphome) de l'iléon terminal chez l'adulte.
    Gastroentérol Clin Biol, 1985; 9: 630-633.

15. RUBIN A, ISAACSON PG
    Florid reactive lymphoid hyperplasia of the terminal ileum in adults: a condition bearing a close resemblance to low-grade malignant lymphoma.
    Histopathology, 1990; 17: 19-26.

16. FLEJOU FF, POTET F, BOGOMOLETZ W et al.
    Lymphoid follicular proctitis. A condition different from ulcerative proctitis ?
    Dig Dis Sci, 1988; 33: 314-320.

17. MYHRE MH, ISAACSON PG

    Primary B-cell gastric lymphoma- A reassessment of histogenesis.

    J Pathol, 1987; 152: 1-11.

18. SPENCER J, DISS TC, ISAACSON PG

    Primary B-cell gastric lymphoma. A genotypic analysis.

    Am J Pathol, 1989; 135: 557-564.

19. PAN L, DISS TC, CUNNINGHAM D, ISAACSON PG

    The bcl-2 gene in primary B-cell lymphoma of mucosa-associated lymphoid tissue (MALT).

    Am J Pathol, 1989; 135: 7-11.

20. CHAN JKC, NG CS, ISAACSON PG

    Relationship between high-grade lymphoma and low-grade B-cell mucosa-associated lymphoid. tissue lymphoma (MALToma) of the stomach.

    Am J Pathol, 1990; 136: 1153-1164.

21. CORNES JS

    Multiple lymphomatous polyposis of the gastrointestinal tract.

    Cancer, 1961; 14: 249-257.

22. ISAACSON PG, McLENNAN KA, SUBBUSWAMY SG

    Multiple lymphomatous polyposis of the gastrointestinal tract.

    Histopathology, 1984; 8: 641-656.

23. AMOUYAL G, BROUSSE N, JARRY A, et al.

    Polypose lymphomateuse digestive : étude d'une observation diagnostiquée par biopsie rectale.

    Gastroenterol Clin Biol, 1988; 12: 255-258.

24. RANCHOD M, LEWIN KJ, DORFMAN RF

    Lymphoid hyperplasia of the gastrointestinal tract. A study of 26 cases and review of the litterature.

    Am J Surg Pathol, 1978; 2: 384-400.

25. MATUCHANSKY C, TOUCHARD G, LEMAIRE M et al.

    Malignant lymphoma of the small bowel associated with diffuse nodular lymphoid hyperplasia.

    N Engl J Med, 1985; 313: 166-171.

26. HARRIS M, BLEWITT RW, DAVIES VJ, STEWART WP

    High-grade non-Hodgkin's lymphoma complicating polypoid nodular lymphoid hyperplasia and multiple lymphomatous polyposis of the intestine.

    Histopathology, 1989; 15: 339-350.

27. GALIAN A, LECESTRE MJ, SCOTTO J, BOGNEL C, MATUCHANSKY C, RAMBAUD JC

    Pathological study of alpha-chain disease with special emphasis on evolution.

    Cancer, 1977; 39: 2081-2101.

28. GALIAN A, LE CHARPENTIER Y, RAMBAUD JC

    La maladie des chaînes lourdes alpha.

    In Nezelof C. (ed): Nouvelles acquisitions en pathologie. Paris, Hermann, 1983; 73-112.

29. SPENCER JO, ISAACSON PG

    Immunology of gastrointestinal lymphoma.

    Clin Gastroenterol, 1987; 1: 605-621.

30. ISAACSON PG, DOGAN A, PRICE SK, SPENCER J

    Immunoproliferative small-intestinal disease. An immunohistochemical study.

    Am J Surg Pathol, 1989; 13: 1023-1033.

31. ISAACSON PG, WRIGHT DH

    Intestinal lymphoma associated with malabsorption. Malignant histiocytosis of the intestine.

    Lancet, 1978; i: 67-70.

32. ISAACSON PG, WRIGHT DH

    Malignant histiocytosis of the intestine.

    Hum Pathol, 1978; 9: 661-677.

33. ISAACSON PG, O'CONNOR NTJ, SPENCER J et al.

    Malignant histiocytosis of the intestine: a T-cell lymphoma.

    Lancet, 1985; ii: 688-691.

34. SPENCER J, CERF-BENSUSSAN N, JARRY A, et al.

    Enteropathy-associated T-cell lymphoma (malignant histiocytosis of the intestine) is recognized by a monoclonal antibody (HLM-1) that defines a membrane molecule on human mucosal lymphocytes.

    Am J Pathol, 1988; 132: 1-5.

35. CERF-BENSUSSAN N, JARRY A, BROUSSE N, LISOWSKA-GROSPIERRE B, GUY-GRAND D, GRISCELLI C

    A monoclonal antibody (HLM-1) defining a novel membrane molecule present on human intestinal lymphocytes.

    Eur J Immunol, 1987; 17: 1279-1285.

36. WRIGHT DH, JONES DB, CLARK H, MEAD GM, HODGES E, HOWELL WM

    Is adult-onset coeliac disease due to a low-grade lymphoma of intraepithelial T lymphocytes?

    Lancet, 1991; 337: 1373-1374.

37. SHEPHERD NA, BLACKSHAW AJ, HALL PA et al.

    Malignant lymphoma with eosinophilia of the gastrointestinal tract.

    Histopathology, 1987; 11: 115-130.

38. KANAVAROS P, LAVERGNE A, GALIAN A, et al.

A primary immunoblastic malignant T lymphoma of the small bowel, with azurophilic intracytoplasmic granules. A histologic, immunologic, and electron microscopy study.

Am J Surg Pathol, 1988; 12: 641-647.

39. ALFSEN GC, BEISKE K, BELL H, MARTON PF

Low-grade intestinal lymphoma of intraepithelial T lymphocytes with concomitant enteropathy-associated T-cell lymphoma: case report suggesting a possible histogenetic relationship.

Hum Pathol, 1989; 20: 909-913.

Cutaneous lymphomas

M. SIGAL-NAHUM, N. BROUSSE, S. BELAICH

The skin, as an organ, presents highly important clinical, pathological and immunological peculiarities. New pathogenic considerations have focused on the peculiar microenvironment of the skin and introduced the concept of skin-associated lymphoid tissue (SALT) (1). Recently, it has been suggested that cutaneous lymphoid cells differ from non-cutaneous lymphoid cells because of the expression of an epitope defined by the HECA-452 antibody. This molecule would seem to play a role either in the homing of lymphoid cells to the skin or in the lymphocyte-epidermis interactions (2).

Secondary cutaneous involvement of a well-known lymphoma is not a matter of diagnosis. But true primary cutaneous lymphomas, especially of low-grade malignancy, may be difficult to distinguish from benign infiltration of the skin.

There is a great variation in terminology and classification of cutaneous lymphomas. Various dermatological classifications have been proposed: morphological classification (monomorphous versus polymorphous cutaneous lymphomas), classification referring to the epidermal migration capacity of lym-

TABLE I

Some clinical criteria for the differentiation of cutaneous T-cell lymphomas from B-cell lymphomas
[from G. Burg (4)]

Small **T**-cell lymphoma	Small **B**-cell lymphoma
Long history (5-20 years)	Short history (1-2 years)
Polymorphous lesions	Uniform lesions
Eczematous lesions, erythema, plaques and tumours	Nodules, tumours
Usually multiple, widespread lesion	Often solitary or sporadic tumours in a given area
Yellowish-brown or pinkish	Deep red, purplish
Eczematous changes with scaling	Smooth surface, without scaling
Late neoplastic lymph-node involvement	Frequent and early neoplastic lymph node involvement

TABLE II

Comparison between cutaneous follicular centre-cell lymphoma and follicular hyperplasia
[from G. Burg (5)]

	Follicular lymphoma	Follicular hyperplasia
Type and distribution	Nodular infiltrate in the deep dermis, often in subcutis	Nodular infiltrate in upper dermis, lower tendency for lower dermis and subcutis
Tingible body macrophages	Often absent	Generally present
Polymorphous population	Present in FCC lymphoma monomorphic in other types	Always present
Immunoglobulin expression	Restricted to one light chain when positive, in and between follicles	Weakly positive, polytypic
Follicular mantle	Variably present	Wide mantles generally present
Reactive cells	Abundant T cells between follicles	Abundant T cells between follicles
Epidermis	Atrophy variably present. Acanthosis rare	Acanthosis or atrophy variably present

phoid cells (epidermotropic cutaneous lymphomas such as mycosis fungoides and non-epidermotropic lymphomas). This topographical classification is easily accessible to a standard histology. More recent immunological classification separates (3) cutaneous T-cell lymphomas usually epidermotropic, from cutaneous B-cell lymphomas.

Some clinical criteria differentiate T-cell from B-cell cutaneous lymphomas (*Table I*) (4). The histological architecture of primary cutaneous lymphomas may, theoretically, be suggestive of the cellular phenotype (*Table II*) (5). A band-like pattern with infiltration of the upper dermis, and exocytosis into the epidermis of single cells or Pautrier microabcesses, are more suggestive of T-cell cutaneous lymphoma, i.e. mycosis fungoides and some adult T-cell leukaemia-lymphoma (ATLL) (6) There is, in fact, a great clinical, cytological and phenotypical

heterogeneity in cutaneous T-cell lymphomas (7,8). A nodular pattern characterized by a sharply demarcated monomorphous infiltrate of the middle and deep dermis and sparing the upper dermis is more evocative of B-cell cutaneous lymphoma. A diffuse, generally non-epidermotropic pattern may be related to any phenotype. Under such conditions, in standard histology, most diagnostically reliable information is given by the morphology of the cells.

In fact, no clear-cut correspondence can be established between histological architecture and cellular phenotype. Consequently, the absence of epidermotropism cannot exclude a cutaneous T-cell lymphoma (i.e. tumoral mycosis fungoides). New immunohistological and genetic methods allow a better classification of T- (9) and B-lymphoid infiltrates, whose malignancy was not easily proved with standard histology.

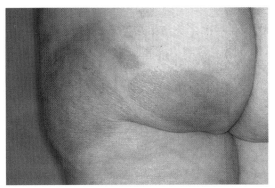

Fig. 1: "Parapsoriasis en plaques". Large erythematous and scaling, well-delineated lesion

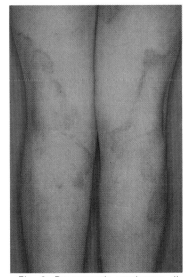

Fig. 2: Pre-mycotic erythema: distinctive and well-delineated lesions

Cutaneous T-cell lymphomas

Primary skin involvement occurs principally in the mycosis fungoides group. In other T-cell lymphomas, primary skin localization may be seen, but staging generally reveals visceral involvement.

Mycosis fungoides, Sézary syndrome and related disorders

Mycosis fungoides (MF)

Clinical presentation

In the MF group, primary cutaneous presentation is the rule and usually remains the only presentation for months and years, so diagnosis is dermatological.

Incidence of this group appears at least equal to that of Hodgkin's disease (10). MF occurs more frequently in men (74% of cases) and 80% of patients are 45 years old or more. Clinical course is generally indolent. After the onset of cutaneous lesions, the median survival is about 10 years (0.8 to 52 years) (11), but only 3.5 years after histological confirmation. More recent studies report a longer median survival period, possibly reflecting improved management and earlier diagnosis (12).

Pathogeny

Determination of the main cell-type involved in MF is essential in understanding the disease. More often, this T cell has functional properties of the T-helper cell (CD4). Like the thymus, the epidermis may be a site for T-cell maturation or differentiation. Epidermis and dermis contain Langerhans cells, lymphoid cells and macrophages. The T cell and peculiar skin micro-environment are involved in immune-response exposure, and certainly in the pathogeny of MF. Likewise, malignant T cells migrate preferentially to lymph-node T zones.

Aetiological factors in MF are unknown: they may be genetic, infectious, oncogenic, or environmental, etc. A viral origin has recently been suggested, and particularly the HTLV-1 retrovirus which is implicated in adult T-cell leukaemia-lymphoma (ATL). Clinical similarities between late-stage aggressive mycosis fungoides and ATL are remarkable. HTLV-1 antibodies were discovered in 11% of cutaneous T-cell lymphomas in Europe (13). This suggests that HTLV-1 may have a role in the pathogenesis of MF (14).

Cutaneous presentation (15,16)

Three clinical presentations are described:

1. The classical form of MF develops over many years through three defined stages: the patch stage, the plaque stage and the tumour stage (11). Initial lesions arise at around 40-60 years and are usually non-specific. Lesions of the patch stage are non-

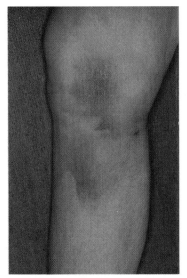

Fig. 3: Mycosis fungoides.
Plaque stage

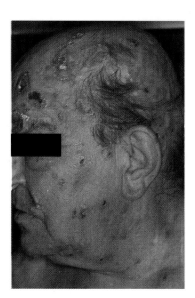

Fig. 5:
Mycosis fungoides. Tumour
stage: ulcerated nodules
and itching lesions

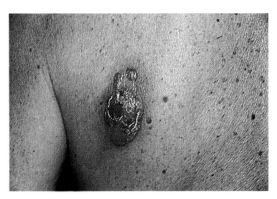

Fig. 4: Mycosis fungoides. Tumour stage

specific, and are described as eczematous or psoriariform dermatitis: these macular lesions are slightly erythematous with a discrete scaling. The premycotic lesions may be associated with severe itching. Present for years, these initial lesions may wax and wane. If MF is suspected, multiple skin biopsies are necessary, but in most cases they remain non-specific. The duration of skin lesions before a definite diagnosis is 4-10 years (range 1 to 48 years) (15,16).

Two cutaneous presentations are more suggestive of the early stage of MF. "Parapsoriasis en plaques" is a large erythematous, and scaling lesion with a well-defined border (fig. 1). In poikiloderma vasculare atrophicans, atrophy with hypo- and hyperpigmentation are associated with telangiectasias.

This classical form progresses in three stages:

- The first stage, **premycotic erythema,** is characterized by well-defined and persistent scaling macules generally of large size and associated with itching. Clear demarcation and figurative forms are highly evocative (fig. 2).

- The erythematous stage then progresses to the **plaque stage** (fig. 3). It is characterized by sharply demarcated papular lesions, oval or circular in shape. These plaques tend to be more stable, and gradually extend. Healing of the centre may give rise to annular figures. These erythematous plaques may be covered with scales or crusts. Itching is frequently a prominent symptom. The plaque stage may occur de novo. At the plaque stage there may appear a peculiar type of follicular degeneration, leading to alopecia: it is characterized by oedema and the presence of mucin in hair follicles. This alopecia mucinosa results from invasion by epidermotropic cells (17).

- **Tumours** or nodules occur late in the course of the patch and plaque stage. They may occur anywhere, on pre-existing lesions or on healthy skin, but have a predilection for the face and body folds. The tumours (fig. 4) are dome-shaped and firm, sometimes ulcerated. Generalization is more or less rapid. Ulceration is not uncommon. Itching may diminish

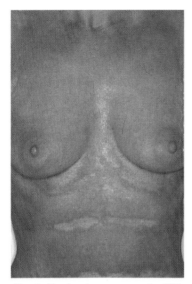

Fig. 6: Erythroderma mycosis (SS): spared areas of normal skin

chromatic, hyperconvoluted, mononuclear cells). However, abnormal circulating cells may be observed in other forms of MF and may be of prognostic significance (24).

Extracutaneous disease

Systemic dissemination is often associated with the evolution from an epidermotropic to a non-epidermotropic phase, and is associated with a poor prognosis. Extracutaneous disease is common at autopsy (72% of cases) (15). Clinically apparent extracutaneous disease is much less commonly detected. Nearly every organ may be involved. The most reliable sign is the enlargement of peripheral lymph nodes. Hepatic, splenic and pulmonary involvement are present in 43 to 52% of patients, and gastrointestinal, kidney, heart and CNS involvement in 18 to 32% of patients (15,18). Bone-marrow involvement is limited and often a late finding (10,19).

Extension

The Ann Arbor classification is not applicable to the MF group since the different subclasses do not reflect the prognostic and clinical course of the disease. Many staging systems have been proposed (20-22). The American MF cooperative group has adapted a uniform staging system (TNM) (4).

Skin involvement (T) (23)

T0: clinically and/or histopathologically suspicious lesions
T1: premycotic lesions, papules or plaques on less than 10% of the skin
T2: premycotic lesions, papules or plaques on more than 10% of the skin
T3: one or more tumours of the skin
T4: extensive, often generalized erythroderma

Peripheral lymph nodes (N)

N0: clinically normal. Pathologically not involved
N1: clinically abnormal. Pathologically not involved
N2: clinically normal. Pathologically involved
N3: clinically abnormal. Pathologically involved

or disappear. This presentation is usually associated with rapid spreading of the disease.

The progressive form is the more usual (11). Median survival after the appearance of the first lesions is about 10 years. Prognosis is worse when tumours are numerous and/or infiltrated areas are large.

2. The presentation of the tumour stage *de novo* (*fig. 5*) may be misdiagnosed for another type of lymphoma, and immunological typing allows correct identification. Prognosis is worse than in the progressive form.

3. Erythroderma MF may be the presenting sign or may occur in the course of a classical form. Clinically, most of the skin surface is involved, and spared areas of seemingly normal skin are highly suggestive (*fig. 6*). Exfoliation or redness may predominate. Lymphadenopathy, itching, alopecia, ectropion, and onychopathy are frequent. Prognosis is unfavourable, with the spontaneous onset of a fatal course within 1 to 2 years.

Sézary syndrome

In the Sézary syndrome (SS), patients have circulating Sézary cells (abnormal hyper-

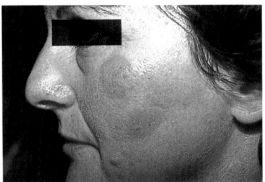

Fig. 7: Pagetoid reticulosis (Woringer-Kolopp disease): erythematous and scaly lesions

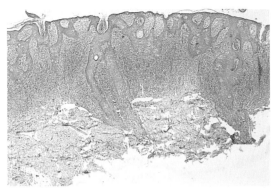

Fig. 9: Mycosis fungoides: band-like infiltrate of the upper dermis

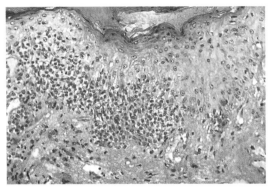

Fig. 8: Pagetoid reticulosis: epidermotropic infiltrate located in deep part of the epidermis

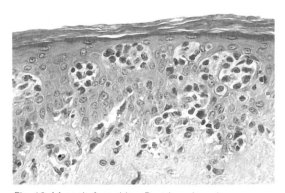

Fig. 10: Mycosis fungoides: Pautrier micro-abcesses

Peripheral blood (B)

B0: atypical circulating cells not present
B1: atypical circulating cells present

Visceral organs (metastasis) (M)

M0: pathologically not involved
M1: pathologically involved

MF-related skin diseases

Other rare skin disorders have been integrated into the MF group. They probably represent a part of the disease spectrum (25-30).

- Pagetoid reticulosis (Woringer-Kolopp disease) (25,27)

This localized form is characterized by a chronic and solitary lesion that is erythematous and scaly (*fig. 7*), with a polycyclic configuration and a sharply demarcated edge. Visceral involvement never occurs. Histopathological study discloses a marked epidermotropic infiltration of a hyperplastic epidermis (*fig. 8*).

Some cases differ by the widespread dissemination of lesions. These cases (the Ketron-Goodman variant) (28) are now considered as MF with extreme epidermotropism (29).

- Granulomatous slack skin

This condition is characterized by progressively appearing pendulous skin folds in flexural areas. Some cases at least are true MF. The superficial dermis and epidermis show histological features indistinguishable from those of MF. There is a granulomatous infiltrate (containing giant cells and granulomatous tubercles) of the deep cutis, and loss of elastic tissue throughout the full thickness of the dermis (26). The disease is indolent, and possibly phagocytosis of lymphocytes by giant cells may limit expansion. Clonality of the T-lymphocyte population was recently demonstrated (30).

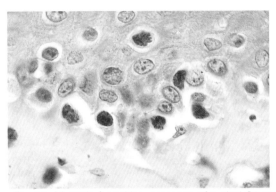

Fig. 11: Mycosis fungoides: presence of typical Sézary cells in epidermis

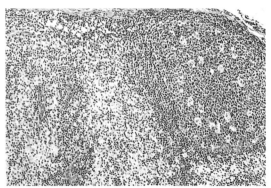

Fig. 12: Mycosis fungoides: tumoral infiltration of para-cortical zones in lymph node

Histopathological manifestations

MF diagnosis requires clinical and histopathological confrontation (4):

a. Typical histological changes associate:

- a band-like infiltrate of the upper dermis extending to the epidermis. One can see single-cell epidermotropism or Pautrier micro-abcesses *(figs. 9,10).*

- cellular infiltrate in MF, typically pleomorphic, and consisting of small to medium-sized lymphoid cells or large blast cells with cerebriform or indented nuclei. Admixture of varying numbers of plasma cells, eosinophils, neutrophils, monocytes and macrophages may be seen. There are small- and large-cell variants of this typical cytomorphological feature. Usually there is an increased number of dilated post-capillary venules within the infiltrate, with prominent endothelial cells.

- Sézary cells *(fig. 11)* with hyperchromatic cerebriform nuclei, typically numerous and highly suggestive, but not specific (31).

b. Histology may be less typical: it may be non-specific, especially at the early stage, or epidermotropism may be absent (at the tumoral stage particularly).

c. Histology may change during the course of the disease: at a late tumoral stage, it often has the aspect of a high-grade malignant T-cell lymphoma (32,33).

Light microscopic diagnosis of MF in the early stage of the disease can be very diffi-

cult. Frequently, skin manifestations are not controversial but standard histological criteria are lacking. Similarly, the unreliability of light microscopic examination in detecting focal invasion in lymph nodes has been recognized by many investigators. Histological changes are attributed to dermatopathic lymphadenopathy (34, 34bis). Lymph node biopsy is mandatory if there is lymph node enlargement. In fact, immunohistochemical (35,36), ultrastructural (37,38) and *in situ* hybridization (39,40) studies have found tumoral cells in histologically non-specific infiltrates in lymph nodes. Initial lesions are found in paracortical T zones *(fig. 12)*. At the stage of lymph-node invasion, MF behaves differently from most other lymphomas (extension along lymphatic chain) (11). However, once the disease leaves the skin, generalized visceral dissemination can be expected. Lymph node invasion seems to occur earlier than previously established: about 27 months after establishment of diagnosis (18). Lymph node invasion is not homogeneous: tumoral lymph node next to lymph nodes wich are simply inflamed.

Various procedures have been used to resolve problems of diagnosis.

1. Electron microscopy

In 1968, Lutzner described the ultrastructural aspects of the Sézary cell in the blood (38). But these cells are not specific and have been detected in skin and lymph-node biopsies during chronic benign dermatitis (41,42).

2. Other methods include morphometric quantification of the nuclear index (43), flow cytometry (44) and cytogenetics (45,46).

All methods are time-consuming and not very sensitive. More recent immunohisto-chemical and genetic methods (39,40) have determined the T-cell nature of the infiltrate and the monoclonality of the cellular prolif-eration.

Immunohistochemical aspects

Mycosis fungoides is a T-cell lymphoma. Blood (Sézary cells), skin and lymph-node tumoral cells usually have a homogeneous phenotype CD3+, CD4+, CD8-, CD1-, mIg- (*fig. 13*). This phenotype corresponds to the phenotype of the normal helper T lympho-cytes (47-52). However, there are few dif-ferences of phenotype related to the involved site; cutaneous tumoral cells are CD7+ DR+ and express transferrin receptor CD71 but blood tumoral cells are CD7- DR- and do not express CD71. DR+ and CD71+ expression seem necessary for a T-lymphoid cell to migrate to the skin (51,53). In fact, MF infiltrates may be heterogenous and T CD8 cells may represent 25% of all cells (55). Moreover, in a few cases, cells express no T-cell antigens (56). For some authors, T CD8 cells predominate at the initial stage of MF (57). When the appearance is heteroge-neous it can be difficult to diffentiate tumoral T-cells from reactive T-cells. More-over, Langerhans CD1+ cells are increased in the dermis and epidermis of patients with MF (49, 58-60). The T CD4 phenotype of cutaneous lymphoid cells is not specific to MF and can be seen in numerous benign cutaneous infiltrates (contact dermatitis, annular granuloma).

In cases of difficult clinical and histological diagnosis, immunohistochemical techniques can establish the diagnosis of lymphoma, if there is either an abnormal antigenic expression or an absence of expression of one or several antigens usually expressed on mature T lymphocytes.

Molecular studies

Rearrangement of genes for the antigen receptor of T cells is a marker of lineage and

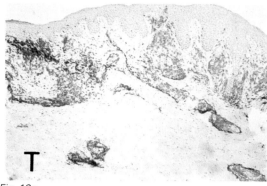

Fig. 13a

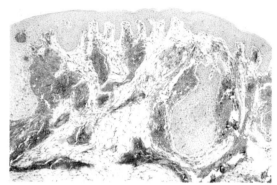

Fig. 13b

Fig. 13: Mycosis fungoides: immunohistochemical aspects. Immunoperoxidase staining using monoclonal antibodies directed against pan-T (CD3, 13a) and Thelper cells (CD4, 13b). The epidermal and dermal infiltrate expresses CD3 and CD4

clonality of a T-lymphoid infiltrate (39,40). This technique is very useful in the diagnosis of lymphoid infiltrates, in differentiating pseudolymphoma from lymphoma and in detecting a minority clonal population among a polyclonal lymphoid infiltrate.

Differential diagnosis

Two major differential diagnoses may be encountered:

- **Actinic reticuloid** is a severe persistent photodermatitis of old patients. It consists of an eczematous, lichenified dermatitis on a sun-exposed area, which may extend to covered skin, forming an erythroderma.

Histology shows a dense polymorphous infiltrate containing atypical lymphocytes with hyperchromatic indented nuclei. Aggregates of mononuclear cells within the epidermis resembling Pautrier's microabcesses can be seen. Furthermore, some cases of actinic reticuloid developing into MF have been published (61). It is uncertain whether chronic actinic dermatitis can lead to induction of an autonomous malignant clone or if these cases are coincidental. A recent immunohistological study shows a predominance of CD8+ cells in the infiltrate of actinic reticuloid (62): this is rarely seen in true MF.

- **Pseudo-lymphomatous** skin reactions resembling MF have been described with drugs (63). Clinically and/or histologically, they are more or less similar to malignant lymphoma. Histology may show cerebriform mononuclear cells and structures Pautrier's micro abcess resembling. However, these structures differ from true structures Pautrier's micro abcess in being composed of histiocytes (63). Moreover, the epidermis shows spongiosis. Cessation of the causative drug results in disappearance of the lesions. Most anticonvulsant drugs can produce the pseudolymphoma syndrome. The most common is diphenylhydantoin.

Other T-cell lymphomas

The other T-cell lymphomas represent a heterogeneous group of neoplasms. Frequency of skin involvement is variable and may reflect patient selection: from 13 to 80% of cases (64-66). These lymphomas may be extra-nodal at the time of presentation (64); however, primary cutaneous presentation is exceptional and staging usually reveals another involved site, especially in high-grade lymphomas (lymphoblastic lymphoma, immunoblastic lymphoma, anaplastic large-cell Ki-1 lymphoma).

We will focus on T-cell chronic lymphocytic leukaemia, adult T-cell leukaemia-lymphoma and anaplastic large-cell lymphoma because of semiological particularities and problems of diagnosis with MF.

T-cell chronic lymphocytic leukaemia (T-CLL)

Cutaneous manifestations are frequently observed in T-CLL (50% of patients) and may appear at the onset of the disease (67). Diffuse erythema or erythroderma are the most common manifestations, and simulates the Sézary syndrome but lesions appear more yellowish. Papulo-nodular lesions and plaques have been described.

Differentiation from the Sézary syndrome may be difficult, but there are no Sézary cells in the peripheral blood and bone-marrow involvement is more frequently found and more extensive in T-CLL than in the Sézary syndrome or MF, where it is commonly absent.

Histopathological study discloses a moderate-to-dense infiltrate in the mid-dermis, but location in the upper dermis with epidermotropism may be seen: lymphocytic cells show round nuclei and lack typical morphological features of Sézary cells (4).

Adult T-cell leukaemia-lymphoma (ATL) (pleomorphic lymphoma related to HTLV-1)

ATL is a peculiar form of peripheral T-cell neoplasia that is related to HTLV-1 infection. It appears to be endemic in certain areas of south-western Japan and clusters have been observed in the Caribbean basin. It has many characteristics common to Sézary syndrome and MF. However, it may be differentiated by its poor prognosis and the presence of viral genome in tumour cells.

Cutaneous manifestations (68) are frequent (43 to 72% of cases) and may be an initial symptom. The dermatological manifestations are polymorphous and vary from papulous to plaque, erythroderma, nodular or tumoral lesions. They may, on rare occasions, become poikilodermic (8). The commonest presentation is a generalized papulous eruption.

Histological features include a dense infiltration of lymphoid cells, most commonly of the pleomorphic type, in the dermis. Epidermotropic infiltrates of neoplastic cells with Pautrier's microabcesses are seen in 17% to 56% of cases (8). Infiltration of the dermis is perivascular, superficial, diffuse or massive in form.

Other symptoms include lymphadenopathy, hepato- and splenomegaly. Hypercalcaemia is quite frequent. This disease is usually leukaemic but a type of lymphoma without leukaemia can occur. Bone-marrow disease is usually mild. Death occurs in less than a year, because of hypercalcaemia, visceral involvement or opportunistic infections. Chronic forms have been reported, often with cutaneous manifestation; hypercalcaemia is absent.

Most cases of ATL belong to the T-helper/inducer subset, CD4 (69), but the T cells appear to function as suppressors of immunoglobulin synthesis *in vitro*. ATL is finally characterized by its association with HTLV-1 retrovirus: HTLV-1-antibodies are present in all cases (13,14). The viral genome has been demonstrated in the nucleus of the pathological cells. It is one of the first cases of neoplasm attributed to a virus in human pathology. However, not all seropositive patients develop a lymphoma: the role of immune supervision has not been clearly established.

Anaplastic large-cell Ki-1 lymphoma (CD30)

Cutaneous presentation is the rule, especially in paediatric series (70,71). Recently, primitive cutaneous anaplastic large-cell Ki-1 lymphoma have been described (72,73). They can remain localized on the skin or they can involve the lymph nodes. Some authors have suggested a more favourable prognosis in the case of primitive cutaneous presentation with a CD30 phenotype. Conversely, a negative CD30 phenotype would seem to correspond to a poor prognosis and rapid generalized dissemination (73). Anaplastic large-cell Ki-1 lymphoma and lymphomatoid papulosis could represent clinical variants of the same entity (72).

Cutaneous T-cell infiltrates: pseudo-, pre- or T lymphomas

The term lymphomatoid vasculitis was proposed (74) to encompass three disorders characterized by infiltration by "dysplastic" lymphocytes associated with vascular injury: lymphomatoid papulosis (LP), lymphomatoid granulomatosis (LG) and angio-immunoblastic lymphadenopathy (AIL). Though they were considered to be "dysplastic" conditions, many authors have reported subsequent evolution to systemic lymphomas. Recently, immunohistochemical and genetic studies have demonstrated the T-lymphomatous nature of most of these cases.

Lymphomatoid papulosis (LP)

This disorder of the skin, described by Macaulay in 1968, is characterized by a continuing self-healing eruption that is clinically benign, but histologically suggestive of malignant lymphoma (75). Clinically, crops of papules and nodules appear (*fig. 14*), become necrotic and heal with scarring in two to six weeks (76). This disease has a chronic course marked by repetitive episodes of healing lesions, often over a period of many years. Histology may differ even in the same patient: schematically, the infiltrate has a tendency for lichenoid distribution and lies in the upper and deep dermis. Infiltration of the epidermis by atypical cerebriform lymphoid cells may occur. Moreover, there is a prominent population of large atypical cells

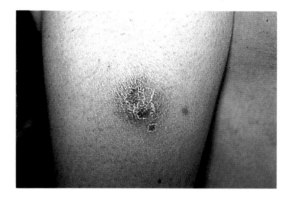

Fig. 14: Lymphomatoid papulosis: necrotic papules

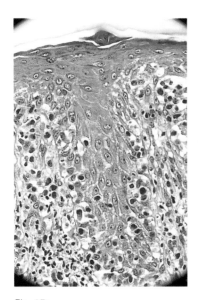

Fig. 15a

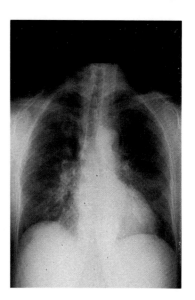

Fig. 17:
Lymphomatoid granulo-
matosis: lung infiltration

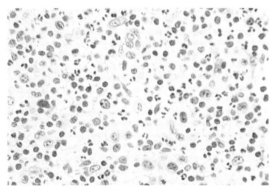

Fig. 15b

Fig. 15: Lymphomatoid papulosis: polymorphous epidermotropic infiltrate. Low (15a) and high (15b) magnification

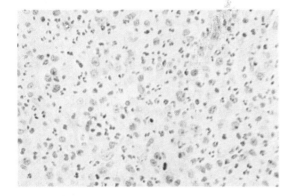

Fig. 16: Lymphomatoid papulosis: immunoperoxidase staining using monoclonal antibody against CD30: large atypical cells express CD30

(fig. 15) that contain cerebriform nuclei or resemble the Reed-Sternberg cells of Hodgkin's disease. In spite of its alarming pathological appearance, the disease generally pursues a benign protracted course. However, there have been several reports of the subsequent emergence of systemic lymphomas in patients with LP (77). Although this entity was first considered to be a pseudo- or a pre-lymphoma (78), molecular studies have identified clonal populations of T cells in a majority of patients with LP (79,80). This result may explain the progression of LP to a "true" lymphoma in about 10 to 20% of cases (76-79). In LP, cells express the Interleukin-2 receptor CD25 (79,81) (fig. 16) that is generally expressed by activated T-lymphoid cells and some lymphomas, and sometimes by Hodgkin's cells (82). A common activated T-helper cell origin for LP, the Reed-Sternberg cells of Hodgkin's disease and some T-cell lymphomas has been proposed (82). In fact, the prognostic significance of immunophenotype and clonality in LP has yet to be defined (79).

Lymphomatoid granulomatosis (LG) and midline granuloma

Liebow's lymphomatoid granulomatosis was initially described as an angiocentric and angiodestructrive lymphoreticular proliferative and granulomatous disease involving predominantly the lungs (fig. 17). It

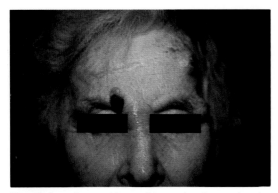

Fig. 18: Lymphomatoid granulomatosis: ulcerated nodular skin lesion

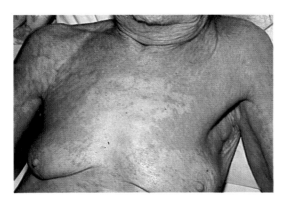

Fig. 19: Angio-immunoblastic lymphadenopathy: cutaneous rash

frequently shows extrapulmonary manifestations when first seen: the most common is cutaneous, occurring in about 20% of cases (83): skin lesions are violaceous plaques or nodules of varying diameter. Necrosis is frequent (*fig. 18*). Systemic involvement occurs months to years later, but prognosis is extremely unfavourable when it appears. Skin histology shows the peculiar feature of invasion of blood vessel walls, nerves and epithelial appendages by an atypical polymorphous infiltrate. LG and midline granuloma are now considered as true peripheral T-cell lymphomas, with T-helper cell phenotype (64,84) and they are classified among the pleomorphic T-cell lymphomas (9).

Angio-immunoblastic lymphadenopathy

In more than 30% of cases, skin lesions are observed (*fig. 19*) and they often precede the development of lymph-node enlargement. The clinical lesions include macu-

lopapular rashes, papular and nodular eruptions (85). Cutaneous necrotizing vasculitis is of unfavourable prognosis (86). Histologically, three cutaneous variants are described (74): a lymphohistiocytic vasculitis, a non-specific peri-vascular infiltrate or a highly characteristic angio-immunoblastic pattern. In fact, this entity is not merely an abnormal immune reaction, but a clonal T-cell proliferation and thus may be interpreted as a T-cell lymphoma (87,88). The proliferating cells are predominantly of CD4 T-helper cell phenotype.

Cutaneous B-cell lymphomas

Cutaneous involvement occurs in about 5% of B-cell lymphomas (89), generally late in the disease. In 1.5 to 2% of cases (90) cutaneous manifestations reveal the disease and remain the sole presentation in about half of the cases (91,92).

Clinical manifestations

These are described in Table 1. Most often these are papules, nodules (*fig. 20*) or plaques and tumours. Even in lymphoma confined to the skin, lesions can be numer-

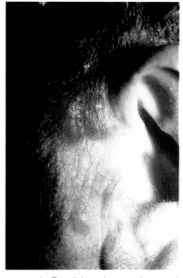

Fig. 20: Non-epidermotropic B-cell lymphoma: deep red cutaneous nodules

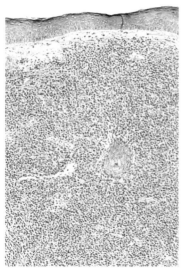

Fig. 21: B-cell lymphoma: non-epi-dermotropic infiltration with sparing of the upper dermis

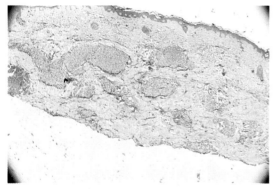

Fig. 22: B-cell lymphoma: "nodular" infiltration located in the mid and deep dermis, predominantly around the vessels and epithelial appendages.

ous and disseminated. Unlike cutaneous T-cell lymphomas, erythema, pruritus and desquamation are rare. Tumoral lesions do not occur on pre-existing lesions.

Staging and prognosis

Primitive B-cell lymphoma confined to the skin has a more favourable prognosis than lymphoma with secondary cutaneous manifestations (92,93). Primitive cutaneous localizations are classified as Ann Arbor stage IE.

Histological aspects

Tumoral infiltration is nodular or diffuse. A

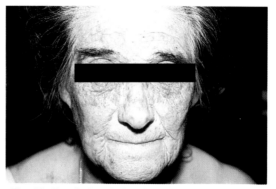

Fig. 23: B-cell chronic lymphocytic leukaemia: papulo-nodular lesions

diffuse pattern, with massive infiltration of the dermis, more or less sparing the papillary dermis (fig. 21), is generally observed in high-grade B-cell lymphomas.

Nodular infiltration is generally encountered in low-grade B-cell lymphomas. With this pattern, differentiation from lymphoid non-tumorous hyperplasia or pseudo-lymphoma may be very difficult. A nodular pattern (fig. 22) in the skin is not synonymous with follicular lymphoma, as it may be in lymph nodes. Other techniques such as immunology or genetic methods are mandatory to confirm the clonality of a nodular infiltrate in the skin (94,95).

Cutaneous B-cell lymphomas of low-grade malignancy

Primary cutaneous involvement is not infrequent in B-cell lymphomas of low-grade malignancy. Differentiation from pseudo-lymphomas may be very difficult on histopathology alone, when the infiltrate is composed of small lymphocytes or mixed-cell population.

B-cell chronic lymphocytic leukaemia

When primary manifestations occur in the skin, patients are usually not leukaemic. Skin lesions (fig. 23) develop in about 20% of patients (96). The presence of nodules on the face may result in the so called "facies leonina". Histologically, small lymphocytic lymphoma of the skin displays the B-cell pattern. The lymphoid population is monomorphous, composed of small lymphocytes, and larger lymphoid cells are inconspicuous. There is no formation of germinal centres. Eosinophils and plasma cells are usually absent. The lymphoid cells are immunologically characterized by a low density of surface immunoglobulins often with coexpression of μ and δ heavy-chain types and are almost always CD5+ (97).

Follicular centre-cell lymphoma

These cutaneous lymphomas are estimated to account for between 18 and 35% of all cutaneous lymphomas (4,7). Primary cutaneous involvement without any systemic manifestation is not uncommon (98-101). Clinically, a great number of patients show skin lesions confined to a circumscribed area. There is a predilection for scalp and forehead. Histological examination may reveal a follicular or diffuse pattern. Small cleaved-cell type, mixed small cleaved- and large-cell or large-cell type may be seen. Most of these lymphomas have lost the expression of immunoglobulins, but express B-lineage markers: CD20+, CD22+ (98,100,101). The host infiltrate constitutes a significant amount of the cutaneous lymphoid infiltrate in the papillary dermis and surrounding the malignant B cells.

This follicular centre-cell cutaneous lymphoma has a low tendency to extracutaneous spread and has a very favourable prognosis (98).

Follicular centre-cell cutaneous lymphoma and small lymphocytic lymphoma may be difficult to distinguish from benign infiltrates of the skin (61,102). Clinically, pseudo-lymphomas may occur as plaques or tumours frequently located on head, ear, nose, scrotum or nipples, and may be quite similar to neoplastic lesions. Histomorphological differentiation may be difficult because pseudo-lymphomas show the B-cell pattern. Some features are said to be more reliable indicators of pseudo-lymphomas: infiltrate located in the upper and mid-dermis, follicle formation with germinal centres, polymorphous infiltrate, acanthotic epidermis. In fact, in primary low-grade B-cutaneous lymphomas, immunophenotypic (103) and genetic (104) studies are mandatory to confirm the clonal nature of the B-cell infiltrate.

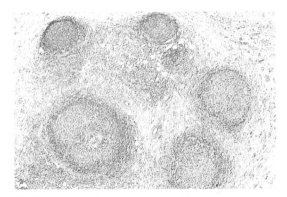

Fig. 24: Skin lymphocytoma/ lymphoid folicles

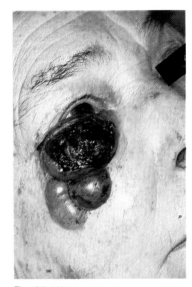

Fig. 25: Waldenström's macroglobulinaemia: ulceronecrotic nodular lessions.

The pseudo-lymphomas simulating B-cell lymphomas are lymphocytoma cutis and Jessner-Kanoff lymphocytic infiltration.

In **lymphocytoma cutis** (*fig. 24*) (cutaneous lymphoid hyperplasia, Spiegler-Fendt sarcoid), the lesions are reddish-brown to purplish, single or multiple. Localized or disseminated nodules occur on the face (ear-lobe particularly) or on the nipples. Histology is characteristic when germinal centres are seen within the infiltrate, giving the appeerence of "a lymph node" in the skin. Some lesions regress spontaneously. The role of spirochaetes (*Borrelia*) is disputed (105).

In **Jessner-Kanoff lymphocytic infiltration**, lesions appear flat, discoid, maculopapular and are pink or red. Their number is variable.

Lesions are located on the face and the back. They tend to regress spontaneously but recurrences may be seen. Borreliosis has been associated with this cutaneous condition (105). Histology has disclosed a predominantly lymphocytic infiltrate around the vessels of the upper and mid-dermis.

Lymphoplasmacytic / cytoid lymphoma, immunocytoma

This group represents 15-20% of all cutaneous neoplasms in Europe (4) but this figure may be less in other parts of the world. Initial skin involvement (*fig. 25*) is frequent, and these cases are more frequent than those with secondary involvement of the skin. Solitary skin tumour is the rule. IgM monoclonal gammopathy is detected in some cases (106,107). Histology shows a B-cell pattern, with a mixed infiltrate of lymphoid and lymphoplasmacytoid cells of different sizes and shapes. Plasma cells are shown to be monoclonal. PAS-positive deposits (IgM) may be seen in the dermis in Waldenström's macroglobulinaemia.

B-cell lymphomas of high-grade malignancy (108)

Primary cutaneous presentation in B-cell lymphomas of high-grade malignancy is exceptional. Involvement of lymph nodes and internal organs develops early in the course of the disease, so diagnosis is not dermatological. These lymphomas include: immunoblastic, lymphoblastic, Burkitt's, and anaplastic large-cell Ki-1 lymphomas.

References

1. SHIMADA S, KATZ SI
   The skin as an immunologic organ.
   Arch Pathol Lab Med, 1988; 112: 231-234.

2. PICKER LJ, MICHIE SA, ROTT LS, BUTCHER EC
   A unique phenotype of skin-associated lymphocytes in humans. Preferential expression of the HECA-452 epitope by benign and malignant T cells at cutaneous sites.
   Am J Pathol, 1990; 136: 1053-1068.

3. EDELSON RL
   Cutaneous T-cell lymphoma. Perspective.
   Ann Intern Med, 1975; 83: 548-552.

4. BURG G, BRAUN-FALCO O
   Cutaneous lymphomas, pseudo-lymphomas and related disorders.
   Springer Verlag, 1983.

5. BURG G, KERL H, PRZYBILLA B, BRAUN-FALCO O
   Some statistical data, diagnosis and staging of cutaneous B-cell lymphomas.
   J Dermatol Surg Oncol, 1984; 10: 256-262.

6. TAKIJAWA M, INOUES F, IWATSUKI K, YAMADA M
   Does adult T-cell leukemia/lymphoma belong to the cutaneous T-cell lymphoma?
   J Am Acad Dermatol, 1988; 18: 379-381.

7. WOOD GS, BURKE JS, HORNING S, DOGGETT RS, LEVY R, WARNKE RA
   The immunologic and clinicopathologic heterogeneity of cutaneous lymphomas other than mycosis fungoides.
   Blood, 1983; 62: 464-472.

8. JIMBOW K, TAKAMI T
   Cutaneous T-cell lymphoma and related disorders. Heterogeneity in clinical, histopathologic, phenotypic and fine structural expressions.
   Int J Dermatol, 1986; 25: 485-497.

9. SUCHI T, LENNERT K, YU LY, KIKUCHI M, SATO E, STANSFELD AG, FELLER AC
   Histopathology and immunochemistry of peripheral T-cell lymphomas. A proposal for their classification.
   J Clin Pathol, 1987; 40: 995-1015.

10. EDELSON RL
    Cutaneous T-cell lymphoma.
    J Dermatol Surg Oncol, 1983; 9: 641-644.

11. EPSTEIN E, LEVIN D, CRAFT J, LUTZNER MA
    Mycosis fungoides: survival, prognostic features, response to therapy and autopsy findings.
    Medicine, 1972; 5: 61-72.

12. TOBACK AC
    Pathogenesis of cutaneous T-cell lymphoma.
    Dermatol Clin, 1985; 3: 605-614.

13. LANGE WANTZIN G, THOMSEN K, NISSEN N
    Occurrence of HTLVI antibodies in cutaneous T-cell lymphoma.
    J Am Acad Dermatol, 1986; 15: 598-602.

14. LANGE WANTZIN G
    Cutaneous T-cell lymphoma and retrovirus infection.
    Dermatologica, 1988; 176: 221-223.

15. BUNN PA, CARNEY DN
    Manifestations of cutaneous T-cell lymphoma.
    J Dermatol Surg Oncol, 1980; 6: 369-377.

16. DEGOS R, CIVATTE J, BELAICH S
Dermatologie.
Flammarion Ed (France), 1981.

17. EMMERSON RW
Follicular mucinosis. A study of 47 patients.
Br J Dermatol, 1969; 81: 395-413.

18. LONG JC, MIHM MC
Mycosis fungoides with extra-cutaneous dissemination: a distinct clinico-pathologic entity.
Cancer, 1974; 34: 1745-1755.

19. SALHANY KE, GREER JP, COUSAR JB, COLLINS RD
Marrow involvement in cutaneous T-cell lymphoma. A clinicopathologic study of 60 cases.
Am J Clin Pathol, 1989; 92: 747-754.

20. FUKS ZY, BAJSHAW MA, FARBER EM
Prognostic signs and the management of mycosis fungoides.
Cancer, 1973; 32: 1385-1395.

21. THOMSEN K
Scandinavian mycosis fungoides trial.
Cancer Treat Rep, 1979; 63: 709-711.

22. VONDERHEID EL
Evaluation and treatment of mycosis fungoides lymphoma.
Int J Dermatol, 1980; 19: 182-188.

23. LAMBERT SI, GREEN SB, BYAR DP et al.
Clinical staging for cutaneous T-cell lymphomas.
Ann Intern Med, 1984; 100: 187-192.

24. SCHECHTER GP, SAUSVILLE EA, FISHMANN B ET AL
Evaluation of circulating malignant cells provides prognostic information in cutaneous T-cell lymphoma.
Blood, 1987; 69: 841-849.

25. WOOD GS, WEISS LM, HU CH, ABEL EA, HOPPE RT, WARNKE RA, SKLAR J
T-cell antigen deficiencies and clonal rearrangements of T-cell receptor genes in pagetoid reticulosis (Woringer-Kolopp disease).
N Engl J Med, 1988; 318: 164-167.

26. LE BOIT PE, ZACKHEIM HS, WHITE CR
Granulomatous variants of cutaneous T-cell lymphoma. The histopathology of granulomatous mycosis fungoides and granulomatous slack skin.
Am J Surg Pathol, 1988; 12: 83-95.

27. WORINGER F, KOLOPP P
Lésion érythémato-squameuse polycyclique de l'avant-bras évoluant depuis 6 ans chez un garçonnet de 13 ans.
Ann Dermatol Syphil, 1939; 10: 945-948.

28. KETRON L, GOODMAN M
Multiple lesions of the skin apparently of epithelial origin resembling clinically mycosis fungoides.
Arch Dermatol Syphil, 1931; 24: 758-785.

29. TAN RSH, MAC LEOD TIF, DEAN SG
Pagetoid reticulosis, epidermotropic mycosis fungoides and mycosis fungoides: a disease spectrum.
Br J Dermatol, 1987; 116: 67-77.

30. LE BOIT PE, BECKSTRAD JH, BOND B
Granulomatous slack skin: T-cell β-chain rearrangements is evidence of the lymphoproliferative nature of a cutaneous elastolytic disorder.
J Invest Dermatol, 1987; 89: 183-186.

31. BENDELAC A, O'CONNOR NJJ, DANIEL MT et al.
Non-neoplastic circulating Sézary-like cells in cutaneous T-cell lymphoma. Ultrastructural, immunologic, and T-cell receptor gene rearrangement studies.
Cancer, 1987; 60: 980-986.

32. SALHANY KE, COUSAR JB, GREER JP, CASEY TT, FIELDS JP, COLLINS RD
Transformation of cutaneous T-cell lymphoma to large-cell lymphoma. A clinico-pathologic and immunologic study.
Am J Pathol, 1988; 132: 265-277.

33. SCHEEN SR, BANKS PM, WINKELMANN RK
Morphologic heterogeneity of malignant lymphoma developing in mycosis fungoides.
Mayo Clin Proc, 1984; 59: 95-106.

34. WECHSLER J, DIEBOLD J, GERARD-MARCHANT R
Les localisations ganglionnaires des lymphomes malins épidermotropes (mycosis fongoïde et syndrome de Sézary).
Bull Cancer (Paris), 1984; 71: 89-99.

34bis VONDERHEID EC, DIAMOND LW, LAI SM, AU F, DELLAVECCHIA MA
Lymph node histopathologic findings in cutaneous T-cell lymphoma. A prognostic classification system based on morphologic assessment.
Am J Clin Pathol, 1992; 97: 121-129

35. SLATER DN, ROONEY N, BLEEHEN S, HAMED A
The lymph node in mycosis fungoides: a light and electron microscopy and immunohistological study supporting the Langerhans' cell-retrovirus hypothesis.
Histopathology, 1985; 9: 587-621.

36. WEISS LM
Immunophenotypic differences between dermatopathic lymphadenopathy and lymph node involvement in mycosis fungoides.
Am J Pathol, 1985; 120: 179-185.

37. LUTZNER MA, HOBBS JW, HORVATH P
Ultrastructure of abnormal cells in Sezary's syndrome, mycosis fungoides and para psoriasis en plaque.
Arch Dermatol, 1971; 103: 375-386.

38. LUTZNER MA, JORDAN HW
The ultrastructure of an abnormal cell in Sézary's syndrome.
Blood, 1968; 31: 719-736.

39. WALDMANN TA, DAVIS MM, BONGIOVANNI KF, KORSMEYER SJ

Rearrangements of genes for the antigen receptor of T cells as markers of lineage and clonality in human lymphoid neoplasms.

N Engl J Med, 1985; 313: 776-783.

40. WEISS LM, HU E, WOOD GS, MOULDS C, CLEARY ML, WARNKE R, SKLAR J

Clonal rearrangements of T-cell receptor genes in mycosis fungoides and dermatopathic lymphadenopathy.

N Engl J Med, 1985; 313: 539-544.

41. GUCCION JG, FISCHMANN AB, BUNN PA, SCHECHTER GP, PATTERSON RH, MATTHEWS MS

Ultrastructural appearance of cutaneous T-cell lymphomas in skin, lymph nodes and peripheral blood.

Cancer Treat Rep, 1979; 63: 565-580.

42. VAN DER PUTTE SCJ, VAN DER MEER JB

Mycosis fungoides: a morphological study.

Clin Exp Dermatol, 1981; 6: 57-67

43. VAN DER LOO EM, VAN VLOTEN WA, CORNELISSE CJ, SCHEFFER E, MEIJER C

The relevance of morphometry in the differential diagnosis of cutaneous T-cell lymphomas.

Br J Dermatol, 1981; 104: 257-269.

44. VAN VLOTEN WA, SCHABERG A, VAN DER PLOEG M

Cytophotometric studies on mycosis fungoides and other cutaneous reticuloses.

Bull Cancer, 1977; 64: 249-258.

45. WHANG-PENZ J, BUNN PA, KNUSTEN T et al.

Cytogenetic abnormalities in patients with T-cell lymphoma.

Cancer Treat Rep, 1979; 63: 575-580.

46. JOHNSON GA, DEWALD GW, STRAND WR, WINKELMANN RK

Chromosome studies in 17 patients with Sézary syndrome.

Cancer, 1985; 55: 2426-2433.

47. NASU K, SAID J, VONDERHEID E, OLERUD J, SAKO D, KADIN M

Immunopathology of cutaneous T-cell lymphomas.

Am J Pathol, 1985; 119: 436-447.

48. KUNG PC, BERGER CL, GOLDSTEIN G, LOGERFO P, EDELSON RL

Cutaneous T-cell lymphoma. Characterization by monoclonal antibodies.

Blood, 1981; 57: 261-266.

49. CHU A, PATTERSON J, BERGER C, VONDERHEID E, EDELSON R

In situ study of T-cell subpopulations in cutaneous T-cell lymphoma. Diagnostic criteria.

Cancer, 1984; 54: 2414-2422.

50. THIVOLET J, SCHMITT D, SOUTEYRAND P, BROCHIER J

Les cellules des lymphomes épidermotropes (mycosis fongoïde et syndrome de Sézary). Etude grâce aux anticorps monoclonaux.

Nouv Presse Med, 1982; 11: 3033-3038.

51. SCHMITT D, THIVOLET J

Use of monoclonal antibodies specific for T-cell subsets in cutaneous disorders: II. Immunomorphological studies in blood and skin lesions.

J Clin Immunol, 1982; suppl. 2, 3: 111-119.

52. RALFKIAER E, WANTZIN GL, MASON DY, HOU JENSEN H, STEIN H, THOMSEN K

Phenotypic characterization of lymphocyte subsets in mycosis fungoides. Comparison with large plaque parapsoriasis and benign chronic dermatoses.

Am J Clin Pathol, 1985; 84: 610-619.

53. HAYNES BF, HENSLEY LL, JEGASOTHY BV

Phenotypic characterization of skin infiltrating T cells in cutaneous T-cell lymphoma: comparison with benign cutaneous T-cell infiltrates.

Blood, 1982; 60: 463-473.

54. HARDEN EA, HAYNES BF

Phenotypic and functional characterization of human malignant T-cells.

Semin Hematol, 1985; 22: 13-26.

55. HOLDEN CA, MORGAN EW, Mc DONALD DM

The cell population in the cutaneous infiltrates of mycosis fungoides: in situ studies using monoclonal antisera.

Br J Dermatol, 1982; 106: 385-392.

56. Mc MILLIAN EM, WASIK R, BEEMAN K, EVERETT MA

In situ *immunologic phenotyping of mycosis fungoides.*

J Am Acad Dermatol, 1982; 6: 888-897.

57. IWAHARA K, HASHIMOTO K

T-cell subsets and nuclear contour index of skin infiltrating T cells in cutaneous T-cell lymphoma.

Cancer, 1984; 54: 440-446.

58. SHAMOTO M

Langerhans cells increase in the dermal lesions of adult T-cell leukaemia in Japan.

J Clin Pathol, 1983, 36, 307-311.

59. Mc KIE RM

A monoclonal antibody technique to demonstrate an increase in Langerhans cells in cutaneous lesions of mycosis fungoides.

Clin Exp Dermatol, 1982; 7: 43-47.

60. ROWDEN G, LEWIS MG

Langerhans cell-involvement in the pathogenesis of mycosis fungoides.

Br J Dermatol, 1976; 95: 665-672.

61. BRODELL RT, SANTA CRUZ DJ

Cutaneous pseudo-lymphomas.

Dermatol Clinics, 1985; 3: 719-734.

62. NORRIS PG, MORRIS J, SMITH NP, CHU AC, HAWK LJM

    Chronic actinic dermatitis: an immunohistologic and photobiologic study.

    J Am Acad Dermatol, 1989; 21: 966-970.

63. KARDAUN SH, SCHEFFER E, VERMEER BJ

    Drug-induced pseudolymphomatous skin reactions.

    Br J Dermatol, 1988; 118: 545-552.

64. WEIS JW, WINTER MW, PHYLIKY RL, BANKS PM

    Peripheral T-cell lymphomas. Histologic, immunohistologic and clinical characterization.

    Mayo Clin Proc, 1986; 61: 411-426.

65. HORNING SJ, WEISS LM, CRABTREE GS

    Clinical and phenotypic diversity of T-cell lymphomas.

    Blood, 1986; 67: 1578-1582.

66. ARMITAGE JO, GREEN JP, LEVINE AM et al.

    Peripheral T-cell lymphoma.

    Cancer, 1989; 63: 158-163.

67. BONVALET D, FOLDES C, CIVATTE J

    Cutaneous manifestations in chronic lymphocytic leukemia.

    J Dermatol Surg Oncol, 1984; 10: 278-282.

68. CHAN HL, SU IJ, KUO TT ET AL

    Cutaneous manifestations of adult T-cell leukemia/lymphoma: report of three different forms.

    J Am Acad Dermatol, 1985; 13: 213-219.

69. MAEDA K, TAKAHASHI M

    Characterization of skin infiltrating cells in adult T-cell leukaemia/lymphoma (ATLL): clinical, histological and immunohistochemical studies on eight cases.

    Br J Dermatol, 1989; 121: 603-612.

70. KADIN ME, SAKO D, BERLINER ET AL

    Childhood Ki-1 lymphoma presenting with skin lesions and peripheral lymphadenopathy.

    Blood, 1986; 68: 1042-1049.

71. SCHNITZER B, ROTH MS, HYDER DM, GINSBURG D

    Ki-1 lymphomas in children.

    Cancer, 1988; 61: 1213-1221.

72 KAUDEWITZ P, STEIN H, DALLENBACH F et al.

    Primary and secondary cutaneous Ki-1+ (CD30) anaplastic large-cell lymphomas.

    Am J Pathol, 1989; 135: 359-367.

73 BELJAARDS RC, MEIJER CJLM, SCHEFFER E ET AL

    Prognostic significance of CD30 (Ki-1/Ber-H2). Expression in primary cutaneous large-cell lymphomas of T-cell origin. A clinicopathologic and immunohistochemical study in 20 patients.

    Am J Pathol, 1989; 135: 1169-1178.

74. MURPHY GF, MIHM MC

    Benign, dysplastic and malignant lymphoid infiltrates of the skin: an approach based on pattern analysis. In lymphoproliferative disorders of the skin.

    Murphy G.F., Mihm M.C. Eds. Butterworths 1986; pp. 123-141.

75. MACAULAY WL

    Lymphomatoid papulosis: a continuing self-healing eruption, clinically benign-histologically malignant.

    Arch Dermatol, 1968; 97: 23-30.

76. SANCHEZ NP, PITTELKOW MR, MULLER SA, BANKS PM, WINKELMANN RK

    The clinicopathologic spectrum of lymphomatoid papulosis: study of 31 cases.

    J Am Acad Dermatol, 1983; 8: 81-94.

77. WANTZIN GL, THOMSEN K, BRANDUP F, LARSEN JK

    Lymphomatoid papulosis. Development into cutaneous T-cell lymphoma.

    Arch Dermatol, 1985; 121: 792-794.

78. ESPINOZA CG, ERKMAN-BALIS B, FENSKE NA

    Lymphomatoid papulosis: a pre-malignant T-cell disorder.

    J Am Acad Dermatol, 1985; 13: 736-743.

79. HARRINGTON DS, BRADDOCK SW, BLOCHER KS, WEISENBURGER DD, SANGER W, ARMITAGE JO

    Lymphomatoid papulosis and progression to T-cell lymphoma: an immunophenotypic and genotypic analysis.

    J Am Acad Dermatol, 1989; 21: 951-957.

80. WEISS LM, WOOD GS, TRELA M, WARNKE RA, SKLAR J

    Clonal T-cell populations in lymphomatoid papulosis.

    N Engl J Med, 1986; 315: 475-479.

81. VARGA FJ, VONDERHEID EC, OLBRICHT SM, KADIN ME

    Immunohistochemical distinction of lymphomatoid papulosis and pityriasis lichenoides et varioliformis acuta.

    Am J Pathol, 1990; 136: 979-987.

82. KADIN M, NASU K, SAKO D, SAID J, VONDERHEID E

    Lymphomatoid papulosis: a cutaneous proliferation of activated helper-T cells expressing Hodgkin's disease-associated antigens.

    Am J Pathol, 1985; 119: 315-325.

83. JAMBROSIC J, FROM L, ASSAAD DA, LIPA M, SIBBALD RG, WALTER JB

    Lymphomatoid granulomatosis.

    J Am Acad Dermatol, 1987; 17: 621-631.

84. FOLEY JF, LINDER J, KOH J, SEVERSON G, PURTILO D

    Cutaneous necrotizing granulomatous vasculitis with evolution to T-cell lymphoma.

    Am J Med, 1987; 82: 839-844.

85. LESSANA-LEIBOWITCH M, MIGNOT L, BLOCH C

Manifestations cutanées des lymphadénopathies angio-immunoblastiques.

Ann Dermatol Venereol, 1977; 104: 603-610.

86. ARCHIMBAUD E, COIFFIER B, BRYON P et al.

Prognostic factors in angioimmunoblastic lymphadenopathy.

Cancer, 1987; 59: 208-212.

87. WEISS LM, STRICKLER JG, DORFMAN RF, HORNING SJ, WARNKE RA, SKLAR J

Clonal T-cell populations in angio-immunoblastic lymphadenopathy and angio-immunoblastic lymphadenopathy-like lymphoma.

Am J Pathol, 1986; 122: 392-397.

88. WATANABE S, SAKO Y, SHIMOYAMA M, MINATO K, SHIMOSATO Y

Immunoblastic lymphadenopathy, angio-immunoblastic lymphadenopathy and IBL-like T-cell lymphoma. A spectrum of T cell neoplasia.

Cancer, 1986; 58: 2224-2232.

89. RISDALL R, HOPPE RT, WARNKE R

Non-Hodgkin's lymphoma. A study of the evolution of the disease based upon 92 autopsied cases.

Cancer, 1979; 44: 529-542.

90. KIM H, DORFMAN RF

Morphological studies of 84 untreated patients subjected to laparotomy for the staging of non-Hodgkin's lymphoma.

Cancer, 1974; 33: 657.

91. EVANS HL, WINKELMANN RK, BANKS GS

Differential diagnosis of malignant and benign cutaneous lymphoid infiltrates.

Cancer, 1979; 44: 699-717.

92. BURKE JS, HOPPE RT, CIBULL MC, DORFMAN RF

Cutaneous malignant lymphoma: a pathologic study of 50 cases with clinical analysis of 37.

Cancer, 1981; 47: 300-310.

93. LONG JC, MIHM MC, QAZI R

Malignant lymphoma of the skin. A clinicopathologic study of lymphoma other than mycosis fungoides diagnosed by skin biopsy.

Cancer, 1976; 38: 1282-1296.

94. ARNOLD A, COSSMAN J, BAKHSHI A, JAFFE ES, WALDMANN TA, KORSMEYER SJ

Immunoglobulin gene rearrangements as unique clonal markers in human lymphoid neoplasms.

N Engl J Med, 1983; 309: 1593-1598.

95. KURTIN P, MURPHY GF, MIHM MC

Lymphoma cutis: B-cell pattern in lymphoproliferative disorders of the skin.

Murphy G.F., Mihm M.C. Ed, Butterworths 1986, 142-159.

96. BURG G, KANDEWITZ R, KLEPZIG K, PRZYBILLA B, BRAUN-FALCO O

Cutaneous B-cell lymphoma.

Dermatol Clin, 1985; 3: 689-704.

97. BROUET J, SELIGMANN M

Chronic lymphocytic leukaemia as an immunoproliferative disorder.

Clin Hematol, 1977; 6: 169.

98. WILLEMZE R, MEIJER CJLM, SENTIS HJ et al.

Primary cutaneous large cell lymphomas of follicular center-cell origin.

J Am Acad Dermatol, 1987; 16: 518-526.

99. KERL H, KRESBACH H

Germinal center-cell-derived lymphomas of the skin.

J Dermatol Surg Oncol, 1984; 10: 291-295.

100. GARCIA CF, WEISS LM, WARNKE RA, WOOD GS

Cutaneous follicular lymphomas.

Am J Surg Pathol, 1986; 10. 454-463.

101. PIMPINELLI N, SANTUCCI M, BOSI A et al.

Primary cutaneous follicular center-cell lymphoma. A lymphoproliferative disease with favourable prognosis.

Clin Exp Dermatol, 1989; 14: 12-19.

102. BURG G, KERL H, SCHMOECKEL C

Differentiation between malignant B cell lymphomas and pseudo-lymphomas of the skin.

J Dermatol Surg Oncol, 1984; 10: 271-275.

103. MEDEIROS LJ, PICKER LJ, ABEL FA et al.

Cutaneous lymphoid hyperplasia. Immunologic characteristics and assessment of criteria recently proposed as diagnosis of malignant lymphoma.

J Am Acad Dermatol, 1989; 21: 929-942.

104. WOOD GS, NGAN BY, TUNG R et al.

Clonal rearrangements of immunoglobulin genes and progression to B-cell lymphoma in cutaneous lymphoid hyperplasia.

Am J Pathol, 1989; 135: 13-19.

105. ABELE DC, ANDERS KH

The many faces and phases of borreliosis II.

J Am Acad Dermatol, 1990; 23: 401-410.

106. SIGAL M, FOLDES C, GROSSIN M, POCIDALO MA, BASSET F, BELAICH S

Localisations cutanées spécifiques d'une maladie de Waldenström.

Ann Dermatol Vénéréol, 1985; 112: 763-764.

107. SWANSON NA, KEREN DF, HEADINGTON JT

Extramedullary IgM plasmocytoma presenting in skin.

Am J Dermatopathol, 1981; 3: 79-83.

108. STANSFELD AG, DIEBOLD J, NOEL H et al.

Updated Kiel classification for lymphomas.

Lancet, 1988; i: 292-293.

Non-Hodgkin's lymphomas of the mediastinum

P. SOLAL-CÉLIGNY, M. PEUCHMAUR, N. BROUSSE

Primary non-Hodgkin's lymphoma (NHL) of the mediastinum has been defined as disease within the mediastinum in patients presenting with symptoms due to an enlarging mediastinal mass (1). Patients in whom staging procedures disclose extra-thoracic NHL involvement are included in some series (2,3,5) but not in others (1,4). The incidence of primary NHL of the mediastinum is about 10 % of all NHL [17 out of 184 NHL patients (9 %) in ref. 1, 25 out of 215 (12 %) in ref. 2]. Two histological groups are largely predominant among primary NHL of the mediastinum : lymphoblastic lymphomas which share all the clinical, histological and immunological features of this category *(see pp. 107-156)* and a more recently described group of diffuse large-cell lymphomas with sclerosis.

This latter group has several clinical, histological and immunological specificities. Patients are predominantly young females. In the largest series of 60 cases (5), the median age was 25 years with 85 % of the patients 35 years or younger. The male-to-female ratio was 1:2.5. Other series confirm these demographic data (1-11,14,16). Symptoms at presentation are rapid in onset and most often associate several of the following: shortness of breath, dry cough, chest and/or back pain, dysphagia, weight loss. Superior vena cava syndrome is the most frequent sign [30 % to 52 % of patients (5,8,9)]. Among patients with superior vena cava syndrome secondary to NHL, 64 % had diffuse large-cell NHL (10). Chest radiographs and CT scans usually show a bulky and rapidly enlarging mediastinal mass. Proximity invasion of chest wall, pec-

toralis muscles, pericardium, pulmonary parenchyma and/or pleura is frequent (2,4,5). Extrathoracic sites are rare at presentation; they are more frequent in relapsing patients, especially affecting kidneys (5-8), adrenal cortex (8) and/or retroperitoneal lymph nodes (5-8). Bone-marrow infiltration is usually not found at presentation (7,8). This most patients [73 % in the series of 60 patients reported by Perrone and colleagues (5)] show no evidence of extrathoracic disease at presentation and are in clinical stage I or II±E of the Ann Arbor staging system.

The diagnosis of diffuse large-cell lymphoma may be difficult to establish on a specimen obtained by mediastinoscopy or thoracotomy because of the extent of associated sclerosis. It has sometimes been misdiagno-

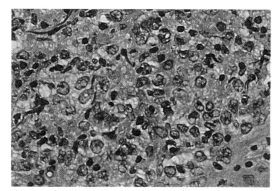

Fig. 1 : *Medistinal lymphoma : infiltration by large tumour cells with a clear cytoplasm*

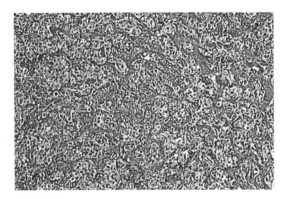

Fig. 2 Mediastinal lymphoma compartmentalization of tumour cells by collagen fibres

sed (5) and considered as malignant thymoma, seminoma or Hodgkin's disease. Immunohistological studies confirm the lymphoid origin of this tumour. Tumour cells are large, often with a clear cytoplasm. The nuclei are round, cleaved or multilobated. Sclerosis is always present to a varying degree. A typical aspect of "compartmentalization" of tumour cells by bundles of collagen has been described *(Fig.1)*. This fibrous stroma separates cells into nests thus mimicking carcinoma.

Immunohistochemical studies allow confirmation of the diagnosis. Tumour cells always have a B-cell phenotype (6,7,11). It is now known that normal thymus contains a B-cell subpopulation. These normal B-cells are present within the medulla and extraparenchymal septa. They have a unique immunophenotype, being uniformly reactive with antibodies to CD19, CD20, CD22 and immunoglobulin heavy chain μ and δ, uniformly non-reactive with antibodies to complement receptors (CD21 and CD35) and reactive with antibodies to κ or imunoglobulin light chains (11,12,15,17). Neo-plastic B-cells have a very similar immunophenotype and these intrathymic B-cells may be the normal counterpart of the malignant cells of mediastinal diffuse large-cell lymphomas (6,9,11).

Recently, 2 cases of low-grade NHL of the thymus with typical histological features of MALT lymphomas have been reported (13). These lymphomas may arise from lymphoid cells associated with the epithelium of Hassal's corpuscles which can be considered as a mucosal organ.

Results of the treatment of patients with primary large-cell NHL of the mediastinum remain controversial. All the published series are retrospective and patients were treated either with radiotherapy alone or, in most cases, with chemotherapy and radiotherapy. In all the reported series, radiotherapy alone appeared inadequate, especially in patients with bulky disease. In some series, the prognosis appeared poor (1,3,7), with median survival between 13 (1) and 23 months (7) as most patients relapsed even after combined modality treatment. In other series (2,8), combined chemotherapy and radiotherapy produced better results: long-term complete remission in 8/12 patients (8), and a 59 % disease-free 5-year actuarial survival in another series of 30 patients (2). These discrepancies in the results of similar treatments remain unexplained. In all these series, the chemotherapy regimens used belong to the so-called first generation regimens (CHOP and/or variants). Results of the treatment of primary NHL of the mediastinum using more aggressive chemotherapy regimens have recently been reported. In one small series of 15 patients treated with an aggressive regimen (MACOP-B or M-BACOD), CR was obtained in 13 cases with only one relapse and a disease-free survival plateau of 90 %.

The role of radiotherapy combined with chemotherapy has still to be ascertained. In a non-randomized series (10), the survival of patients treated with chemotherapy and radiotherapy was similar to that of patients treated with chemotherapy alone but the frequency of local relapses was lower.

References

1. LICHTENSTEIN AK, LEVINE A, TAYLOR CR et al.
   Primary mediastinal lymphoma in adults.
   Am J Med, 1980; 68: 509-514.
2. YOUSEM SA, WEISS LM, WARNKE RA
   Primary mediastinal non-Hodgkin's lymphomas: a morphologic and immunologic study of 19 cases.
   Am J Clin Pathol, 1985; 83: 676-680.

3. TRUMP DL, MANN RB

   Diffuse large cell and undifferentiated lymphoma with prominent mediastinal involvement. A poor prognostic subset of patients with non-Hodgkin's lymphoma.

   Cancer, 1982; 50: 277-282.

4. LEVITT LJ, AISENBERG AC, HARRIS NL, LINGGOOD RM, POPPEMA S

   Primary non-Hodgkin's lymphoma of the mediastinum.

   Cancer, 1982; 50: 2486-2492.

5. PERRONE T, FRIZZERA G, ROSAI J

   Mediastinal diffuse large-cell lymphoma with sclerosis: a clinicopathologic study of 60 cases.

   Am J Surg Pathol, 1986; 10: 176-191.

6. ADDIS BJ, ISAACSON PG

   Large-cell lymphoma of the mediastinum: a B-cell tumor of probable thymic origin.

   Histopathology, 1986; 10: 379-390.

7. HAIOUN C, GAULARD P, ROUDOT-THORA-VAL F et al.

   Mediastinal diffuse large-cell lymphoma with sclerosis: a condition with a poor prognosis.

   Am. J Clin Oncol, 1989 ; 12: 425-432.

8. TODESCHINI G, AMBROSETTI A, MENEGHI-NI V et al.

   Mediastinal large B-cell lymphoma with sclerosis: a clinical study of 21 patients.

   J Clin Oncol, 1990; 8: 804-808

9. LAMARRE L, JACOBSON J, AISENBERG AC et al.

   Primary large-cell lymphoma of the mediastinum: a histologic and immunophenotypic study of 29 cases.

   Am J Surg Pathol, 1989; 13: 730-739.

10. PEREZ-SOLER R, Mc LAUGHLIN P, VELAS-QUEZ WS et al.

    Clinical features and results of management of superior vena cava syndrome secondary to lymphoma.

    J Clin Oncol, 1984; 2: 260-266

11. DAVIS RE, DORFMAN RF, WARNKE RA

    Primary large-cell lymphomas of the thymus: a diffuse B-cell neoplasm presenting as primary mediastinal lymphoma.

    Hum Pathol, 1990; 21: 1262-1268.

12. ISAACSON RG, NORTON AJ, ADDIS BJ

    The human thymus contains a novel population of B lymphocytes.

    Lancet, 1987; 2: 1488-1491.

13. ISAACSON PG, CHAN JKG, TANG D, ADDIS BJ

    Low-grade B-cell lymphoma of Mucosa-Associated Lymphoid Tissue arising in the thymus. A thymic lymphoma mimicking myoepithelial sialadenitis.

    Am J Surg Pathol, 1990; 14: 342-351.

14. JACOBSON JO, AISENBERG AC, LAMARRE L et al.

    Mediastinal large-cell lymphoma. An uncommon subset of adult lymphoma curable with combined modality therapy.

    Cancer, 1988; 62: 1893-1898.

15. MOLLER P, MOLDENHAUER G, MOMBURG F et al

    Mediastinal lymphoma of clear cell type is a tumor corresponding to terminal steps of B-cell differentiation.

    Blood, 1987; 69: 1087-1095.

16. MILLER JB, WARIAKOJIS D, BITRAN JD et al.

    Diffuse histiocytic lymphoma with sclerosis: a clinico-pathologic entity frequently causing superior venocaval obstruction.

    Cancer, 1981; 47: 748-756.

17. HOFMANN WJ, MOMBURG F, MOLLER P

    Thymic medullary cells expressing B-lymphocyte antigens.

    Hum Pathol, 1988; 19: 1280-1287.

Non-Hodgkin's lymphomas of the lung

P. SOLAL-CÉLIGNY, C. DARNE, N. BROUSSE

Pulmonary involvement in NHL

Almost all reports on pulmonary involvement in NHL were published during the years 1970-80 and used plain chest radiography for diagnosis. Reported incidences were 3.7% in previously untreated patients (1) and higher figures [19% (2) to 31% (3)] if patients at presentation and in relapse were included. Using more sensitive diagnosis techniques such as CT scan, prevalence may be even higher. Lung involvement has been considered as the most frequent extranodal localization in cutaneous T-cell lymphomas (4-6).

Histological and immunohistochemical studies of pulmonary involvement disclose a spectrum of NHL similar to nodal NHL.

According to a recent study, there is a relationship between cytogenetic aberrations and lung involvement. Eight out of ten patients (80%) with chromosome 9 abnormalities showed clinical evidence of pulmonary involvement versus 8% of patients without chromosome 9 abnormalities (7).

As in all extranodal sites, pulmonary involvement is frequent in HIV-associated non-Hodgkin's lymphoma. It was diagnosed in 8 out of 88 patients *ante-mortem* (8) and found in 8 out of 12 patients at autopsy (9).

Usually, pulmonary sites are asymptomatic or may be revealed by non-specific symptoms: dry cough, dyspnoea, chest pain. In rare cases, there was acute respiratory failure due to the rapid onset of pulmonary involvement of an aggressive NHL (10,11). The radiographic pattern of lung-NHL involvement partly depends on NHL histological type. In small lymphocytic NHL, predominantly basal reticulonodular infiltrates (3) or well-differentiated, solitary or multiple, nodules (12,13) are the most usual pattern. In diffuse aggressive NHL, multiple nodules, with or without cavitation, lung consolidation or patchy infiltrates may be seen (1-3,5,6,14). Unlike Hodgkin's disease, mediastinal adenopathies are not always associated with lung involvement, even in previously untreated patients (1,14).

Clinical and radiographic patterns of pulmonary NHL sites are not specific. If a diagnosis of NHL lung involvement is suspected in a given patient, several tests must be performed:

- to gather arguments for the diagnosis of pulmonary NHL involvement;

- to rule out other diseases which can simulate pulmonary NHL involvement: bacterial, viral (cytomegalovirus) or mycotic infections, drug-induced hypersensitivity, pneumonitis (bleomycin, methotrexate), radiation pneumonitis, etc.

These tests may include :

- sputum cytodiagnosis (15,16);

- fibreoptic bronchoscopy with biopsy of endobronchial lesions (17-19), bronchial brushing and bronchoalveolar lavage (20-23) with cytopathological, immunopathological and molecular biological (24) studies of bronchoalveolar fluid and cells;

- surgical or transbronchial or trephine-needle lung biopsy using both routine histological methods and, whenever possible, immunophenotyping of an immediately frozen specimen (25).

Primary pulmonary lymphomas

The most simple and practical definition of primary pulmonary lymphomas (PPL) of the lungs has been given by Weiss et al. (25) i.e. lymphomas that clinically present in the lung. More restrictive definitions - requiring especially negative extra-thoracic staging - have been proposed (26,27). Primary pulmonary lymphomas are rare tumours (0.5 to 1% of primary malignant pulmonary tumours).

Until recently, PPL had to be distinguished from two other primary pulmonary lymphoid proliferations which were considered to be non-neoplastic, i.e. pseudolymphoma, a localized lesion, and its diffuse counterpart, lymphoid interstitial pneumonia (LIP) (25,26,28-35). More recent studies suggest that pseudolymphoma and some cases of LIP are monoclonal lymphoid proliferations (27,34) derived from the Bronchial-Associated Lymphoid Tissue (BALT) (36) and must be considered to be PPL.

Several patients, before developing PPL, have a previous history of auto-immune disease, the most frequent being Sjögren's syndrome (38,40). Patients with PPL are middle-aged [mean = 57 yrs, n = 146 (26)], without sex predominance. About half of the reported patients were asymptomatic, PPL being discovered on a routine chest X-ray. The other half had non-specific pulmonary symptoms (cough, dyspnoea, chest pain) with or without B symptoms (26).

The most common radiographic finding is a solitary ill-defined parenchymal nodule, predominantly in the lower lobes, often containing an air bronchogram (12,26,37, 41). Other patterns may be seen: multiple nodules, fluffy infiltrates, lobar consolidation, etc. Mediastinal adenopathies are extremely rare. Pleural effusion was recorded in 13% of the patients in the series (26).
At CT scan examination, most patients have multiple nodules - 1 to 8 cm in diameter - with shaggy borders (41).
A serum M component may be found in some PPL patients, whose tumour often has a plasmacytic component (26,30). Clinical and radiographic aspects of cases reported as "pseudo-lymphoma" were indistinguishable from those considered as PPL except that pleural effusion and hilar adenopathies were not recorded (28,30,33).
The diagnosis of PPL can be made on a transbronchial or surgical lung biopsy. Fibreoptic endoscopy is usually normal but can show a diffuse thickening of bronchial mucosa or localized stenoses. Macroscopical aspects of PPL are similar, whatever the histological type. The tumour forms a nodule, often large (5 to 10 cm), whitish or greyish, homogeneous or ill-defined and infiltrating surrounding parenchyma. It may be associated with pleural invasion or compression of broncho-vascular structures (26-28).

Approximately 70 to 90% PPL are low-grade non-Hodgkin's lymphomas. Low-grade PPL share all the features of low-grade NHL of Mucosa-Associated Lymphoid Tissue (MALT) *(see figs 1 & 2, pp. 171-172)*. Malignant cells are monomorphous and have the morphological appearance of so-called centrocyte-like cells, similar to those described in gastric NHL. Lympho-epithelial lesions are rare but have been described (34,35). Polytypic follicles with germinal centres and plasma cells are numerous.

In their review of cases considered as "pseudolymphomas", Addis et al. (34) thus concluded that the classical morphological criteria used to separate PPL from pseudolymphomas such as those proposed by Saltzstein (28) or Colby and Carrington (29) appeared unreliable. Besides, immuno-histochemical studies have demonstrated the monotypic nature of the lymphoid infiltrate in almost all of these cases, thus justifying their inclusion in the group of low-grade PPL.

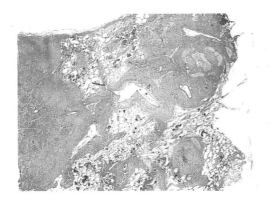

Fig. 1: Primary pulmonary lymphoma, low-grade. Low magnification (acknowledgments to Dr. O. Groussard)

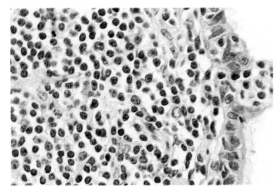

Fig. 2: Primary pulmonary lymphoma, small-cell type

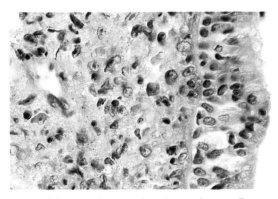

Fig. 3: Primary pulmonary lymphoma, large-cell type. Identical magnification to fig. 2

Low-grade PPL arising from the BALT have an indolent course similar to that described in patients considered to have a "pseudolymphoma" (26,30,33). Either patients are cured after surgical removal or there is a relapse in the lungs after a long period of latency. Nevertheless, several authors have reported cases with transformation into a high-grade lymphoma in patients initially diagnosed either as PPL (34,42) or "pseudolymphoma" (33,39). Patients may also relapse at other sites of MALT such as the gastro-intestinal tract, salivary glands, etc. (35-42).

High-grade primary pulmonary NHL are less frequent (10 to 30% of primary pulmonary NHL). Macroscopically, they form well-delineated nodules, often with necrosis. They can invade arteriole and/or venule wall. They emcompass all the histological subtypes of high-grade NHL *(fig. 3)*. Most of them are large-cell NHL and have a B-cell phenotype.

Among lymphoid proliferations of the lungs, **lymphomatoid granulomatosis** (LG) is an uncommon but well-described entity which is now recognized as a primary high-grade T-cell NHL (43). LG was described in 1972 by Liebow et al. (44) as an angiocentric and angiodestructive lymphoreticular proliferative and granulomatous disease. Lethal midline granuloma (or polymorphic reticulosis) has similar histological features (45). The former predominantly involves the lungs, while the latter is a disease of the nose and the upper respiratory tract. Both diseases have therefore been classified together under the term "angiocentric immunoproliferative lesions" (46).

Most patients with LG are middle-aged males. They complain of respiratory symptoms (dry or productive cough, dyspnoea) and malaise (44,47,48). In occasional patients, symptoms rapidly progress to respiratory failure (47). Multiple bilateral nodules, peripheral and predominant in the lower lobes, are the most usual radiographic finding. Diffuse reticulonodular or patchy infiltrates or lung consolidation with air bronchogram may also be seen (44,47,48). Mild pleural effusions are frequent. Besides the lungs, LG may also affect other organs, especially skin [43% (44)], central nervous system [22% (44)] and kidneys. Erythematous, macular or plaque-like lesions are the most usual cutaneous manifestation (47). Neurological symptoms are polymorphic: ataxia, hemiparesis, aphasia, cranial nerve palsy, etc.

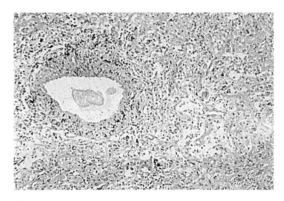

Fig. 4: Lymphomatoid granulomatosis of the lung: lung infiltration with vascular involvement (acknowledgments to Dr. J.F. Mosnier)

Histologically, LG is characterized by a diffuse lymphoid infiltration of the lungs, also involving vessel walls *(fig. 4)*. The infiltrate is polymorphous, with lymphocytes, plasma cells, histiocytes and, in some cases, epithelioid and giant cells. Polymorphonuclear cells are rare. Lymphoid cells are heterogeneous in size, with small cells and large cells, with a large nucleus and multiple nucleoli, described by Liebow under the term "atypical lymphoreticular cells". The infiltrate involves alveolar walls and extends to the walls of arteries and veins. This vascular involvement is the cause of the parenchymal necrosis often observed (44,47-50).

Nosology and pathogenesis of LG and related disorders have long been discussed. Some useful insights into their pathogenesis have been recently gained by immunophenotyping and molecular biology.

Since the first reports, a possible evolution of LG towards high-grade NHL has been seen [5 out of the first 40 patients described by Liebow et al. (44)]. It was then suggested that most cases - if not all - of LG could be T-cell NHL since proliferating cells had mature T-cell characteristics (29,49,50). A clonal rearrangement of the ß chain of the T-cell receptor gene was found in most (43,51), but not all (52), of the cases that have been studied. Whether LG is from its onset a malignant T-cell disorder or a non-malignant disorder which secondarily evolves towards a T-cell NHL is unknown.

The prognosis of LG is unfavourable, with a median survival period of 14 months (47). The optimal therapy is unknown. On the basis of a prospective trial, Fauci et al. (53) suggested that treatment with cyclophosphamide and prednisone of patients at a so-called "granulomatous" phase of the disease may improve the prognosis and delay the development of malignant lymphoma. Nevertheless, the criteria distinguishing the "granulomatous" phase from the "lymphomatous" phase are unclear. Lipford et al. suggested that a long survival period can only be obtained by the achievement of an initial complete response and that previous immunosuppressive treatment (cyclophosphamide and prednisone) may compromise the results of aggressive chemotherapy in the "lymphomatous" phase (51).

No optimal therapy can be proposed and only trends suggested. At diagnosis, a thorough search for a malignant T-cell clone, if possible using molecular biology, must be made. If it is present, aggressive chemotherapy is warranted. If not demonstrated, watchful waiting or treatment with cyclophosphamide and prednisone may be proposed.

Lymphoid interstitial pneumonitis (LIP)

Nosology and pathogenesis of LIP, as initially described by Carrington and Liebow (54), is uncertain. Previously, LIP was considered as a benign diffuse lymphoid hyperplasia of the lungs.

LIP occurs either in previously healthy subjects or in patients with immune diseases such as hypogammaglobulinaemia (55-57), Sjögren's syndrome (38,58) or active chronic hepatitis (59). Patients with LIP complain of progressively increasing dyspnoea, often with a dry cough. Radiographically, LIP appears as a bilateral, diffuse, reticulonodular pattern, predominant in the lower lobes. Some pulmonary consolidation may be seen with air bronchogram. Hilar adenopathies and pleural effusions are not usually found. After a long-lasting evolution, lungs may have a "honeycomb" radiological pattern (41,42, 54,60-62). Pulmonary function tests usually show restrictive or mixed abnormalities.

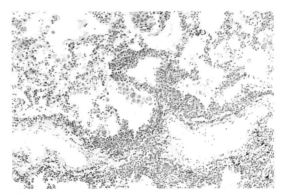

Fig. 5: Lymphoid interstitial pneumonitis: interstitial lymphoid infiltrate

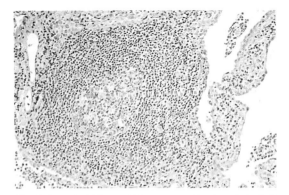

Fig. 6: Lymphoid interstitial pneumonitis: lymphoid follicle with germinal centre

tological and immunological characteristics, LIP has long been considered as a benign, non-lymphomatous, polyclonal lymphoid hyperplasia. Nevertheless, in two cases of LIP associated with Sjögren's syndrome, immunohistochemical studies showed a monotypic lymphoid infiltrate and the course of the disease was rapid. In some other cases, a histological transformation of an LIP into a high-grade NHL had been suggested but initial immuno histochemical studies had not been performed (33,60-62). Thus the term LIP must be defined more precisely. Faced with a diffuse lymphoid infiltration of the lungs, immunohistochemical studies must be performed to assess the polytypy or monotypy of the infiltrate. If it appears to be a monomorphous population of small B lymphocytes, a diagnosis of low-grade diffuse small-cell NHL can be made. On the other hand, if the infiltrate is polymorphous and formed of polytypic B and T cells, a diagnosis of LIP can be reached.

LIP has a severe course. In the 13 cases of Strimlan et al. (63), 5 patients died from respiratory failure after a mean period of 8.6 months. Response to steroids appeared rather poor.

More recently, several cases of LIP associated with HIV infection have been reported. This occurs mostly in children (64,65) but has also been reported in 16 adults (33,66-69). For unknown reasons, 15 of them were black. The nature of LIP in HIV infection is uncertain. Besides LIP, patients have generalized lymphoid hyperplasia involving lymph nodes, liver, spleen, salivary glands. In these patients, LIP may be a reaction to direct infection of lungs by HIV (69) and/or by Epstein-Barr virus (70).

LIP has also been reported:
- in chronic active Epstein-Barr virus infection (71); and
- after allogenic bone-marrow transplantation (72).

LIP may accordingly be considered to be a syndrome most probably including monoclonal and non-monoclonal (poly- or oligoclonal) lymphoid proliferations.

In patients with LIP, there is a diffuse lymphoid infiltrate of pulmonary interstitium associated with a thickening of alveolar walls (fig. 6). This infiltrate is polymorphous with lymphocytes, plasma cells and histiocytes. Co-existing with this infiltrate, there are often lymphoid follicles with germinal centres (fig. 5). Follicles are located either in the thickened alveolar walls or in the vicinity of broncho-vascular axes. There is neither infiltration, nor destruction of vessel and bronchus walls. Other lesions may be observed: sarcoid-like granulomas and amyloid deposits. Immunohistochemical studies show simultaneous presence of B cells - with kappa and lambda light chains and all heavy-chain classes - and T cells (fig. 7) (33,56,61,62). Because of these his-

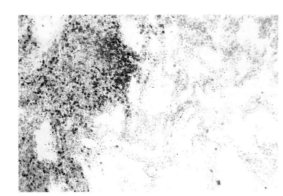

Fig. 7a

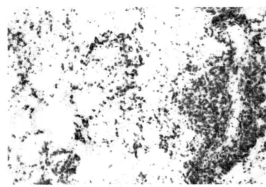

Fig. 7b

Fig. 7: Immunohistochemical analysis of a lymphoid interstitial pneumonitis:
7a: immunoperoxidase staining with anti-pan B antibody (CD22) showing some scattered or clustered B cells
7b: interstitial T-cell infiltrate staining with anti-CD23 antibody

References

1. FILLY R, BLANK N, CASTELLINO RA
   Radiographic distribution of intrathoracic disease in previously untreated patients with Hodgkin's disease and non-Hodgkin's lymphoma.
   Radiology, 1979; 120: 277-281.

2. MANHOHARAN A, PITNEY WR, SCHONELL ME, BADER LV
   Intrathoracic manifestations in non-Hodgkin's lymphomas.
   Thorax, 1979; 34: 29-32.

3. JENKINS PF, WARD MJ, DAVIES M, FLETCHER J
   Non-Hodgkin's lymphomas, chronic lymphatic leukemia and the lung.
   Br J Dis Chest, 1981; 75: 22-30.

4. RAPPAPORT H, THOMAS LB
   Mycosis fungoides: the pathology of extracutaneous involvement.
   Cancer, 1974; 34: 1198-1229.

5. WOLFE JD, TREVOR ED, KJELDSBERG CR
   Pulmonary manifestations of mycosis fungoides.
   Cancer, 1980; 46: 2648-2653.

6. STOKAR LM, VONDERHEID EC, ABELL E, DIAMOND LW, ROSEN SE, GOLDWEIN MI
   Clinical manifestations of intrathoracic cutaneous T-cell lymphoma.
   Cancer, 1985; 56: 2694-2702.

7. OFFIT K, RICHARDSON ME, QUANGUANG C et al.
   Non-random chromosomal aberrations are associated with sites of tissue involvement in non-Hodgkin's lymphoma.
   Cancer Genet Cytogenet, 1989; 37: 85-93.

8. ZIEGLER JL, BACKSTEAD JA, VOLBERDING PA et al.
   Non-Hodgkin's lymphoma in 90 homosexual men.
   N Engl J Med, 1984; 311: 565-570.

9. LOUREIRO C, GILL PS, MEYER PR, RHODES R, RARICK MU, LEVINE AM
   Autopsy findings in AIDS-related lymphoma.
   Cancer, 1988; 62: 735-739.

10. CATHCART-RAKE W, BONE RC, SOBANYA RE, STEPHENS RC
    Rapid development of diffuse pulmonary infiltrates in histiocytic lymphoma.
    Am Rev Resp Dis, 1978; 117: 587-592.

11. MILLER K, SAHN S
    Mycosis fungoides presenting as ARDS and diagnosed by bronchoalveolar lavage.
    Chest, 1986; 89: 312-314.

12. JULSRUD PR, BROWN LR, CHIN-YANG L, ROSENOW EC, CROWE JK
    Pulmonary processes of mature-appearing lymphocytes: pseudolymphoma, well-differentiated lymphocytic lymphoma and lymphocytic interstitial pneumonitis.
    Radiology, 1978; 127: 289-296.

13. TURNER RR, COLBY TV, DOGGETT RS
    Well-differentiated lymphocytic lymphoma. A study of 47 patients with primary manifestation in the lung.
    Cancer, 1984; 54: 2088-2096.

14. BALIKIAN JP, HERMAN PG
    Non-Hodgkin's lymphomas in the lungs.
    Radiology, 1979; 132: 569-576.

15. SCHUMANN GB, DI FIORE K, JOHNSTON JL
Sputum cytodiagnosis of disseminated histiocytic lymphoma: a case report.
Acta Cytol, 1983; 27: 262-266.

16. MANHOHARAN A, FORO J, HILL J, PAINTER D, MILLER D
Sputum cytology in the diagnosis of pulmonary non-Hodgkin's lymphomas.
Thorax, 1984; 39: 392-393.

17. GRIBETZ AR, CHUANG MT, TEIRSTEIN AS
Fiberoptic bronchoscopy in patients with Hodgkin's and non-Hodgkin's lymphomas.
Cancer, 1980; 46: 1476-1478.

18. RICHERT-BOE KE, BAGBY GC
Burkitt's lymphoma presenting as an endobronchial lesion.
Am J Med, 1988; 85: 864-866.

19. ROSE RM, GRIGAS D, STRATTEMEIR E, HARRIS NL, LINGGOODE RM
Endobronchial involvement in non-Hodgkin's lymphoma.
Cancer, 1986; 57: 1750-1755.

20. GALLAGHER CJ, KNOWLES GK, HABESHAW JA, GREEN M, MALPAS JS, LISTER TA
Early involvement of the bronchi in patients with malignant lymphoma.
Br J Cancer, 1983; 48: 777-781.

21. MYERS JL, FULMER JD
Bronchoalveolar lavage in the diagnosis of pulmonary lymphomas.
Chest, 1987; 91: 642-643.

22. LORENZETTI E, NARDI F
Diagnostic value of bronchial washing in a case of primary pulmonary non-Hodgkin's lymphoma.
Appl Pathol, 1984; 2: 277-281.

23. DAVIS WB, GADEK JE
Detection of pulmonary lymphoma by bronchoalveolar lavage.
Chest, 1987; 91: 787-790.

24. PISANI RJ, WITZIG TE, LI CY, MORRIS MA, THIBODEAU S
Confirmation of lymphomatous pulmonary involvement by immunophenotypic and gene rearrangement analysis of bronchoalveolar lavage fluid.
Mayo Clin Proc, 1990; 65: 651-656.

25. WEISS LM, YOUSEM SA, WARNKE RA
Non-Hodgkin's lymphomas of the lung. A study of nineteen cases emphasizing the utility of frozen section immunologic studies in differential diagnosis.
Am J Surg Pathol, 1985; 9: 480-490.

26. KOSS MN, HOCHHOLZER L, NICHOLS PW, WEHUNT WD, LAZARUS AA
Primary non-Hodgkin's lymphomas and pseudolymphoma of lung: a study of 161 patients.
Hum Pathol, 1983; 14: 1024-1038.

27. HERBERT A, WRIGHT DH, ISAACSON PG, SMITH JL
Primary malignant lymphoma of the lung: histopathologic and immunologic evaluation of nine cases.
Hum Pathol, 1984; 15: 415-422.

28. SALTZSTEIN SL
Pulmonary lymphomas and pseudolymphomas: classification, therapy and prognosis.
Cancer, 1963; 16: 928-954.

29. COLBY TV, CARRINGTON CB
Pulmonary lymphomas: current concepts.
Hum Pathol, 1983; 14: 884-887.

30. CORDIER JF, BERNAUDIN JF, MARY P et al.
Pseudolymphomes et lymphomes pulmonaires primitifs. 4 observations.
Rev Mal Resp, 1984; 1: 105-111.

31. KENNEDY JL, NATHWANI BN, BURKE JS, HILL LR, RAPPAPORT H
Pulmonary lymphomas and other pulmonary lymphoid lesions.
Cancer, 1985; 56: 539-552.

32. LETOURNEAU A, AUDOUIN J, GARBE L et al.
Primary pulmonary malignant lymphoma, clinical and pathological findings, immunocytochemical and ultrastructural studies in 15 cases.
Hematol Oncol, 1983; 1: 49-60.

33. KRADIN RL, MARK EJ
Benign lymphoid disorders of the lung with a theory regarding their development.
Hum Pathol, 1983; 14: 857-867.

34. ADDIS BJ, HYJEK E, ISAACSON PG
Primary pulmonary lymphoma: a re-appraisal of its histogenesis and its relationship to pseudolymphoma and lymphoid interstitial pneumonia.
Histopathology, 1988; 13: 1-17.

35. LI G, HANSMANN ML, ZWINGERS T, LENNERT K
Primary lymphomas of the lung: morphological, immunohistochemical and clinical features.
Histopathology, 1990; 16: 519-531.

36. BIENENSTOCK J, JOHNSTON N, PEREY DYE
Bronchial lymphoid tissue. I. Morphologic characteristics.
Lab Invest, 1973; 28: 686-692.

37. L'HOSTE RJ, FILIPPA DA, LIEBERMAN PH, BRETSKY S
Primary pulmonary lymphomas. A clinicopathologic analysis of 36 cases.
Cancer, 1984; 54: 1397-1406.

38. FAGUET GB, WEBB HH, AGEE JF, RICHS WI, SHARBOUGH AH
Immunologically diagnosed malignancy in Sjögren's pseudolymphoma.
Am J Med, 1978; 65: 424-429.

39. KRADIN RL, YOUNG RH, KRADIN LA, MARK EJ

Immunoblastic lymphoma arising in chronic lymphoid hyperplasia of the pulmonary interstitium.

Cancer, 1982; 50: 1339-1343.

40. STRIMLAN CV, ROSENOW EC, DIVERTIE MB, HARRISON EG

Pulmonary manifestations of Sjögren's syndrome.

Chest, 1976; 70: 354-361.

41. PETERSON H, SNIDER HL, YANN LT, BOWLDS CF, ARNU EH, LI CY

Primary pulmonary lymphomas: a clinical and immunohistochemical study of six cases.

Cancer, 1985; 56: 805-813.

42. ISAACSON PG, SPENCER J

Malignant lymphoma of mucosa-associated lymphoid tissue.

Histopathology, 1987; 11: 445-462.

43. GAULARD P, HENNI T, MAROLLEAU JP et al.

Lethal midline granuloma (polymorphic reticulosis) and lymphomatoid granulomatosis. Evidence for a monoclonal T-cell lymphoproliferative disorder.

Cancer, 1988; 62: 705-710.

44. LIEBOW AA, CARRINGTON CB, FRIEDMAN PJ

Lymphomatoid granulomatosis.

Hum Pathol, 1972; 3: 457-458.

45. DE REMEE RA, WEILAND LH, Mc DONALD TJ

Polymorphic reticulosis, lymphomatoid granulomatosis: two diseases or one?

Mayo Clin Proc, 1978; 53: 634-640.

46. COSTA J, MARTIN SE

Pulmonary lymphoreticular disorders, in JAFFE ES Ed. Surgical pathology of lymph nodes and related organs.

Philadelphia. WB Saunders 1985: 282-289.

47. KATZENSTEIN AA, CARRINGTON CB, LIEBOW AA

Lymphomatoid granulomatosis. A clinicopathologic study of 152 cases.

Cancer, 1979; 43: 360-376.

48. PATTON WF, LYNCH JP

Lymphomatoid granulomatosis. Clinicopathologic study of four cases and literature review.

Medicine, 1982; 61: 1-11.

49. COLBY TV, CARRINGTON CB

Pulmonary lymphomas simulating lymphomatoid granulomatosis.

Am J Surg pathol, 1982; 6: 19-32.

50. NICHOLS P, KOSS M, LEVINE AM, LUKES RH

Lymphomatoid granulomatosis. A T-cell disorder?

Am J Med, 1982; 72: 467-471.

51. LIPFORD EH, MARGOLICK JB, LONGO DL, FAUCI AS, JAFFE ES

Angiocentric immunoproliferative lesions: a clinicopathologic spectrum of post-thymic T-cell proliferations.

Blood, 1988; 72: 1674-1681.

52. BLEIWEISS IJ, STAUCHEN JA

Lymphomatoid granulomatosis of the lung: report of a case and gene rearrangement studies.

Hum Pathol, 1988; 19: 1109-1112.

53. FAUCI AS, HAYNES BF, COSTA J, KATZ P, WOLFF SM

Lymphomatoid granulomatosis. Prospective clinical and therapeutic experience over 10 years.

N Engl J Med, 1982; 306: 68-74.

54. CARRINGTON CB, LIEBOW AA

Lymphocytic interstitial pneumonia.

Am J Pathol, 1966; 48: 36a.

55. CHURCH JA, ISSACS H, SAXON A, KEENS TG, RICHARDS WR

Lymphoid interstitial pneumonitis and hypogammaglobulinemia in children.

Am Rev Respir Dis, 1981; 124: 491-496.

56. LIEBOW AA, CARRINGTON CB

Diffuse pulmonary lymphoreticular infiltrations associated with dysproteinemia.

Med Clin North Amer, 1973; 57: 809-843.

57. LEVINSON AI, HOPEWELL PC, STITES DP, SPITLER LE, FUDENBERG H

Coexistent lymphoid interstitial pneumonia, pernicious anemia and agammaglobulinemia.

Arch Intern Med, 1976; 136: 213-216.

58. SCHUURMAN HJ, GOOSZEN HC, TAN IWN, KLUIN PM, WAGENAAR SS, VAN UNNIK JAM

Low-grade lymphoma of immature T-cell phenotype in a case of lymphocytic interstitial pneumonia and Sjögren's syndrome.

Histopathology, 1987; 11: 1193-1204.

59. HELMAN CA, KEETON GR, BENATAR SR

Lymphoid interstitial pneumonia with associated chronic active hepatitis and renal tubular acidosis.

Am Rev Resp Dis, 1977; 115: 161-164.

60. HERBERT A, WALTERS MT, CAWLEY MID, GODFREY RC

Lymphocytic interstitial pneumonia identified as lymphoma of Mucosa-Associated Lymphoid Tissue.

J Pathol, 1985; 146: 129-138.

61. WAUGHN-STRIMLAN C, ROSENOW EC, WEILAND LH, BROWN LR

Lymphocytic interstitial pneumonitis. Review of 13 cases.

Ann Intern Med, 1978; 88: 616-621.

62. HALPRIN GM, RAMIREZ J, PRATT PC
    Lymphoid interstitial pneumonia.
    Chest, 1972; 62: 418-423.

63. STRIMLAN CV, ROSENOW EC, WEILAND LH, BROWN LR
    Lymphocytic interstitial pneumonitis.
    Ann Intern Med, 1978; 88: 616-621.

64. FALLOON J, EDDY J, WIENER L, PIZZO PA
    Human immundeficiency virus infection in children.
    J Pediatr, 1989; 114: 1-30.

65. RUBINSTEIN A, MORECKI R, SILVERMANN B et al.
    Pulmonary disease in children with acquired immunodeficiency syndrome and AIDS-related complex.
    J Pediatr, 1986; 108: 498-503.

66. SOLAL-CELIGNY Ph, COUDERC LJ, HERMANN D et al.
    Lymphoid interstitial pneumonitis in acquired immunodeficiency syndrome-related complex.
    Am Rev Resp Dis, 1985; 131: 956-960.

67. GRIECO MH, CHINAY-ACHARYA P
    Lymphocytic interstitial pneumonia associated with the acquired immunodeficiency syndrome.
    Am Rev Resp Dis, 1985; 131: 952-955.

68. MORRIS JC, ROSEN MJ, MARCHEVSKY A, TEIRSTEIN AS
    Lymphocytic interstitial pneumonia in patients at risk for the Acquired Immune Deficiency Syndrome.
    Chest, 1987; 91: 63-67.

69. ZIZA JM, BRUN-VEZINET F, VENET A et al.
    Lymphadenopathy-associated virus isolated from bronchoalveolar lavage fluid in AIDS-related complex with lymphoid interstitial pneumonitis.
    N Engl J Med, 1985; 313: 183.

70. ANDIMAN WA, MARTIN K, RUBINSTEIN A et al.
    Opportunistic lymphoproliferations associated with Epstein-Barr viral DNA in infants and children with AIDS.
    Lancet, 1985; 2: 1390-1393.

71. SCHOOLEY RT, CAREY RW, MILLER G et al.
    Chronic Epstein-Barr virus infection associated with fever and interstitial pneumonitis.
    Ann Intern Med, 1986; 104: 636-643.

72. PERREAULT C, COUSINEAU C, D'ANGELO G
    Lymphoid interstitial pneumonia after allogenic bone marrow transplantation. A possible manifestation of chronic graft-versus-host disease.
    Cancer, 1985; 55: 1-9.

Bone-marrow involvement in non-Hodgkin's lymphomas

J. Y. SCOAZEC, N. BROUSSE

Bone-marrow involvement is frequent in NHL *(Table I)* and its overall incidence has been estimated to account for up to 75% of cases (1-11). As regards its prognostic significance, two situations must be clearly distinguished. In NHL of low-grade malignancy, bone-marrow involvement is the rule and indicates the "systemic" character of these proliferations. In contrast, in NHL of high-grade malignancy, bone-marrow involvement is much rarer; its occurrence testifies to the secondary dissemination of the disease from its primary site and has an unfavourable prognostic significance.

Bone-marrow involvement in NHL is rarely accompanied by peripheral blood abnormalities (7). Cytopenias are infrequent, and the existence of abnormal circulating lymphoid cells is not uniform. Systematic biopsy is therefore necessary to assess the diagnosis. Bone-marrow biopsy may also give addi-tional information: **(a)** assessment of the diagnosis in the absence of tumours easily accessible to surgical biopsy (as, for example, in cases of primary splenic presentation); **(b)** evaluation of the functional status of myeloid tissue; and **(c)** monitoring of the treatment and control of its long-term consequences.

Diagnostic methods

Transcutaneous bone-marrow biopsy is the technique currently used for diagnosis of bone-marrow involvement in NHL. Its sensitivity is much higher than that of bone-marrow aspiration. However, the latter allows better analysis of the cytological characteristics of lymphoid cells. Bilateral transcuta-

TABLE I

Frequency of bone-marrow involvement in various series

References	Number of patients	BM involved (%)
Jones et al. (1)	205	18
Dick et al. (2)	108	37
Stein et al. (3)	121	36
Goffinet et al. (4)	423	32
Chabner et al. (5)	170	34
Coller et al. (6)	85	42
Ribas-Mundo et al. (7)	200	45
Foucar et al. (8)	176	53
Anderson et al. (9)	473	36
Bartl et al. (10)	678	69
International Working Formulation (11)	1014	29

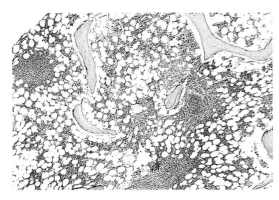

Fig. 1: Bone-marrow involvement in NHL, small lympho-cytic: nodular infiltration.

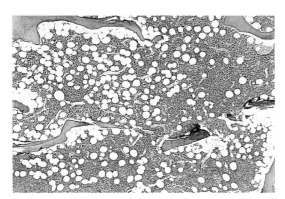

Fig. 3: Bone-marrow involvement in NHL, small lympho-cytic: interstitial infiltration.

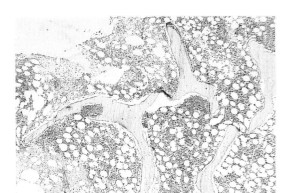

Fig. 2: Bone-marrow involvement in follicular NHL, small cleaved cell: paratrabecular infiltration.

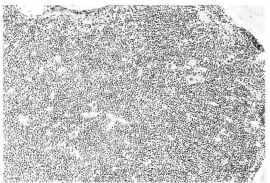

Fig. 4: Bone-marrow involvement in NHL, small lympho-cytic: diffuse infiltration.

neous biopsies may increase detection of bone-marrow involvement in NHL: in about 20% of cases, involvement is found in only one of the biopsy specimens (6,12). This feature is more characteristic of large-cell NHL. Magnetic resonance imaging (MRI) of vertebral, pelvic and femoral marrow may complement blind bone-marrow biopsy (13,14). MRI is less sensitive than biopsy in the detection of diffuse and minimal infiltration (15,16). Conversely, it may detect foci of infiltration located elsewhere than in the iliac crests and may thus guide biopsy (13-16).

Bone-marrow manifestations of NHL

Four architectural types of bone-marrow involvement in NHL are to be distinguished: the nodular, the paratrabecular, the interstitial and the diffuse dense.

Nodular lesions *(fig. 1)* comprise round aggregates of neoplastic lymphoid cells scattered among the myeloid tissue. They vary in size and number. Most often, they are large and numerous. They are located in the centre of medullary spaces and have no contact with osseous trabeculae. Several lymphoid aggregates may fuse into larger masses invading large parts of the biopsy. Nodular lesions are poorly delineated: at high magnification, neoplastic cells are seen infiltrating the adjacent haematopoietic tissue. Paratrabecular infiltrates *(fig. 2)* are constituted of poorly defined aggregates of neoplastic lymphoid cells situated along osseous trabeculae. Interstitial infiltrations *(fig. 3)* are composed of neoplastic lymphoid cells scattered amongst the normal myeloid cells. Neoplastic lymphoid cells may be isolated or may form small aggregates. The density of the infiltration usually varies from one medullary space to another. Diffuse dense infiltrations *(fig. 4)* are characterized by the disappearance of the nor-

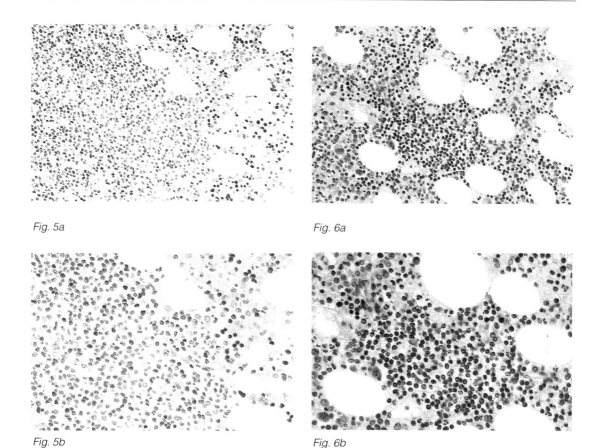

Fig. 5a

Fig. 6a

Fig. 5b

Fig. 6b

Fig. 5: Bone-marrow involvement in diffuse NHL, small cleaved cell: this lymphomatous nodule is ill-defined (5a) and constituted by a monomorphic population of small cleaved cells (5b).

Fig. 6: Benign lymphoid nodule: small nodule, well-circumscribed (6a), polymorphous, with lymphocytes, plasma cells and some mast cells (6b).

mal myeloid architecture. Medullary spaces are filled with a dense lymphoid proliferation which takes the place of haematopoietic cells and adipocytes. Coexistence of two types of infiltration on the same biopsy is frequent: for instance, nodular and paratrabecular lesions are often associated with a certain degree of interstitial infiltration.

Lymphoid infiltrations of the bone marrow are frequently accompanied by a moderate or mild increase in the fibrillar network. Myelofibrosis may be associated with interstitial and diffuse dense infiltrations. Lymphoid infiltration of the bone marrow is generally accompanied by a reactive cellular population, comprising variable proportions of eosinophils, mast cells and plasma cells. Myeloid tissue is usually hypoplastic. Granular hypoplasia may occur early in the course of disease while megacaryocytes generally

persist at later stages, even amongst diffuse dense infiltrations.

Diagnostic difficulties

Diagnostic difficulties in the assessment of lymphoid infiltrations of the bone marrow are mainly of two types. The first is the identificaton moderate interstitial infiltrations, especially in the case of lymphoblastic and small non-cleaved lymphomas. The detection of such moderate infiltrations necessitates careful examination of all sections of the biopsy at high magnification. A second difficulty, more frequently encountered, is the evaluation of the malignant character of an infiltration of the bone marrow constituted of small lymphoid cells.

TABLE II

Comparison between lymphomatous nodules and benign lymphoid nodules

	Lymphomatous nodules	**Benign nodules**
Size	Often large	Often small
Number	Usually multiple	Single or multiple
Localization	Not specially related to sinuses; often paratrabecular	Perivascular
Limits	Ill-defined	Well-defined
Cell population	Usually monomorphic	Polymorphic
Germinal centers	Never	Possible (rare)
Immunohistochemistry	Monoclonal B cells with rare T cells	Numerous T cells with polyclonal B cells

When marrow infiltration is paratrabecular, interstitial or diffuse dense, its lymphomatous nature is easy to ascertain, since reactive lesions are almost always nodular and perivascular. The sole exception is HIV-1 infection, in which paratrabecular lymphoid aggregates of uncertain significance may be observed (17). Nodular lesions may be more difficult to interpret, since lymphoid nodules may be discovered in the bone marrow of about 10% of healthy subjects after 60 years of age (10). Such "benign" or "reactive" nodules *(fig. 6)* may be confused with marrow involvement in small lymphocytic NHL *(fig. 5)*. Several histological arguments, summarized in *Table II,* favour the diagnosis of malignant lymphoid infiltration of the bone marrow (6,18). In contrast to "benign" lymphoid nodules, malignant ones are multiple on the same section (or in the same biopsy, as shown by serial sections). Malignant lymphoid nodules are usually larger. They are not well-defined. Their cytological aspect is much more monomorphous, while benign lymphoid nodules comprise variable proportions of small lymphocytes, eosinophils, histiocytes and plasma cells. Benign nodules are often perivascular, but this sign has no absolute value.

A particular problem is represented by cases of uncertain significance and behaviour, known as nodular lymphoid hyperplasias of the bone marrow (18). Such lesions are characterized by the presence of multiple, benign-appearing lymphoid nodules in the bone marrow. They have been described in various conditions, including diabetes and connective-tissue diseases. Their relationship to NHL, which they may precede, has not been clarified.

Correlations between bone-marrow involvement and histological type of NHL

The frequency of bone-marrow involvement in NHL varies according to the histological type *(Table III)* (1-3,6,8,11,19,20). Among B-cell lymphomas, one may schematically distinguish:

TABLE III

Correlations between histological type and frequency of bone-marrow involvement

	Working Formulation (11)	Rappaport classification				Lukes-Collins classification	
		Jones. et al. (1)	Dick. et al. (2)	Rosen-berg (19)	Stein et al. (3)	Coller (6)	Foucar et al. (8)
Low-grade							
Small lymphocytic	71%		100%	33%	100%	100%	89%
Plasmacytoid							100%
Follicular, SCC	51%	30%	57%	55%	59%	39%	57%
Follicular, mixed	30%	15%		19%	0%	100%	25%
Intermediate-grade							
Follicular, LC	34%		67%	4%			30%
Diffuse, SCC	32%	29%	27%	29%	61%	56%	45%
Diffuse, mixed	14%	21%		26%	0%	23%	60%
Diffuse, LC	10%	5%		7%	5%	25%	25%
High-grade							
Immunoblastic	12%						B: 0%
Lymphoblastic	50%						T: 50%
Small non-cleaved cell	14%						10%
SCC : small cleaved cell ; LC: large cell							

- a first group in which bone-marrow involvement is almost constant: diffuse small lymphocytic lymphomas;

- a second group in which bone-marrow involvement occurs in at least 70% of cases: the small cleaved and mixed-cell types, follicular and diffuse;

- a third group in which bone-marrow involvement occurs in less than 50% of cases: the large-cell and immunoblastic types.

In T-cell lymphomas, bone-marrow involvement has been said to occur with a higher

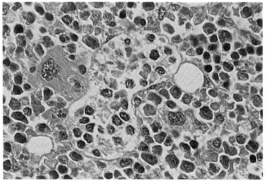

Fig. 7: Bone-marrow infiltration by T-cell lymphoma: intra-sinusal involvement (Photograph by Dr. P. Gaulard).

TABLE IV

**Correlations between histological type and
pattern of infiltration in 101 cases**

	Total number of patients vs number of patients of with BM involved	Pattern of infiltration				
		Nodular	Paratrabecular	Interstitial	Mixed	Diffuse
Follicular lymphomas						
- small cleaved cell	9/9	2	3	1	3	0
- mixed	4/0	0	0	0	0	0
- large-cell	1/0	0	0	0	0	0
- mantle-cell	1/1	1	0	0	0	0
Diffuse lymphomas						
- small lymphocytic	13/13	4	0	0	6	3
- plasmacytoid	8/8	1	0	2	2	3
- small cleaved cell	20/17	2	2	3	6	4
- mixed	9/4	0	1	0	2	1
- large-cell	26/11	4	1	1	1	4
- immunoblastic	6/2	2	0	0	0	0
- small non-cleaved cell, Burkitt-type	1/0	0	0	0	0	0
- lymphoblastic	3/1	0	0	1	0	0

frequency than in B-cell lymphomas. However, the various series reported do not concur. Figures varying between 30 and 70% have been reported for the T-cell lymphomas classified as mixed- and large-cell, and immunoblastic in the Working Formulation (21-23). This frequency is higher (more than 80% of cases) in adult T-cell leukaemia/lymphoma associated with HTLV-1 (*see pp. 31-39*) (24,25). This syndrome must be distinguished from chronic T-lymphocytic leukaemia, in which bone-marrow infiltration is constant (22).

Histological characters of marrow infiltration also vary with the type of NHL. Preferential modes of infiltration may be recog-nized (*Table IV*). For instance, paratrabecular infiltrates are characteristic of follicular small cleaved- and mixed-cell lymphomas. In the same way, bone-marrow involvement in peripheral T-cell lymphomas presents distinctive characters (*fig. 7*) (22). Generally, infiltrates are nodular or paratrabecular. Their cellular composition is polymorphous: the lesions comprise a variable proportion of neoplastic lymphoid cells, usually often pleomorphic, accompanied by small lymphocytes, eosinophils, and histiocytes. T-cell infiltrates are usually accompanied by a dense, hypervascularized stroma. Such lesions are therefore similar to involvement of the bone marrow in Hodgkin's disease.

In a few cases, the cytological appearance of marrow infiltration differs from that observed in the initial nodal site NHL classified as mixed on the basis of a lymph node biopsy may be accompanied by marrow infiltrations consisting of only small lymphoid cells. In the same way, NHL classified as large-cell on the basis of a lymph node biopsy may be accompanied by marrow infiltrations of small-cell or mixed cytological appearance. The frequency of these site-related variations has been estimated to be up to 25% (8,26).

Immunohistochemical features

Immunohistochemical investigations have shown that bone-marrow infiltrations by B-cell lymphomas have the same phenotype as initial nodal sites (27-29). Immunohistochemistry also reveals that certain non-lymphoid cells, such as follicular dendritic reticulum cells, normally absent from the bone marrow (30), may be found among marrow infiltrations by follicular B-cell NHL.

As at other sites, neoplastic T cells infiltrating bone marrow frequently lose expression of one or several differentiation antigens (31,32). This may represent a useful diagnostic sign, if an immunohistochemical study of frozen bone marrow biopsies is necessary to assess the diagnosis of peripheral T-cell lymphoma. Indeed, certain cases of peripheral T-cell lymphoma have the particularity of being confined to bone marrow at initial presentation and sometimes during the entire course of the disease (31,33).

References

1. JONES SE, ROSENBERG SA, KAPLAN AS
   Non-Hodgkin's lymphoma. I. Bone-marrow involvement.
   Cancer, 1972; 29: 954-960.

2. DICK F, BLOOMFIELD CD, BRUNNING RD
   Incidence, cytology and histopathology of non-Hodgkin's lymphomas in the bone marrow.
   Cancer, 1974; 83: 1382-1398.

3. STEIN RS, ULTMANN JE, BYRNE GE et al.
   Bone-marrow involvement in non-Hodgkin's lymphomas.
   Cancer, 1976; 37: 629-636.

4. GOFFINET DR, WARNKE R, DUNNICK NR et al.
   Clinical and surgical (laparotomy) evaluation of patients with non-Hodgkin's lymphomas.
   Cancer Treat Rep, 1977; 61: 981-992.

5. CHABNER BA, JOHNSON RE, DE VITA VT JR et al.
   Sequential staging in non-Hodgkin's lymphomas.
   Cancer Treat Rep, 1977; 61: 993-997.

6. COLLER BS, CHABNER BA, GRALNICK HR
   Frequencies and patterns of bone-marrow involvement in non-Hodgkin's lymphomas: observations on the value of bilateral biopsies.
   A J Hematol, 1977; 3: 105-119.

7. RIBAS-MUNDO M, ROSENBERG SA
   The value of sequential bone-marrow biopsy and laparotomy and splenectomy in a series of 200 consecutive untreated patients with non-Hodgkin's lymphomas.
   Eur J Cancer, 1979; 15: 941-952.

8. FOUCAR K, McKENNA RW, FRIZZERA G, BRUNNING RD
   Bone-marrow and blood involvement by lymphoma in relationship to the Lukes-Collins classification.
   Cancer, 1982; 49: 888-897.

9. ANDERSON T, CHABNER BA, YOUNG RC et al.
   Malignant lymphoma. I. The histology and staging of 473 patients at the National Cancer Institute.
   Cancer, 1982; 50: 2699-2707.

10. BARTL R, FRISCH F, BURKHARDT R et al.
    Assessment of bone-marrow histology in the malignant lymphomas (non-Hodgkin's): correlation with clinical factors for diagnosis, prognosis, classification and staging.
    Br J Haematol, 1982; 51: 511-530.

11. The non-Hodgkin's lymphoma pathologic classification project:
    National Cancer Institute sponsored study of classifications of non-Hodgkin's lymphomas. Summary and description of a Working Formulation for Clinical Usage.
    Cancer, 1982; 49: 2112-2135.

12. BRUNNING RD, BLOOMFIELD CD, McKENNA RW, PETERSON L
    Bilateral trephine bone-marrow biopsies in lymphomas and other neoplastic diseases.
    Ann Intern Med, 1975; 82: 365-366.

13. SHIELDS AF, PORTER BA, CHURCHLEY S, OLSON DO, APPELBAUM FR, THOMAS ED
    The detection of bone-marrow involvement by lymphoma using magnetic resonance imaging.
    J Clin Oncol, 1987; 5: 225-232.

14. RICHARDS MA, WEBB JAW, JEWELL SE, AMESS JAL, WRIGLEY PFM, LISTER TA

Low-field strength magnetic resonance imaging of bone marrow in patients with malignant lymphoma.

Br J Cancer, 1988; 57: 412-417.

15. DOHNER H, GUCKEL F, KNAUF W et al.

Magnetic resonance imaging of bone marrow in lymphoproliferative disorders: correlation with bone marrow biopsy.

Br J Haematol, 1989; 73: 12-17.

16. HOANE BR, SHIELDS AF, PORTER BA, SHULMAN HM

Detection of lymphomatous bone-marrow involvement with magnetic resonance imaging.

Blood, 1991; 78: 728-738.

17. OSBORNE BM, GUARDA LA, BUTLER JJ

Bone-marrow biopsies in patients with the acquired immunodeficiency syndrome.

Hum Pathol, 1984; 15: 1048-1053.

18. RYWLIN A, ORTEGA RS, DOMINGUEZ GJ

Lymphoid nodules of bone-marrow, normal and abnormal.

Blood, 1974; 43: 389-400.

19. ROSENBERG SA

Bone-marrow involvement in the non-Hodgkin's lymphomata.

Br J Cancer (supplt 2), 1975; 31: 261-264.

20. The Kiel Lymphoma Study Group:

Clinical and prognostic relevance of the Kiel Classification of non-Hodgkin's lymphomas: results of a prospective multicenter study by the Kiel Lymphoma Study Group.

Hematol Oncol, 1984; 2: 269-306.

21. GREER JP, YORK JC, COUSAR JB, MITCHELL RT, FLEXNER JM, COLLINS RD, STEIN RA

Peripheral T-cell lymphoma: a clinicopathologic study of 42 cases.

J Clin Oncol, 1984; 2: 788-798.

22. HANSON CA, BRUNNING RD, GAJL-PECZALSKA KJ, FRIZZERA G, McKENNA RW

Bone-marrow manifestations of peripheral T-cell lymphoma. A study of 30 cases.

Am J Clin Pathol, 1986; 86: 449-460.

23. COIFFIER B, BERGER F, BRYON PA, MAGAUD JP

T-cell lymphoma: immunologic, histologic, clinical and therapeutic analysis of 63 cases.

J Clin Oncol, 1988; 6: 1584-1589.

24. KADIN ME, BERARD CW, NANBA K, WAKASA H

Lymphoproliferative diseases in Japan and Western Countries: Proceedings of the United States-Japan seminar.

Hum Pathol, 1983; 14: 745-772.

25. BLAYNEY DW, JAFFE ES, BLATTNER WA et al.

The human T-cell leukemia/lymphoma virus (HTLV1) associated with American adult T-cell leukemia/lymphoma (ATL).

Blood, 1983; 62: 401-405.

26. FISHER DE, JACOBSON JO, AULT KA, HARRIS NL

Diffuse large-cell lymphoma with discordant bone-marrow histology. Clinical features and biological implications.

Cancer, 1989; 64: 1879-1887.

27. WOOD GS, WARNKE RA

The immunologic phenotyping of bone-marrow biopsies and aspirates: frozen section techniques.

Blood, 1982; 59: 913-922.

28. PIZZOLO G, CHILOSI M, CETTO GL, FIORE-DONATI L, JANOSSY G

Immuno-histological analysis of bone-marrow involvement in lymphoproliferative disorders.

Br J Haematol, 1982; 50: 95-100.

29. CHILOSI M, PIZZOLO G, CALIGARIS-CAPPIO F et al.

Immunohistochemical demonstration of follicular dendritic cells in bone-marrow involvement of B-cell chronic lymphocytic leukemia.

Cancer, 1985; 56: 328-332.

30. CHILOSI M, PIZZOLO G, FIORE-DONATI L, BOFILL M, JANOSSY G

Routine immunofluorescent and histochemical analysis of bone-marrow involvement of lymphoma/leukaemia: the use of cryostat sections.

Br J Cancer, 1983; 48: 763-775.

31. WHITE DM, SMITH AS, WHITEHOUSE JMA, SMITH JL

Peripheral T-cell lymphoma: value of bone-marrow trephine immunophenotyping.

J Clin Pathol, 1989; 42: 403-408.

32. GAULARD P, KANAVAROS P, FARCET JP et al.

Bone marrow histological and immunohistological findings in peripheral T-cell lymphomas. A study of 38 cases.

Hum Pathol, 1991; 22: 331-338.

33. CARTON JC, CONRAD ME, VOGLER LB, PARMLEY RT

Isolated marrow lymphoma: an entity of possible T-cell derivation.

Cancer, 1980; 46: 1767-1774.

Blood involvement in chronic (mature) B- and T-lymphoproliferative syndromes

G. FLANDRIN

The clinical manifestations of chronic lymphoid leukaemias (CLL), as well as morphological aspects of peripheral blood lymphoid cells, are various. During the course of some non-Hodgkin's lymphomas (NHL), especially follicular NHL, abnormal lymphoid blood cells may be difficult to distinguish from CLL cells. Since the 1970s, new immunological techniques which allow the typing of membrane molecules (most often glycoproteins) and of some cytoplasmic molecules have greatly improved our understanding of the immune system and contributed useful information on the origin of lymphoproliferative syndromes.

The first contribution was confirmation of the validity of the distinction upon cytological criteria between lymphoblasts and mature lymphocytic cells. The former have an "immature" phenotype and the latter a "mature" one according to the known normal maturation pathway of B and T cells.

The second contribution was to strengthen the correspondence that cytological and clinical criteria had previously established between an immature phenotype and a rapid course (acute lymphoblastic leukaemias) or a mature phenotype and a more benign course (chronic lymphoproliferative syndromes). It has been further shown that the division into T- and B- lymphoproliferative syndromes improved the validity of subclassification. For instance, almost all cases of CLL were monoclonal proliferations of B cells. Conversely, Sézary cells have been shown to be T cells. The cells of hairy-cell leukaemia, whose origin was controversial for many years, were finally accepted as B cells. For some other entities, morphological and immunological data have to be taken into account for establishing a diagnosis.

The discriminating power of immunological techniques was greatly strengthened by the use of monoclonal antibodies against many cell-surface epitopes. These antibodies are presently used:

- for identifying **the B- or T-cell origin** of tumour cells;

- for specifying their **maturation stage,** especially for T cells; and

TABLE I

Immunological methods for B-cell markers

Reagent	Methods*	Designation	Specificity
Anti-human Ig	Cell suspensions Fixed cells	SmIg	B lymphocytes (light-chain restricted)
		CyIg	
Mouse erythrocytes	Spontaneous rosetting	M-rosettes	B-CLL cells
Monoclonal antibodies	Cells in suspension or smeared on slides	Immunofluorescence Immunoperoxidase Immunoalkaline phosphatase	(Table II)
* Cryopreserved cells may also be used			

- for recognizing some "activation" antigens.

The concomitant application of morphological and immunological methods has reinforced the value of cytomorphology and has proved advantageous in increasing our understanding of the heterogeneity of B-CLL itself.

Nevertheless, in clinical practice the cytological diagnosis of the chronic lymphoid leukaemias and allied conditions remains difficult because of their extreme variability.

A classification can now be proposed for "mature" lymphoproliferative syndromes, without taking into account acute lymphoproliferative syndromes (which have an "immature" immunological phenotype) such as acute lymphoblastic leukaemias. Only "mature" lymphoproliferative syndromes will be considered. This classification, although incomplete, can be considered as a basis for improving our knowledge of immunology, cytogenetics and molecular biology as well as for establishing causality, prognosis and therapy relationships. This classification is based upon the blood picture of these diseases, since this is the most usual mode of presentation for clinicians and biologists. The diagnosis suggested by

the blood picture may be modified, in particular if a lymph-node biopsy has been secondarily performed. Lymph-node morphological analysis relies upon another classification scheme (Working Formulation for Clinical Usage, for instance). These two diagnoses may be either identical or apparently divergent for terminology reasons.

Markers for T and B lymphocytes

The identification of specific markers for B and T cells has provided the basis for two broad categories of lymphoid leukaemias. Two markers for B and T lymphocytes were the first to be categorised - membrane immunoglobulins (SmIg), also shown in the cytoplasm (CyIg), and a rosette test with sheep erythrocytes, E-rosette, also recognised by monoclonal antibodies (CD2). These methods and an increasing range of monoclonal antibodies are now essential for the classification of leukaemias and lymphomas. In addition to "pan-B" or "pan-T" reagents, which define the two main lines of

TABLE II

Monoclonal antibodies for the study of B-cell disorders

CD N°	Reactivity	Commonly used monoclonal antibodies
CD5	Mature T cells (strong) B-CLL cells and some NHL cells (weak expression)	Leu1, T101, T1, OKCLL, UCHT2
CD10	Common ALL antigen, early B cells, and some NHL (follicular)	J5, OKB-CALLA, VIL-A1, NU-N1, anti-CALLA
CD19	All B lymphocytes from early to late maturation stages	B4, Leu12
CD20	Most B lymphocytes	B1, Leu16, RFB7, NU-B2
CD21	Restricted to intermediate maturation stages of B cells	B2, RFB6, BA-5
CD22	Late B cells, hairy cells	B3, Leu14, TO15, RFB4, CLB/BLy1
FMC7*	Late B cells, hairy cells, B prolymphocytes	FMC7
CD24	Most B lymphocytes	BA1
CD25	Activated B and T cells; hairy cells	Anti-Tac, Tac1, IL-2R1
CD38	Activated B and T cells; plasma cells	OKT10
Anti-class II MHC antigens*	All B lymphocytes up to plasma cells; activated T cells and haemopoietic precursors	HLA-Dr , OLIa, GRB1, FMC4

* Not allocated to a particular cluster of differentiation ; FMC7 is probably distinct from CD22, although findings in some of the B-cell leukaemias suggest that both appear on the cell membrane at a relatively late stage of B-cell maturation *(Table III)*.

differentiation, some antigens are restricted to some maturation stages and therefore fulfil a useful role for the subclassification. For example, B lymphocytes of CLL are characterised by a distinct pattern of reactivity (1) that consists of the expression of SmIg (weakly) and of the CD5 antigen, high affinity for binding mouse erythrocytes (M-rosettes), and low expression of B maturation antigens such as those detected by monoclonal antibodies FMC7 or the CD22 group on the cell membrane.

The methods to be used and the choice of reagents will depend on the availability and experience of individual laboratories and are beyond the scope of this report. Viable cells are stained in suspension by immunofluorescence methods and observations made by flow cytometry or fluorescence microscopy. The detection of antigens or immunoglobulins on the cell surface and cytoplasm is also possible on fixed-cell preparations - for example, those prepared by a cytocentrifuge, or on frozen sections of

TABLE III

Markers in chronic B-cell leukaemias

Marker	CLL	PLL	HCL	NHL* Follicular lymphoma	Intermediate	SLVL	Plasma-cell tumours**
SmIg	Weak	Strong	Strong	Strong	Moderate	Strong	Negative
CyIg	-	-/+	-/+	-	-	-/+	++
M-rosettes	++	-	-/+	-/+	-/+	-	-
CD5	++	-/+	-	-	++	-	-
CD19/20/24	++	++	++	++	++	++	-
Anti-class II	++	++	++	++	++	++	
FMC7/CD22	-/+	++	++	+	+	++	
CD10	-	-/+	-	+	-/+	-	-/+
CD25	-	-	++	-	-	-/+	-
CD38	-	-	-/+	-/+	-	-/+	++

+ Indicates incidence at which a marker is positive in > 30% of cells in a particular B-cell tumour (++ = 80-100%; + = 40-80%; -/+ = 10-40%; - = 0-9% of cases)

* Non-Hodgkin's lymphomas (NHL) with a high incidence of peripheral-blood or bone-marrow disease.

** Myelomatosis and plasma-cell leukaemia: Waldenström's macroglobulinaemia cells show a similar phenotype except for sharing some features with PLL, HCL and NHL (expression of FMC7, CD22 and some other B-cell antigens).

lymphoid organs prepared by immunocytochemical methods. The proposals for phenotyping B- and T-cell disorders are continually improving with the introduction of new monoclonal antibodies.

B-lymphoid leukaemias

This group of disorders has well-characterised clinical, morphological, and histological features. The defining criterion for diagnosis is the demonstration of a monoclonal population of B cells, shown by immunoglobulin light-chain restriction, and evidence of B-lineage differentiation shown by one or more specific monoclonal antibodies such as CD19, CD20 or CD24 (2).

The markers recommended for the diagnosis of chronic B-cell leukaemias, listed in *Tables I* and *II,* are intended only as guidelines. The patterns of reactivity observed in the most common forms of B-cell leukaemia and NHL with peripheral blood and bone marrow disease are summarised in *Table III.* The phenotype of a chronic B-cell leukaemia is immunologically mature and should be distinguished from that of early B-lineage acute lymphoblastic leukaemias which are immunologically immature - for

TABLE IV

Monoclonal antibodies for the study of T-cell disorders

CD N°	Reactivity	Commonly used monoclonal antibodies
CD1a	Cortical thymocytes; T lymphoblasts	Leu6, T6, OKT6, NA134, NU-T2
CD2	Receptor for sheep erythrocytes; most T cells	T11, OKT11, Leu5
CD3	Mature T lymphocytes	OKT3, Leu4, UCHT1, T3
CD4	Helper/inducer subset	OKT4, T4, Leu3, NU-TH/1
CD5	*(Table II)*	
CD7	Mature and immature T cells	3AI, WT1, Leu9, OKT16
CD8	Cytotoxic/suppressor subset	T8, OKT8, Leu2, NU-T5/Cn UCHT4
CD25	*(Table II)*	

example, positive for the enzyme terminal deoxynucleotidyl transferase (TdT). At the other extreme, plasma cells are associated with the loss of B-cell antigens and class II molecules and the appearance of new antigens such as those detected by CD38 and other monoclonal antibodies such as PCA-1 (2) or BU11 (3). Other reagents not included in *Table III* are anti-HC2 (4) and LeuM5 (CD11c) (5) which react with hairy cells. Because LeuM5 is also positive in monocytes, its value for detecting hairy cells may depend on the simultaneous demonstration of a B-cell antigen, such as CD20 or CD24.

CLL is the B-cell leukaemia which can best be defined by immunological phenotyping *(Table III)*. Cells of some NHL (intermediate or diffuse small cleaved), however, share with CLL lymphocytes the expression of CD5 and have a weaker expression of SmIg than other NHL and B-cell PLL. "Deviation" from typical CLL phenotype is seen in cases with an increased proportion of prolymphocytes or CLL/PL (6) in which marker characteristics intermediate between CLL and PLL may be seen - for example, strong expression of SmIg and reactivity with FMC7 (1,6,7). If four positive criteria for B-cell CLL are set; weak SmIg, > 30% M-rosettes, < 50% CD5+ cells and < 30% FMC7+ cells, a combination of three or four of these markers is seen in 80% of typical CLL, in 65% of CLL/PL cases, and in none of those with a diagnosis of B-PLL (8). Two-thirds of cases of B-PLL have a phenotype quite different from that of CLL: strong SmIg, low M-rosettes and CD5, and > 30% of FMC7+ cells (8,9).

From the above it is apparent that immunological phenotyping provides useful information

TABLE V

Markers in chronic (mature) T-cell leukaemias

Marker	T-CLL	T-PLL	ATLL	Sézary syndrome
TdT	-	-	-	-
CD1a	-	-	-	-
E-rosettes	++	++	++	++
CD2	++	++	++	++
CD3	++	+	++	++
CD4	-	+	++	++
CD5	-	++	++	++
CD7	-	++	-	-
CD8	++	-/+	-	-
CD25	-	-	++	-
CD38	-	-	-	-

+ Indicates rate at which a marker is positive in > 30% of cells, in particular T-cell leukaemias (++ = 80-100%; -/+ = 10-40%; - = 0-9% of cases).

about cell lineage and the stage of B-cell maturation. The final diagnosis, however, depends on the composite information derived from clinical features, cell morphology, histology and membrane markers. It should be recognised that even with optimal methods there are always some cases with atypical features that do not fit exactly into any of the named diagnoses, perhaps reflecting the great heterogeneity of the lymphoid system.

T-cell leukaemias

There is considerable heterogeneity in this group of disorders because of the existence of many functional subsets and stages of maturation of T lymphocytes from which the leukaemia may originate. The reagents used for the diagnosis and classification of the T-cell leukaemias are listed in *Table IV*.

The main distinguishing feature between the immature (or thymic derived) and mature (or post-thymic) T-cell disorders is the presence in the former, which comprises acute T-lymphoblastic lymphoma, of TdT and thymic antigens, such as those recognised by CD1a. Neither TdT nor CD1a are found in chronic T-cell leukaemias *(Table V)*. Important for their consistency as pan-T markers are E-rosettes and CD2 and CD3. The pan-T reagents CD5 and CD7 are more consistently positive in thymic than in post-thymic T-cell malignancies *(Table V)*.

Most types of mature T-cell leukaemia involve CD4+ cells; cases of T-CLL and persistent T lymphocytosis are often, but not always, CD8+ proliferations. Even within CD4+ disorders the neoplastic cells may represent different functional subsets. In addition, other reagents may add further diagnostic information: for example, CD25 is characteristically positive in adult T-cell

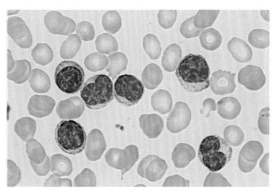

Fig. 1: Peripheral blood film of B-Chronic lymphocytic leukaemia (CLL).

leukaemia/lymphoma (ATLL) cells and rarely in other T-cell leukaemias. Monoclonal antibodies such as Leu7, CD16, and CD11b, which react with large granular lymphocytes and cytotoxic cells, including natural killer cells, can further identify rare types of T-cell leukaemia, which often come under the designation of T-CLL.

As with the B-cell disorders, immunological methods are necessary to define T-cell leukaemias and provide guidance to specific diagnoses, but are not sufficient to define clinicopathological entities. For this, the immunological features need to be integrated with cytomorphological and histopathological findings. Furthermore, monoclonal antibodies cannot establish whether a T-cell proliferation is clonal. This is now possible by analysis of the rearrangement of the T-cell receptor β, δ- and γ-chain genes and by chromosome studies.

Proposals for a classification of the cytomorphology of chronic (mature) lymphoproliferative disorders

First, T- and B- lymphoproliferative disorders have to be studied separately (10). For some categories, such as CLL, hairy-cell leukaemia, ATL, diagnosis may be made only from cytological examination since the cells have specific morphological characteristics. For all other T- and B- lymphoproliferative disorders, the origin of tumour cells must be specified using specific immunological markers. Cytogenetic studies may also provide information on pathogenesis and prognosis.

B-cell leukaemias: cell morphology

The characteristics of the various types of lymphocytes seen in the most common B-cell leukaemias allow distinction between the small lymphocytes of typical CLL and the large lymphocytes and pro-lymphocytes seen in CLL of mixed-cell type. A subtle distinction can be made between the pleomorphic prolymphocytes seen in CLL/PL and the more uniform ones seen characteristically in B-cell PLL. In the leukaemic forms of NHL clea-ved or cleft cells are characteristic of fol-licular lymphoma, and cells of variable morphology and some degree of nuclear irregularity are a feature of other types of NHL.

Chronic lymphocytic leukaemia

Peripheral blood

Defining criteria using the current staging systems for the disease suggest that a persistent lymphocytosis of $> 10 \times 10^9/l$ is sufficient for a diagnosis of CLL. In adults with lymphocytosis between 5 and $10 \times 10^9/l$, cell-marker studies are necessary to confirm the presence of monoclonal B cells. In typical cases of CLL the cells are small with a conspicuous though narrow rim of cytoplasm *(fig. 1)*. Both the nuclear and cytoplasmic outlines are regular, although a small degree of nuclear irregularity with a kidney shape or a small indentation is seen in some cases *(fig. 2)*.

The cytoplasm is homogeneous and weakly basophilic and granules are not seen.

The nuclear/cytoplasmic ratio is high. The nuclear chromatin is characteristically dense with clumps of dark chromatin separated by narrow pale spaces. With the standard Romanovsky stains the nucleoli are either not visible or are inconspicuous and small. Some morphological variation is seen from patient to patient. In some, the cytoplasm tends to be a little more abundant. When more than 10% of the lymphocytes are large or are prolymphocytes the diagnosis of mixed-cell type CLL should be considered. Smudge cells are artefacts of blood films, which are not diagnostic, but nevertheless are characteristic of B-cell CLL and in general tend to be more conspicuous with a high white-cell count.

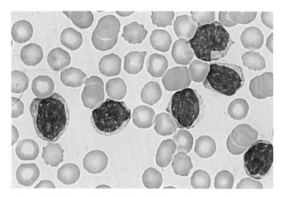

Fig. 2: Peripheral blood film of CLL with more than 10% prolymphocytes (CLL/PL).

Bone marrow

Aspirates are generaly hypercellular and show lymphocytic infiltration. Bone-marrow biopsy specimens are necessary to define the various patterns of infiltration and to exclude the diagnosis of NHL such as follicular lymphoma. The extent of infiltration, which may be interstitial, nodular, mixed or diffuse, correlates with the clinical stage (19,20).

Lymph-node biopsy

Although lymph-node disease in CLL is common, biopsies are not performed routinely. They are necessary in cases with low lymphocyte counts or when the membrane phenotype departs considerably from the typical pattern described in *Table III*, and, when the counts are high, if the morphology suggests a diagnosis of NHL.

CLL, mixed-cell types

In several cases diagnosed as CLL the morphological features are different from those described above. Two types of this form of CLL may be found: (**i**) a mixture (dimorphic picture) of small lymphocytes and prolymphocytes (> 10% and less than 55%) designated CLL/PL; and (**ii**) a spectrum of small-to-large lymphocytes with occasional (less than 10%) prolymphocytes. There is currently no clear evidence for a biological disadvantage in the latter group with respect to typical CLL, but data are accumulating which suggest refractoriness to treatment and a worse prognosis for the CLL/PL group (21,22).

In two-thirds of cases of CLL/PL the composite membrane phenotype of B-CLL is found, and in one-third only one or two of the CLL markers (usually CD5 or high M-rosettes) are demonstrable (8).

Although clinical and laboratory features of CLL/PL are at least in some respects intermediate between those of CLL and PLL, marker studies suggest a closer affinity with CLL (6,8). The small lymphocytes of CLL/PL tend to have a larger volume than those of CLL (21) and the prolymphocytes tend to be more pleomorphic than those seen in PLL *(fig. 2)*. These cases are clinically heterogeneous and include patients with typical CLL which evolves into a more aggressive form, described as CLL in "prolymphocytoid" transformation (22) and others who present with an increased proportion of prolymphocytes and whose course may not be progressive.

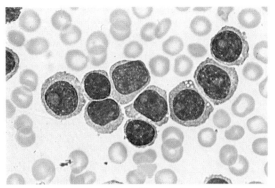

Fig. 3: Peripheral blood film of B-prolymphocytic leukaemia (B-PLL).

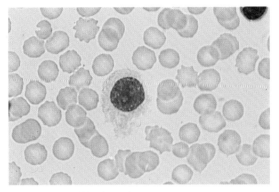

Fig. 4: Hairy-cell leukaemia.

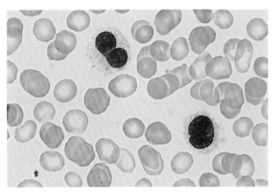

Fig. 5: Hairy-cell leukaemia. Hairy cells with indented or kidney-shaped nuclei.

The cases in the second group of CLL of mixed-cell type are less well-defined and less common. These are characterised by larger cells than those seen in typical CLL, tend to have a lower nuclear/cytoplasmic ratio, and show a trend towards increased cytoplasmic basophilia. A clear distinction between two cell populations by size (small and large) is not usually possible. The percentage of prolymphocytes is less than 10%. Histological studies of lymph-nodes and bone-marrow biopsy specimens are important to distinguish these cases from some forms of NHL.

Prolymphocytic leukaemia

PLL is a distinct disorder characterised by a high white-cell count and splenomegaly without lymphadenopathy (23). The membrane phenotype of the prolymphocyte is quite distinct from that of CLL *(Table III)* but has similarities to that of other B-cell leukaemias. The prolymphocyte is the predominant cell in peripheral blood films (> 55%, usually > 70%) and is characterised *(Table VI)* by its large size, round nucleus with a prominent vesicular nucleolus, relatively well condensed nuclear chromatin and a lower nuclear/cytoplasmic ratio than the small lymphocyte of CLL *(fig. 4)*. These morphological features must be sought in well spread areas of blood films. The bone-marrow infiltration is diffuse, not very different from that of CLL, or has a mixed interstitial-nodular pattern. The histological appearance of lymph nodes shows diffuse disease with or without a pseudo-nodular pattern (24). The histological appearance of the spleen shows white- and red-pulp infiltration, with large proliferative nodules in the white pulp with a characteristic bizonal appearance – dense at the centre and lighter at the periphery (25).

Hairy-cell leukaemia

The hairy cell is the outstanding morphological feature of this disease (26). It has fine, irregular cytoplasmic projections or villi

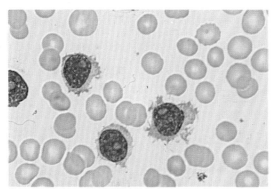

Fig. 6: Hairy-cell variant, with abnormal cells sharing the features of both prolymphocytes (prominent nucleolus), and hairy cells.

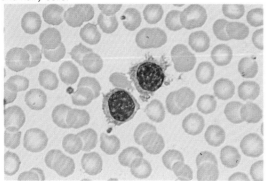

Fig. 7: Peripheral blood of "splenic lymphoma with villous lymphocytes" (SLVL).

and is, overall, larger than most other lymphocytes. On peripheral blood films the cytoplasm stains light blue and has a poorly defined outline *(figs 4 and 5)*. Fine azurophilic granules are seen occasionally. Rod-shaped inclusions with a pale centre correspond to the ribosome-lamellar complexes seen on electron-microscopic examination. The nuclear/cytoplasmic ratio is low and the nucleus is excentrically placed. The nucleus is oval, round, or kidney-shaped. The nuclear chromatin has a fine dispersed pattern and nucleoli are inconspicuous, small, and usually single. The bone marrow is always affected in HCL but may be difficult to aspirate because of associated fibrosis. Material available from scanty aspirates or touch print preparations may be useful to identify hairy cells. Bone-marrow biopsy

sections are essential for diagnosis. These show variable degrees of infiltration by hairy cells which can be identified by nuclear shape, the chromatin pattern, and the clear zone that separates one cell from another resulting from the abundant cytoplasm. The histological appearance of the spleen shows a distinctive pattern of red-pulp infiltration with the formation of pseudo-sinuses and widening of the pulp cords. Membrane markers *(Table III)* support the diagnosis of HCL, in particular combined reactivity with CD25, Leu M5, and HC2. Tartrate-resistant acid phosphatase (TRAP) is a typical cytochemical finding (27).

Hairy-cell variant (HCL-V)

This relatively rare disorder was described as having morphological features which are intermediate between hairy cells and prolymphocytes. The characteristic cells have an abundant cytoplasm, more basophilic than in hairy cells, but with similar villous projections, moderately condensed heterochromatin with a prominent nucleolus as in PLL cells, and have a slightly higher nuclear/cytoplasmic ratio than typical hairy cells *(fig. 6)*. The disease runs a chronic course with splenomegaly and a high white-cell count (usually > 50 x 10^9/l, a rare finding in typical HCL) without monocytopenia. As in HCL, the variant cells infiltrate the spleen mainly in the red pulp. The membrane phenotype is close to that of prolymphocytes. In contrast to typical hairy cells, HCL-V cells do not react with CD25 and HC2 but some cases are LeuM5-positive. Membrane IgG is often found on the cell membrane but in some cases SmIg cannot be demonstrated.

Splenic lymphoma with villous lymphocytes (SLVL)

It has been recognised that some patients suspected on clinical and laboratory grounds (splenomegaly and circulating lymphocytes with villous projections) of having HCL, have, in fact, a predominantly splenic form of NHL, as established by analysis of the histological appearance of the spleen (30,31). A small monoclonal band is shown in the serum or urine in two-thirds of cases. The white-cell count is usually between 3 and 38 x 10^9/l and the circulating lymphocytes, which comprise most of the cells, are larger than CLL lymphocytes and are close to the size of prolymphocytes. The nucleus is round or ovoid, has clumped chromatin, and in half of the cases also has a small, distinct nucleus *(fig. 7)*. The amount of cytoplasm is variable and is moderately basophilic. The main features are the presence of short villi, often situated at one pole of the cell. The nuclear/cytoplasmic ratio is higher than in hairy cells of HCL and HCL-V; a few cells show lymphoplasmacytic features *(fig. 7)*. Membrane markers of SLVL cases are similar to those of B-PLL. Unlike HCL cells, these villous lymphocytes do not react with HC2, CD25, LeuM5, or cytochemically with the TRAP reaction. The differential diagnoses to be considered are CLL, B-PLL, HCL and HCL-variant. The histological appearance of the spleen shows white-pulp disease (in contrast to HCL and HCL-V), with or without clinically important red-pulp infiltration (30,31). The bone marrow is not infiltrated in half of the cases; in others, there is moderate-to-pronounced diffuse or nodular infiltration.

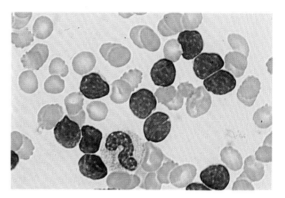

Fig. 8: Leukaemic phase of follicular lymphoma.

Leukaemic manifestations of NHL

Before the era of immunological markers several conditions (B- and T-derived) were broadly described as "lymphosarcoma cell leukaemia" (32). These cases were thought to represent *de novo* lymphoid leukaemias, but it is clear that these are cases of NHL which present in a leukaemic phase of their disease or which have progressed to a leukaemic phase. The most common form is follicular lymphoma in leukaemic phase (33-35). Spiro et al. reported that 38% of cases with histologically confirmed follicular lymphoma presented with a lymphocytosis greater than 5 x 10^9/l which was described as "CLL-like syndrome" (33). In a significant proportion of such cases, however, the morphological features were different from those of CLL.

Whenever it is suspected that a lymphocytosis is associated with a NHL, bone-marrow and lymph-node biopsy sections are an essential part of the investigation. When referring to this group of cases, only those in which the disease presents in a leukaemic phase, which may be arbitrarily defined as > 5 x 10^9/l abnormal lymphocytes, will be considered here. This does not preclude the identification of a small percentage of NHL cells in the peripheral blood. Although the abnormal circulating cells may be derived from several histological subtypes of NHL (34), the most common and best characterised form is the leukaemic phase of follicular lymphoma (35). Cases of stage IV NHL with bone-marrow disease (36) but no peripheral-blood disease will not be discussed.

Leukaemic phase of follicular lymphomas

High lymphocyte counts (45-220 x 10^9/l) (34) simulating a lymphoid leukaemia may be observed at presentation in follicular lymphomas. The morphological features of the circulating cells in follicular lymphoma are small, cleaved lymphocytes (often smaller than CLL lymphocytes) with a high nuclear/cytoplasmic ratio and very scanty cytoplasm, usually confined to a thin rim visible between the concavities of the nucleus *(fig. 8)*. The nuclear chromatin is uniformly condensed without clumping. Prominent but usually very narrow nuclear clefts or fissures are seen in > 30% of cells;

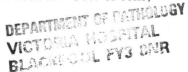

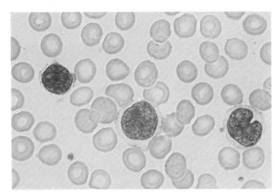

Fig. 9: Leukaemic phase of "intermediate" NHL.

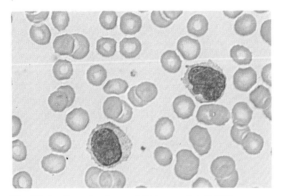

Fig. 10: Leukaemic phase of "intermediate" NHL.

Intermediate NHL or mantle-zone lymphoma

There are no detailed studies of the leukaemic manifestation of this lymphoma (37-40). The most common cell is of medium size, has condensed chromatin, an inconspicuous nucleolus with slight nuclear irregularities best characterised as indentations and clefts *(fig. 9)*. The latter are not as pronounced or as deep as in follicular lymphoma cells. Larger cells with a high nuclear/cytoplasmic ratio and without a prominent nucleolus are seen *(fig. 10)*. In a few cases the appearances are those given above for CLL of mixed-cell types, except that most cases of intermediate NHL have a paucity of small lymphocytes. Bone-marrow biopsy specimens show diffuse disease. The lymphoid population is monotonous and the cells are larger than CLL lymphocytes and tend to have an irregular nuclear outline. The above morphological criteria were derived from the examination of blood and bone-marrow films from cases in which there was a consensus for the diagnosis of NHL-intermediate type in leukaemic phase (37-40). Membrane-marker studies show CD5+ cells (37-40), and SmIg staining of moderate intensity with μ and δ as the main heavy-chain classes (41). CD10 is positive when tested on all cell suspensions but negative by immunocytochemistry.

Lymphoplasmacytic lymphomas

These are cases in which monoclonal immunoglobulin bands are present in the serum and include Waldenström's macroglobulinaemia and also cases of SLVL, described above. In Waldenström's macroglobulinaemia the paraprotein concentrations are > 20 g/l, while in SLVL the IgG or IgM paraprotein band concentrations are < 20 g/l; the white-cell count is usually > 10 x 10⁹/l in SLVL and < 10 x 10⁹/l in Waldenström's macroglobulinaemia. The circulating lymphoid cells in Waldenström macroglo-bulinaemia comprise a mixture of small and large lymphocytes, sometimes with an excentric nucleus and pronounced cytoplasmic basophillia and morphological diversity. The bone marrow is often diseased in Waldenström's macroglobuli-

these clefts often rise at sharp angles to the nuclear surface and when they are deep they divide the nucleus in two. These features of the nucleus are even more apparent on ultrastructural analysis. The cell outline is often angular and nucleoli are either absent or barely visible. Membrane markers *(Table III)* show differences with the findings in B-CLL; SmIg is strong, the percentage of M-rosettes is low, FMC7 is positive, CD5 is usually negative and CD10 is often positive. These findings are helpful when the cytological features described above are not typical and suggest a diagnosis of CLL. Bone-marrow disease is common and typically shows a paratrabecular localisation of lymphocytic infiltration (36), although diffuse infiltration can also be found.

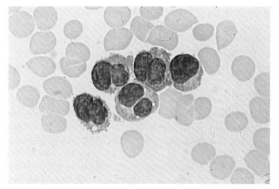

Fig. 11: Plasma cell leukaemia, with small plasma cells.

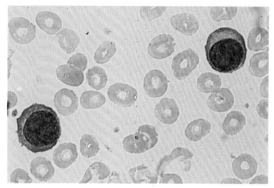

Fig. 12: Plasma cell leukaemia, with blast-like plasma cells.

naemia with a mixture of cells of different nuclear maturity, some with dense chromatin and others with fine chromatin, and variable basophilia. A proportion of plasma cells and of mast cells is characteristic of Waldenström's macroglobulinaemia.

Plasma-cell leukaemia (PCL)

PCL refers to patients with primary leukaemia and not the terminal phase of myelomatosis (multiple myeloma) in which abnormal plasma cells circulate in 2% of cases (42). PCL is usually an acute illness sometimes resembling acute leukaemia. Hepatosplenomegaly is more common and bone lesions are less common than in myelomatosis, while hypercalcaemia and renal failure are common. We recognise two morphological types of PCL. In one, the cells are small and range from lymphocytes with basophilic cytoplasm to plasma cells, and in the other they are blast-like cells. In the former, but not in the latter type, there is nuclear excentricity and a clear Golgi zone. Intense basophilia is a feature mainly of the small plasmacytic type *(figs 11* and *12)*. Membrane-marker studies *(Table III)* are helpful in recognising the plasmablasts. Antigens normally found in B cells are lacking but new late B-cell antigens appear. The presence of monoclonal CyIg and expression of CD38 are diagnostic. Ultrastructural analysis often discloses plasma cell features. Other laboratory investigations

(Bence-Jones proteinuria, hypercalcaemia) may also contribute towards a diagnosis of PCL.

T-cell leukaemias: cell morphology

Once markers have assigned a lymphocytic proliferation to the T-cell series, the next step is to define the morphology of the cells. The cells seen in the mature T-cell leukaemias include lymphocytes with a range of morphological type: (i) large granular lymphocytes, characterised by abundant cytoplasm and azurophil granules; (ii) prolymphocytes with a prominent nucleolus, basophilic cytoplasm, and no azurophil granules; (iii) pleomorphic, polylobed cells; and (iv) small or large cerebriform cells. Lymphocytes with a mature morphology but without azurophil granules are present in normal peripheral blood but are very rarely seen as the predominant cell in T-cell leukaemias (44).

T-cell lymphocytosis and T-CLL

The upper limit of the absolute lymphocyte count in adults is about 4.8 x 10^9/l. Most normal lymphocytes are small- to medium-sized with a high nuclear/cytoplasmic ratio

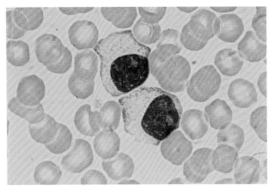

Fig. 13: Peripheral blood film of chronic T-lymphocytic leukaemia (proliferation of large granular lymphocytes).

is likely to be T-CLL; rarely, the white-cell count is > 20 x 10^9/l. In most cases the cells are large granular lymphocytes (45-47). These have a low nuclear/cytoplasmic ratio and show several fine or sometimes coarse azurophil granules in the abundant pale blue cytoplasm; occasional cells with the same morphology are agranular. The nucleus is round or oval, slightly excentric, and has clumped nuclear chromatin; nucleoli are rare *(fig. 13)*. These lymphocytes which consitute 50-93% of the peripheral blood leucocytes, react strongly with cytochemical reactions for acid phosphatase and β-glucuronidase, but weakly or not all with α-naphthyl acetate esterase (ANAE) (48). Ultrastructural analysis shows that the azurophil granules are distinct structures designated as parallel tubular arrays (49).

and a densely clumped nuclear chromatin; nucleoli are usually indistinct. Most cells are agranular with a thin layer of basophilic or colourless cytoplasm. About 80% of the circulating lymphocytes are of T-cell origin. Cases of reactive B-cell lymphocytosis are extremely rare. More frequently, an absolute increase in the number of atypical T lymphocytes is seen as a result of several infective processes. Reactive lymphocytosis is self-limiting and is rarely above 5 x 10^9/l. The most common causes are viral infections, Epstein-Barr virus or cytomegalovirus in adults, and *Bordetella pertussis* in children in which very high counts may occur. The atypical cells have a lower nuclear/cytoplasmic ratio than normal, are often two to four times the size of normal lymphocytes, and have variable cytoplasmic basophilia; sometimes the nucleus is irregular and resembles that of the monocyte but it almost always has the coarsely clumped chromatin characteristic of lymphocytes.

In contrast to reactive lymphocytosis, chronic or persistent (> 3 months) T lymphocytosis of unknown cause occurs and further study shows the proliferation to be clonal. The lymphocytosis tends to increase gradually over the ensuing months or years and is often associated with cytopenias, usually neutropenia. If T lymphocytosis of > 5 x 10^9/l persists for over six months and consists of a relatively uniform population of lymphocytes, the diagnosis

In addition to cases with a chronic course and stable T-lymphocytosis, there are those with more bulky disease of liver and spleen and progressive course with rising white-cell counts. In both types of T-CLL the phenotype is that of the so-called T-γ lymphocyte with a spectrum of antigenic profiles; most cases with a chronic course have a CD3+, CD8+, CD4-, Leu7+, membrane phenotype *(Table V)*. Cases with unusual phenotypes, representing granular lymphocytes rarely seen in normal peripheral blood - for example, CD4+, CD16+, CD8+, CD11b+, etc. - tend to have a more aggressive evolution. DNA analysis with probes for the β- and δ-chain genes of the T-cell receptor shows the genes to be in a rearranged configuration in most cases of chronic T-cell lymphocytosis as defined above, thus justifying the term of T-CLL or large granular lymphocyte leukaemia for this group of patients. Chronic T lymphocytosis can be distinguished from T-CLL only by proving clonality by DNA (10) or cytogenetic analysis in the latter condition (45).

Bone-marrow aspirates in cases of T-CLL show infiltration of variable degree; minor in the early stages, > 50% in later stages (46-47). Bone marrow trephine-biopsy specimens show focal or more diffuse accumulations which do not displace the normal bone-marrow cells. In some cases a maturation arrest of the granulocytic series is seen and in others there is erythroid hypoplasia. The latter features are closely associated with the presence of neutropenia or aregenerative anaemia (46-47).

T-prolymphocytic leukaemia

About 20% of patients who present with clinical and morphological features of PLL have a T-cell malignancy (2). Within the mature T-cell leukaemia, T-PLL may represent up to 40% of cases. As in B-PLL, in T-PLL the white-cell count is usually > 100 x 10^9/l at presentation but, in contrast, there are usually lymphadenopathy, skin lesions, and serous effusions as well as splenomegaly, and the course is aggressive. The circulating cells in half of the cases of T-PLL resemble those of B-PLL and unless cell-marker studies are performed, it may be difficult to distinguish between these two disorders. In other cases, T-PLL cells have less cytoplasm and a higher nuclear/cytoplasmic ratio than B-PLL cells (44). T prolymphocytes may also have an irregular nuclear outline *(fig. 14)*. In some cases the cells are small and the nucleolus is not easily seen by light microscopy. In general, T prolymphocytes have a deep basophilic cytoplasm which sometimes even suggests plasma-cell differentiation. Also characteristic is the presence of large and dense localised granular structures (49) which correlates with the strong positivity with cytochemical reactions for most acid hydrolases, including ANAE (48). The chromosome abnormality inv (14) has been found consistently in two-thirds of the cases studied with identical breakpoints at 14q11 and 14q32 (7). Membrane markers *(Table V)* show that most T-PLL are CD4+, CD8- proliferations; a minority coexpress CD4 and CD8 and a few are CD4-, CD8+ (9,44). Unlike other mature T-cell leukaemias, in particular those with a CD4+ phenotype, T-PLL cells express the CD7 antigen strongly.

There is little information on the histopathological features of T-PLL. The few cases studied showed diffuse infiltration of

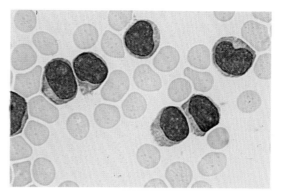

Fig. 14: T-prolymphocytic leukaemia.

the splenic red pulp with obliteration of the white pulp. In lymph-nodes the infiltration is diffuse and affects predominantly paracortical areas. The bone marrow is usually diffusely infiltrated and shows increased fibrosis (50).

Adult T-cell leukaemia/lymphoma

Over a decade ago the first reports of an unusual syndrome in Japanese adults appeared (51,52). The patients had manifestations of generalised lymphadenopathy with circulating abnormal lymphoid cells associated with hypercalcaemia, bone lesions, skin lesions and bone-marrow disease.

The white-cell count ranged widely and the percentage of abnormal cells ranged from 10 to 80% (52,53). The cells varied considerably in size from that of a small lymphocyte to a large mononuclear cell (over 14 μm). The nuclear chromatin was relatively homogeneous and clumped or condensed. The nuclear outline has been variously described as convoluted or "clover-leafed". This conveys the most striking feature of the cells: pronounced polymorphism *(figs. 15 and 16)*. Nucleoli are uncommon and, when present, are small. The cytoplasm is agranular and strongly basophilic. Occasionally it is difficult to distinguish the cells from those seen in Sézary syndrome; electron microscopy

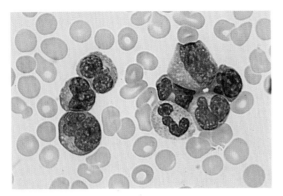

Fig. 15: Peripheral blood of adult T-cell lymphoma/leukaemia (ATL).

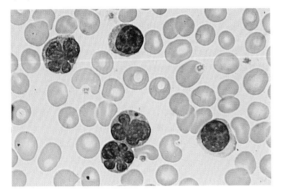

Fig. 16: Peripheral blood of adult T-cell lymphoma/leukaemia (ATL).

chronic ATL the white-cell count is lower, there are fewer circulating abnormal cells, and the survival period is more than one year. The bone marrow is often normal in these cases. Finally, a group of patients have normal white-cell counts and few non-specific symptoms, and a low proportion of abnormal T lymphocytes in the blood films. Evidence of clonality in such cases can be shown by molecular methods with appropriate HTLV-1 probes. This condition has been designated as "smouldering" ATL (54).

ATL has a distinct epidemiology which relates to the distribution of its causative agent, the human type-C retrovirus HTLV-1 (55). The association of HTLV-1 with ATL has been shown by serological and molecular studies. Almost all patients with ATL have a high titre of antibodies to HTLV-1, and DNA analysis shows clonal integration of HTLV-1 in the neoplastic ATL cells. Most cases have been found in south-western Japan (52-54), the Caribbean region, and in Caribbean immigrants who reside in other countries (56).

Sézary syndrome

This disorder is characterised by generalised exfoliative erythroderma and an epidermal infiltrate of atypical mononuclear cells. The abnormal circulating cells in such cases are known as Sézary cells. Sézary syndrome was the first disorder shown to be of T-cell origin (57,58). In peripheral, blood films there are two types of Sézary cells: large (fig. 17) and small (fig. 18). The large Sézary cells, with near tetraploid chromosome number, are less common. They are larger than neutrophils and sometimes also larger than monocytes. The nucleus is large and occupies four-fifths of the cell with a round or oval profile and densely clumped chromatin. A grooved pattern is apparent and this corresponds to the cerebriform nuclear shape shown at ultrastructural level (44). Nucleoli are small and rarely visible. The cytoplasm shows clear basophilia, has a narrow rim around the nucleus, and lacks azurophil granules.

may help for this purpose. There are also instances in which T-PLL may be confused with ATL because the prominent nucleolus normally seen in T-PLL cells can be indistinct and the nuclear outline may be irregular (42). In addition to polylobed cells, some blastic cells with basophilic cytoplasm are almost always seen in blood films of ATL. Positive cytochemical markers include acid phosphatase, β-glucuronidase, and ANAE. The membrane phenotype is summarised in Table IV. The cells are CD4+ and, unlike other T-cell disorders, consistently express the receptor for Interleukin-2 (CD25).

There is a spectrum of clinical syndromes in ATL (54). The most common, acute ATL, presents with a high white-cell count, hypercalcaemia, and the survival period is less than one year. In the more

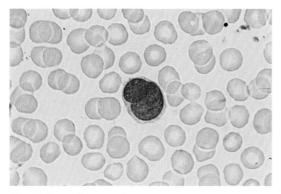

Fig. 17: Large Sézary cell.

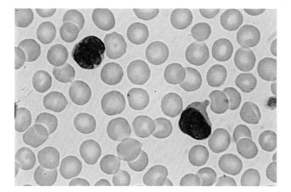

Fig. 18: Peripheral blood of Sézary syndrome, small-cell variant (Lutzner cell).

in the upper dermis with epidermotropism and Pautrier microabscesses. The membrane phenotype of Sézary cells is that of a mature T lymphocyte with CD3+, CD4+, CD8- markers *(Table V)*.

Discussion

The subdivision of chronic (mature) lymphoid blood disorders into several distinct entities requires determination of the membrane phenotype of the neoplastic cells as well as description of their morphological features.

The usefulness of these subdivisions resides in the relationships between morphological patterns and clinical features, especially prognosis. Recent therapeutic improvements have been facilited by this information. For instance, alpha-interferon appeared most active in hairy-cell leukaemia. Clear distinction between CLL and PLL has been justified by the differences in clinical presentation and treatment response. Without a precise analysis of morphological and immunological characteristics there is a clear risk of confusion between CLL, hairy-cell leukaemia and the leukaemic phase of some NHL. For instance, the identification of splenic lymphoma with villous lymphocytes among B-cell lymphoproliferative disorders is most useful because of the risk of confusion with hairy-cell leukaemia.

The recognition of distinct entities within the T-cell leukaemias has important epidemiological and pathophysiological connotations as illustrated by ATL, the T-cell leukaemia caused by HTLV-1 and T-PLL, where a specific chromosome abnormality, inv (14), is often found. A more systematic analysis of chromosome abnormalities and of their relationships with the previously described morpho-immunological entities would further justify such a classification. Cytogenetic studies have proved useful in the study of molecular biology of lymphoid proliferations. Some morphological

The small-cell variant of Sézary cell (also known as the Lutzner cell) is more common (59). The cell is the size of a small lymphocyte *(fig. 18)* but has the same grooved nuclear chromatin pattern as the large Sézary cell *(fig. 19)*. Lutzner cells, however, usually have a higher nuclear/cytoplasmic ratio than small lymphocytes and sometimes show cytoplasmic vacuoles (PAS positive) around the nucleus. Electron microscopical examination is useful for the morphological identification of small and large Sézary cells. Bone-marrow aspirates are either normal or show minimal infiltration; obvious disease is seen when the white-cell count is high. Skin-biopsy sections show the typical pattern of infiltration entities are associated with certain translocations, for instance t(14;18) in follicular lymphomas (62), trisomy 12 in CLL (12-14), t(11;14) in B-PLL (17) and inv (14) in T-PLL.

References

1. CATOVSKY D, MELO JV, MATUTES E

   Biological markers in lymphoproliferative disorders.

   In : Bloomfield CD ed. Chronic and acute leukaemias in adults. The Hague: Martinus Nijhoff Publischers, 1985; 69-112.

2. ANDERSON KC, BATES MP, SLAUGHENHOUPT BL et al.

   Expression of human B cell-associated antigens in leukaemias and lymphomas: a model of human B-cell differentiation.

   Blood, 1984; 63: 1424-1433.

3. NATHAM PD, WALKER L, HARDIE D et al.

   An antigenic study of human plasma cells in normal tissue and in myeloma identification of a novel plasma cell-associated antigen.

   Clin Exp Immunol, 1986; 65: 112-119.

4. POSNETT DN, WANG C-Y, CHIORAZZI N, CROW MK, KUNKEL HG

   An antigen characteristic of hairy-cell leukaemia cells expressed on certain activated B cells.

   J Immunol, 1984; 133: 1635-1640.

5. SCHWARTING R, STEIN H, WANT CY

   The monoclonal antibodies S-HCL1 (Leu-14) and S-HCL3 (Leu-M5) allow the diagnosis of hairy-cell leukaemia.

   Blood, 1985; 65: 974-983.

6. MELO JV, CATOVSKY D, GALTON DAG

   The relationship between chronic lymphocytic leukaemia and prolymphocytic leukaemia. 1 - Clinical and laboratory features of 300 patients and characterisation of an intermediate group.

   Br J Haematol, 1986; 63: 377-387.

7. SCOTT CS, LIMBERT HJ, ROBERTS BE, STARK AN

   Prolymphocytoid variants of chronic lymphocytic leukaemia: an immunological and morphological survey.

   Leuk Res, 1987; 11: 135-140.

8. MELO JV, BRITO-BABAPULLE V, OLIVEIRA MSP, GALTON DAG, CATOVSKY D

   The relationship between chronic lymphocytic leukaemia and prolymphocytic keukaemia.

   In: Gale RP, Rai K, Eds. Chronic lymphocytic leukaemia. Recent progress and future direction. New York: Alan R. Liss Inc, 1987; 205-214.

9. CATOVSKY D, WESCHLER A, MATUTES E et al.

   The membrane phenotype of T-prolymphocytic leukaemia.

   Scand J Haematol, 1982; 29: 398-404.

10. MINDEN MD, MAK TW

    The structure of the T-cell antigen receptor genes in normal and malignant T cells.

    Blood, 1986; 68: 327-336.

11. BENNETT JM, CATOVSKY D, DANIEL MT et al.

    The French American British (F.A.B.) Cooperative Group. Proposals for the classification of chronic (mature) B- and T- lymphoid leukaemias.

    J Clin Path, 1989; 42: 567-584.

12. JULIVSSON G, GAHRTON G

    Chromosome aberrations in B-cell chronic lymphocytic leukemia. Pathogenetic and clinical implications.

    Canc Genet Cytogenet, 1990; 45: 143-160.

13. ROSSEN PE

    Cytogenetic and molecular changes in chronic B-cell leukemia.

    Canc Genet Cytogenet, 1989; 43: 43-50.

14. HURET JL, MOSSAFA H, BRIZARD A et al.

    Karyotypes of 33 patients with clonal aberrations in chronic lymphocytic leukemia. Review of 216 abnormal karyotypes in chronic lymphocytic leukemia.

    Ann Genet, 1989; 32: 155-159.

15. KODURU PRK, FILIPPA DA, RICHARDSON ME et al.

    Cytogenetic and histologic correlations in malignant lymphoma.

    Blood, 1987; 69: 97-102.

16. GAHRTON G, ROBERT K-H, FRIBERG K, ZECH L, BIRD AG

    Non-random chromosomal aberrations in chronic lymphocytic leukaemia revealed by polyclonal B-cell-mitogen stimulation.

    Blood, 1980; 56: 640-647.

17. BRITO-BABAPULLE V, PITTMAN S, MELO JV, POMFRET M, CATOVSKY D

    Cytogenetic studies on prolymphocytic leukaemia. 1-B cell prolymphocytic leukaemia.

    Hematol Pathol, 1987; 1: 27-33.

18. BRITO-BABAPULLE V, POMFRET M, MATUTES E, CATOVSKY D

    Cytogenetic studies on prolymphocytic leukaemia. II-T-cell prolymphocytic leukaemia.

    Blood, 1987; 70: 926-931.

19. ROZMAN C, MONTSERRAT E, RODRIGUEZ-FERNANDEZ JM et al.

Bone marrow histologic pattern. The best single prognostic parameter in chronic lymphocytic leukaemia: a multivariate survival analysis of 329 cases?

Blood, 1984; 64: 642-648.

20. PANGALIS GA, ROUSSOU PA, KITTAS C, KOKKINOU S, FESSAS P

B-chronic lymphocytic leukaemia. Prognostic implication of bone-marrow histology in 120 patients experience from a single hematology unit.

Cancer, 1987; 69: 767-771.

21. MELO JV, CATOVSKY D, GREGORY WM, GALTON DAG

The relationship between chronic lymphocytic leukaemia and prolyphocytic leukaemia. IV - Analysis of survival and prognostic features.

Br J Haematol, 1987; 65: 23-29.

22. VALLESPI T, TORRABADELLA M, JULIA A et al.

Chronic lymphocytic leukaemia: a multivariate survival analysis including morphological types of lymphoid cells in peripheral blood.

In: Gale RP, Rai KR, eds. Chronic lymphocytic leukaemia. Recent progress and future direction. New York: Alan R. Liss. Inc., 1987; 277-288.

23. MELO JV, WARDLE J, CHETTY M et al.

The relationship between chronic lymphocytic leukaemia and prolymphocytic leukaemia III - Evaluation of cell size by morphology and volume measurements.

Br J Haematol, 1986; 64: 469-478.

24. ENNO A, CATOVSKY D, O'BRIEN M et al.

"Prolymphocytoid" transformation of chronic lymphocytic leukaemia.

Br J Haematol, 1979; 41: 9-18.

25. GALTON DAG, GOLDMAN JM, WILTSHAW E, CATOVSKY D, HENRY K, GOLDENBERG GJ

Prolymphocytic leukaemia.

Br J Haematol, 1974; 27: 7-23.

26. OWENS MR, STRAUCHEN JA, ROWE JM, BENNETT JM

Prolymphocytic leukaemia: histologic findings in atypical cases.

Hematol Oncol, 1984; 2: 249-257.

27. LAMPERT I, CATOVSKY D, MARSH GW, CHILD JA, GALTON DAG

The histopathology of prolymphocytic leukaemia with particular reference to the spleen: a comparison with chronic lymphocytic leukaemia.

Histopathology, 1980; 4: 3-19.

28. BOURONCLE BA

Leukemic reticuloendotheliosis (hairy-cell leukaemia).

Blood, 1979; 53: 412-436.

29. YAM LT, JANCKILA AJ, LI C-Y, LAM WKW

Cytochemistry of tartrate-resistant acid phosphatase: 15 years' experience.

Leukaemia, 1987; 1: 285-288.

30. CAWLEY JC, BURNS GF, HAYHOE RGH

A chronic lymphoproliferative disorder with distinctive features: a distinct variant of hairy-cell leukemia.

Leuk Res, 1980; 4: 547-559.

31. CATOVSKY D, O'BRIEN M, MELO JV, WARDLE J, BROZOVIC M

Hairy-cell leukaemia (HCL) variant: an intermediate disease between HCL and B-prolymphocytic leukaemia.

Semin Oncol, 1984, 11. 362-369.

32. MELO JV, HEGDE U, PARREIRA A, THOMPSON I, LAMBERT IA, CATOVSKY D

Splenic B-cell lymphoma with circulating villous lymphocytes: differential diagnosis of B-cell leukaemias with large spleens.

J Clin Pathol, 1987; 40: 642-651.

33. NEIMAN RS, SULLIVAN AL, JAFFE R

Malignant lymphoma simulating leukaemic reticuloendotheliosis. A clinicopathologic study of ten cases.

Cancer, 1979; 43: 329-342.

34. ISAACS R

Lymphosarcoma cell leukaemia.

Ann Intern Med, 1937; 11: 657-662.

35. SPIRO S, GALTON DAG, WILTSHAW E, LOHMANN RC

Follicular lymphoma: a survey of 75 cases with special reference to the syndrome resembling chronic lymphocytic leukaemia.

Br J Cancer, 1975; 31 (suppl. II): 60-72.

36. COME SE, JAFFE ES, ANDERSON JC, MANN RB et al.

Non-Hodgkin's lymphomas in leukemic phase : clinicopathologic correlations.

Am J Med, 1980; 69: 667-674.

37. MELO JV, ROBINSON DSF, DE OLIVEIRA MP et al.

Morphology and immunology of circulating cells in leukaemic phase of follicular lymphoma.

J Clin Pathol, 1988; 41: 951-959.

38. BENNETT JM, CAIN KC, GLICK JH, JOHNSON GT et al.

    The significance of bone-marrow involvement in non-Hodgkin's lymphomas: the Eastern Cooperative Oncology Experience.

    J Clin Oncol, 1986; 4: 1462-1469.

39. SWERDLOW SH, HABESHAW JA, MURRAY LJ, DHALIWAL HS et al.

    Centrocytic lymphoma: a distinct clinicopathologic and immunologic entity. A multiparameter study of 18 cases at diagnosis and relapse.

    Am J Pathol, 1983; 113: 181-197.

40. JAFFE S, BOOKMAN MA, LONGO DL

    Lymphocytic lymphoma of intermediate differentiation-mantle zone lymphoma: a distinct subtype of B-cell lymphoma.

    Hum Pathol, 1987; 18: 877-880.

41. WEISENBURGER DD, SANGER WG, ARMITAGE JO, PURTILO DT

    Intermediate lymphocytic lymphoma: immunophenotypic and cytogenetic findings.

    Blood, 1987; 69: 1617-1621.

42. POMBO DE OLIVEIRA MS, JAFFE H, CATOVSKY D

    Leukaemic phase of mantle-zone (intermediate) lymphoma: its characterization in 11 cases.

    J Clin Path, 1989; 42: 962-972.

43. HARRIS NL, NADLER LM, BHAN AK

    Immunohistologic characterisation of two malignant lymphomas of germinal center type (centroblastic/centrocytic and centrocytic) with monoclonal antibodies.

    Am J Pathol, 1984; 117: 262-272.

44. KYLE RA, MALDONADO JE, BAYRD ED

    Plasma-cell leukemia: report on 17 cases.

    Arch Intern Med, 1974; 133: 813-818.

45. PARREIRA A, ROBINSON DSF, MELO JV et al.

    Primary plasma-cell leukaemia: immunological and ultrastructural studies in 6 cases.

    Scand J Haematol, 1985; 35: 570-578.

46. MATUTES E, GARCIA TALAVERA J, O'BRIEN M, CATOVSKY D

    The morphological spectrum of T-prolymphocytic leukaemia.

    Br J Haematol, 1986; 64: 111-124.

47. BROUET JC, FLANDRIN G, SASPORTES M, PREUD'HOMME JL, SELIGMANN M

    Chronic lymphatic leukaemia of T-cell origin.

    Lancet, 1975; ii: 890-893.

48. NEWLAND AC, CATOVSKY D, LINCH D et al.

    Chronic T-cell lymphocytosis: a review of 21 cases.

    Br J Haematol, 1984; 58: 433-446.

49. LOUHRAN TP JR, KADIN ME, STARKEBAUM G et al.

    Leukemia of large granular lymphocytes: association with clonal chromosomal abnormalities and autoimmune neutropenia, thrombocytopenia and hemolytic anemia.

    Ann Intern Med, 1985; 102: 169-175.

50. COSTELLO C, CATOVSKY D, O'BRIEN M, MORILLAR R, VARADIS

    Chronic T-cell leukaemias. 1 - Morphology, cytochemistry and ultrastructure.

    Leuk Res, 1980; 4: 463-476.

51. CROCKARD AD, CHALMERS D, MATUTES E, CATOVSKY D

    Cytochemistry of acid hydrolases in chronic B- and T-cell leukaemias.

    Am J Clin Pathol, 1982; 78: 437-444.

52. HERNANDEZ NIETO L, LAMBERT IA, CATOVSKY D

    Bone marrow histological patterns in B- and T-pro-lymphocytic leukaemia.

    Hematol Pathol, 1989; 3: 79-84.

53. YODOI J, TAKATSUKI K, MASUDA T

    Two cases of T-cell chronic lymphocytic leukemia in Japan.

    N Engl J Med, 1974; 290: 572-573.

54. UCHIYAMA T, YODOI J, SAGAWA K, TAKATSUKI K, UCHINO H

    Adult T-cell leukemia: clinical and hematologic features of 16 cases.

    Blood, 1977; 50: 481-492.

55. KINOSHITA K, KAMIHIRA S, IKEDA S et al.

    Clinical, hematologic and pathologic features of leukemic T-cell lymphoma.

    Cancer, 1982; 50: 1554-1562.

56. ABRAMS MB, SIDAWY M, NOVICH M

    Smoldering HTLV-associated T-cell leukemia.

    Arch Intern Med, 1985; 145: 2257-2258.

57. POIESZ BJ, RUSCETTI FW, GAZDAR AF et al.

    Detection and isolation of type C retrovirus particles from fresh and cultured lymphocytes of a patient with cutaneous T-cell lymphoma.

    Proc Natl Acad Sci USA, 1980; 77: 7415-7419.

58. BLATTNER WA, BLAYNEY DW, ROBERT-GUROFF M et al.

    Epidemiology of human T-cell leukemia/lymphoma virus.

    J Infec Dis, 1983; 147: 406-416.

59. BROUET JC, FLANDRIN G, SELIGMANN M

    Indications of the thymus-derived nature of the proliferating cells in six patients with Sézary's syndrome.

    N Engl J Med, 1973; 289: 341-344.

60. FLANDRIN G, BROUET JC

    The Sézary cell: cytologic, cytochemical and immunologic studies.

    Mayo Clin Proc, 1974; 49: 575-583.

61. LUTZNER MA, EMERIT I, DUREPAIRE R, FLANDRIN G, GRUPPER CH, PRUNERIAS M

    Cytogenetic, cytophotometric and ultrastructural study of large cerebriform cells of the Sézary syndrome and description of a small-cell variant.

    JNCI, 1973; 50: 1145-1162.

62. CROCE CM, NOWELL PC

    Molecular basis of human B cell neoplasia.

    Blood, 1985; 65: 1-7.

Liver involvement in non-Hodgkin's lymphomas

J.-Y. SCOAZEC, N. BROUSSE

Since secondary involvement of the liver in non-Hodgkin's lymphoma is usually accompanied by only mild clinical and/or biological abnormalities, its incidence is often underestimated. However, systematic histological investigations have shown that liver is one of the most frequent secondary extranodal sites involved in non-Hodgkin's lymphoma (1-3). In contrast to secondary involvement, primary hepatic non-Hodgkin's lymphomas are exceedingly rare.

Secondary liver involvement in non-Hodgkin's lymphomas

Symptoms and signs of secondary liver involvement are usually absent or mild. Liver enlargment is rarely observed. Functional findings are either normal or moderately altered, cholestasis being the most frequent biological abnormality (4). Radiological examination (sonography, computed tomography) only detects the largest lesions and usually fails to diagnose minimal involvement.

Liver biopsy therefore is the only reliable procedure to diagnose secondary hepatic involvement in non-Hodgkin's lymphoma. Three techniques have been used: (a) percutaneous needle biopsy; (b) needle biopsy during laparoscopy; and (c) wedge biopsy during laparotomy. Percutaneous liver biopsy is the least sensitive method (1,4,5).

However, since systematic laparotomy and/or laparoscopy are no longer in use, percutaneous liver biopsy is currently the usual technique for staging purposes.

Overall incidence of secondary liver involvement in non-Hodgkin's lymphoma has been variously estimated. Figures from 15 (6) to 40% (7) have been reported, depending on the sensitivity of the staging procedure. When percutaneous needle biopsy is used alone, liver involvement is detected in about 25% of cases. Incidence of liver involvement also varies with histological type. When systematically sought, liver involvement may be detected in up to 80% of non-Hodgkin's lymphoma, small lymphocytic type (3) and in up to 50% of follicular lymphomas (1,3,4). In contrast, it is observed in less than 15% of large-cell and immunoblastic lymphomas (3).

In some cases, histological diagnosis of secondary liver involvement by non-Hodgkin's lymphoma may be difficult. Diagnostic difficulties depend on the histological type. Most of them are encountered in hepatic lesions due to NHL, small-cell type (figs 1 & 2), which may be confused with dense inflammatory infiltrates, such as those observed in certain cases of chronic hepatitis (fig. 3). The most significant histological features favouring the diagnosis of secondary NHL are: (a) the regular enlargement of involved portal tracts, generally round and well delineated; (b) the monomorphic cytological appearance of the lymphoid infiltrate; (c) the coexistence of

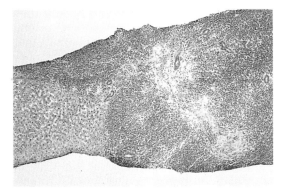

Fig. 1a

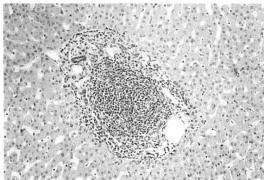

Fig. 2a

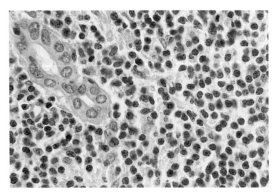

Fig. 1b

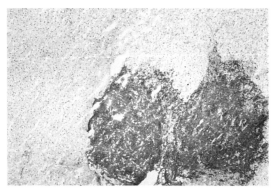

Fig. 2b

Fig. 1: **Lymphoma of the liver, small-cell type**. Morphological aspects at low magnification (1a) and high magnification (1b)

normal and involved portal tracts on the same biopsy; and *(d)* the presence of abnormal lymphoid cells in hepatic parenchyma. In difficult cases, immunohistochemical examination may be useful to show the polyclonality of inflammatory infiltrates *(fig. 4)*, contrasting with the monoclonality of lymphomatous infiltrates *(fig. 3)* (8). Moreover, inflammatory infiltrates consist predominantly of T cells (8), while small-cell NHL are usually of B-cell origin *(figs 1 & 2)*. Specific involvement of the liver in small-cell NHL must also be distinguished from the non-specific lymphoid infiltrates which may be observed in the liver during the course of certain lymphoid malignancies. Non-specific infiltrates are lobular and/or portal. They generally consist of a polymorphous population, comprising small lymphocytes, plasma cells, histiocytes and eosinophils. T lymphocytes are numerous *(fig. 3)* (9). The significance of non-specific infiltrates, which may also be observed in

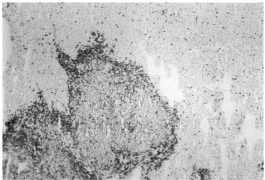

Fig. 2c

Fig. 2: **Lymphoma of the liver, small B-cell type.** Involvement of a portal tract (2a). Immunohistochemical demonstration of the monotypic nature: anti-κ reactivity of lymphoid cells (2b). Absence of reactivity with a pan-T-cell antibody CD3 with small reactive T cells around the nodule (2c)

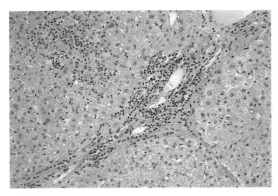

Fig. 3a

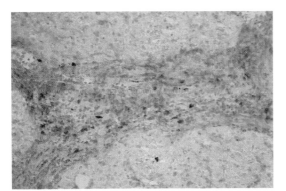

Fig. 3b

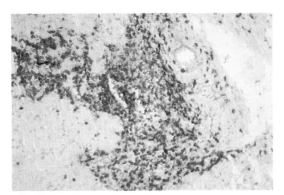

Fig. 3c

Fig. 3: **Lymphoid infiltrate of portal tract and lobule in chronic hepatitis** (3a). Immunohistochemistry shows the differences with hepatic lymphoma: rare B cells (3b, anti-pan-B CD22 antibody) and numerous T cells (3c, CD3 labelling)

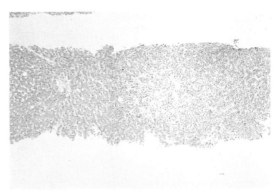

Fig. 4a

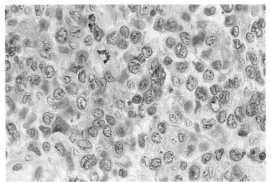

Fig. 4b

Fig. 4: **Primary large-cell lymphoma of the liver,** at low (4a) and high (4b) magnifications

Hodgkin's disease (10), is not clear. It is well established that the existence of such lesions is not correlated with the presence of a specific involvement.

Large-cell NHL (fig. 4) raise another type of diagnostic difficulty: the differential diagnosis with undifferentiated liver carcinoma. In this case, immunohistochemistry using markers specific for lymphoid and epithelial cells (which can be performed on paraffin-embedded sections) is helpful in solving diagnostic problems (8).

Certain cases of T-cell lymphomas, in which neoplastic infiltration is strictly or predominantly intrasinusoidal (fig. 5) (11,12), may be confused with hairy-cell leukaemia. Cytological analysis of neoplastic lymphoid cells and immunohistochemical examination (8) make it possible to reach the correct diagnosis.

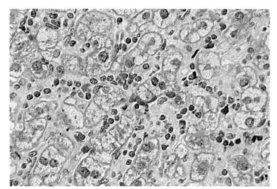

Fig. 5: **Hepatic lymphoma, T-cell type:** *dense lymphoid infiltration of the sinusoids*
(Dr. P. Gaulard)

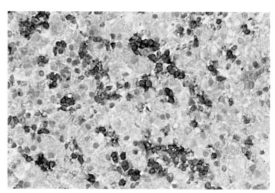

Fig. 6: **Hepatic lymphoma, T-cell type:** *intrasinusoidal lymphoid cells are labelled by CD3 antibody*
(Dr. P. Gaulard)

Non-Hodgkin's lymphomas with primary presentation in the liver

Exceptionally, certain NHL may present as predominant liver disease. Several types of clinical presentation have been observed: acute hepatic failure, isolated hepatic tumour or hepatomegaly.

NHL presenting as acute hepatic failure

Fulminant hepatic failure may reveal various types of malignant haematological disorder and, in particular, various types of NHL, including the small cleaved, the small non-cleaved and the large-cell types (13,14). On clinical examination, the liver is usually enlarged and rapidly expanding. Biological alterations are characterized by an association of cell-lysis signs, paradoxically often moderate, signs of hepatocellular failure, cholestasis and lactic acidosis. On histological examination, hepatic parenchyma is densely infiltrated by neoplastic lymphoid cells, which may be observed in portal tracts, sinusoids, and even portal vascular walls. Hepatic plates are atrophic. Prognosis is unfavourable and the outcome rapidly fatal. However, if chemotherapy is initiated promptly, remission may be achieved (14).

NHL presenting as primary hepatic tumours

The so-called "primary" NHL of the liver are rare: about 60 cases have been reported in the literature (15-18). Their incidence has recently increased since they represent one of the major causes of primary hepatic tumours in the acquired immunodeficiency syndrome (17,18).

Patients usually present with an apparently primary hepatic tumour, which may be accompanied by signs of portal hypertension and by constitutional symptoms (fever, weakness, weight loss). Radiological examinations (sonography, computed tomography, and arteriography) show the existence of one, or more rarely, several intra-hepatic masses, hypo- or hyper-echogenic, hypodense and hypovascularized. In the absence of specific clinical and radiological features, the correct diagnosis is reached only by the histological examination of a guided liver biopsy or of a surgical specimen.

Most cases of "primary" non-Hodgkin's lymphoma of the liver are of the large-cell type. Immunohistochemical examination shows that most of them are of B-cell lineage (16,17); several cases of T-cell lymphoma have been reported (19,20). On biopsy material, differential diagnosis may be difficult with a poorly differentiated carcinoma. Immunohistochemical examination demonstrating the expression of specific cellular markers is helpful in solving such diagnostic problems, even on fixed material.

Prognosis of "primary" NHL of the liver is difficult to ascertain, since the number of reported cases is low. However, it is generally accepted that hepatic lymphomas have a better prognosis than NHL of the same histological type arising in other sites. Local treatment, particularly surgical resection, if possible, may improve the prognosis (17,19).

Peripheral T-cell lymphomas presenting as predominant liver disease

A subset of peripheral T-cell lymphomas is characterized by a distinctive clinical, histological and immunological presentation (21-23). Clinically, patients present with marked liver enlargement, usually associated with splenomegaly, but without detectable superficial lymphadenopathy. Liver findings are usually mildly altered. Histologically, lymphoid tumour cells densely infiltrate sinusoids (fig. 5). In contrast, portal involvement is absent or moderate. Immunologically, intrasinusoidal T-cell lymphomas are characterized by a mature T-cell phenotype (fig. 6), lack of reactivity with the T marker anti-CD5, and expression of the γ/δ-antigen receptor.

References

1. CHABNER BA, JOHNSON RE, DE VITA VT Jr et al.

   Sequential staging in non-Hodgkin's lymphomas.

   Cancer Treat Rep, 1977; 61: 993-997.

2. ANDERSON T, CHABNER BA, YOUNG RC et al.

   Malignant lymphoma. I. The histology and staging of 473 patients at the National Institute.

   Cancer, 1982; 50: 2699-2707.

3. THE KIEL LYMPHOMA STUDY GROUP

   Clinical and prognostic relevance of the Kiel Classification of non-Hodgkin's lymphomas: results of a prospective multicenter study by the Kiel Lymphoma Study Group.

   Hematol Oncol, 1984; 2: 269-306.

4. KIM H, DORFMAN RF, ROSENBERG SA

   Pathology of malignant lymphomas in the liver: application to the staging.

   In: Progress in liver diseases, Grune and Stratton, New-York; vol. 5: p. 683-698.

5. KIM H, DORFMAN RF

   Morphological studies in 84 untreated patients subjected to laparotomy for the staging of non-Hodgkin's lymphomas.

   Cancer, 1974; 33: 657-674.

6. GOFFINET DR, WARNKE R, DUNNICK DR et al.

   Clinical and surgical (laparotomy) evaluation of patients with non-Hodgkin's lymphomas.

   Cancer Treat Rep, 1977; 61: 981-992.

7. KOLARIC K, ROTH A, DOMINIS M, JAKASA V

   The diagnosis value of percutaneous liver biopsy in patients with non-Hodgkin's lymphomas. A preliminary report.

   Acta Hematol Gastroenterol, 1977; 24: 440-443.

8. VOIGT JJ, VINEL JP, CAVERIVIERE P et al.

   Diagnostic immuno-histochimique des localisations hépatiques des hémopathies lymphoïdes malignes. Etude de 80 cas.

   Gastroentérol Clin Biol, 1989; 13: 343-352.

9. VERDI CJ, GROGAN TM, PROTELL R, RICHTER L, RANGER C

   Liver biopsy immunotyping to characterize lymphoid malignancies.

   Hepatology, 1986; 6: 6-13.

10. LESLIE KO, COLBY TV

    Hepatic parenchymal lymphoid aggregates in Hodgkin's disease.

    Hum Pathol, 1984; 15: 808-809

11. DIEBOLD J

    Le sinusoïde hépatique en pathologie hématologique.

    Arch Anat Cytol Pathol, 1984; 32: 301-306.

12. KADIN ME

    T-gamma cells: a missing link between malignant histiocytosis and T-cell leukaemia-lymphoma ?

    Hum Pathol, 1981; 12: 771-773

13. COLBY TV, LABRECQUE DR

    Lymphoreticular malignancy presenting as fulminant hepatic disease.

    Gastroenterol, 1982; 82: 339-345

14. ZAFRANI ES, LECLERCQ B, VERNANT JP, PINAUDEAU Y, CHOMETTE G, DHUMEAUX D
    Massive blastic infiltration of the liver: a cause of fulminant hepatic failure.
    Hepatology, 1983; 3: 428-432.

15. FEKETE F, MOLAS G, TOSSEN JC, DEGOTT C, LANGUILLE O, POTET F
    Lymphome histiocytaire primitif du foie. Etude de deux cas et revue de la littérature.
    Gastroentérol Clin Biol, 1983; 7: 785-791.

16. OSBORNE BM, BUTLER JJ, GUARDA LA
    Primary lymphoma of the liver: ten cases and review of the literature.
    Cancer, 1985; 56: 2902-2910

17. SCOAZEC JY, DEGOTT C, BROUSSE N et al.
    Non-Hodgkin's lymphoma presenting as a primary tumor of the liver: presentation, diagnosis and outcome in eight patients.
    Hepatology, 1991; 13: 870-875.

18. CACCAMO D, PERVES NK, MARCHEVSKY A
    Primary lymphoma of the liver in the acquired immunodeficiency syndrome.
    Arch Pathol Lab Med, 1986; 110: 553-555.

19. ANDREOLA S, AUDISIO RA, MAZZAFERRO V, DOVI R, MAKOWA L, GENNARI L
    Primary lymphoma of the liver showing immunohistochemical evidence of T-cell origin. Successful management by right trisegmentectomy.
    Dig Dis Sci, 1988; 33: 1632-1636.

20. ANTHONY PP, SARSFIELD P, CLARKE T
    Primary lymphoma of the liver: clinical and pathological features of 10 patients.
    J Clin Pathol, 1990; 43: 1007-1013.

21. GAULARD P, ZAFRANI ES, MAVIER P et al.
    Peripheral T-cell lymphoma presenting as predominant liver disease. A report of three cases.
    Hepatology, 1986; 6: 864-868.

22. GAULARD P, BOURQUELOT P, KANAVAROS P et al.
    Expression of the alpha/beta and gamma/delta T-cell receptors in 57 cases of peripheral T-cell lymphomas. Identification of a subset of gamma/delta T-cell lymphomas.
    Am J Pathol, 1990; 137: 617-628.

23. FARCET JP, GAULARD P, MAROLLEAU JP et al.
    Hepatosplenic T-cell lymphoma: sinusal/sinusoidal localization of malignant cells expressing the T-cell receptor gamma/delta.
    Blood, 1990; 75: 2213-2219.

Spleen involvement in non-Hodgkin's lymphomas

J.-Y. SCOAZEC, N. BROUSSE

Secondary splenic involvement has been found in between 40 and 60% of non-Hodgkin's lymphoma cases, irrespective of the histological type (1,2). In contrast, apparently primary splenic lymphomas are exceedingly rare: their frequency has been estimated to be less than 1% of all NHL (3).

Secondary involvement of the spleen in NHL

Secondary involvement of the spleen in NHL is usually revealed by splenomegaly, and in exceptional cases by splenic rupture (4). For staging purposes, splenic involvement is assimilated to lymph-node involvement. Its frequency depends on the histological type. Secondary involvement of the spleen is observed in 50 to 60% of NHL of low or intermediate grades of malignancy (i.e. follicular lymphomas, diffuse lymphomas of small lymphocytic, small cleaved-cell and mixed-cell types). In contrast, splenic involvement occurs in only 20 to 40% of diffuse, large-cell and immunoblastic lymphomas (1,2,5).

Gross features

Spleens involved in NHL are generally of increased size: their weight is usually between 1,500 and 1,700 gr (3,6). However, it must be emphasized that normal-sized spleens can be involved. Examination of autopsy specimens has shown that up to 30% of normal-sized spleens were microscopically involved (3).

Four types of gross involvement are to be distinguished (6-8):

- absence of macroscopically visible lesions, the white pulp being apparently normal;

- diffuse and homogeneous involvement by multiple nodules measuring 1 to 5 mm in diameter;

- focal or diffuse involvement by large and usually confluent nodules measuring 1 to 5 cm in diameter; and

- focal involvement by a single large mass, usually with central necrosis (*fig. 1*).

Histological features

Histological features and diagnostic problems are different for B- and T-cell lymphomas.

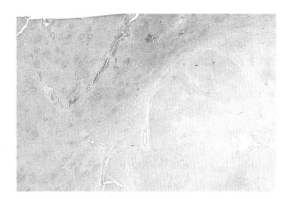

Fig. 1: **Large-cell lymphoma of spleen:** *large single tumour with central necrosis*

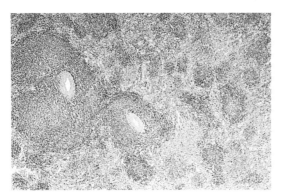

Fig. 2: **Small-cell lymphoma of spleen:** *hypertrophy of the white pulp*

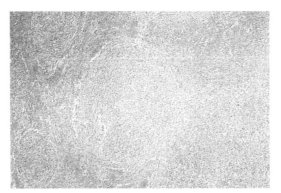

Fig. 3: **Small-cell lymphoma of spleen:** *hypertrophy of the white pulp with infiltration of the red pulp*

Secondary spleen involvement in **B-cell NHL** characteristically affects the white pulp (9,10) (*fig. 2*). Corpuscles are larger and more numerous than in the normal spleen. They are usually of irregular shape and tend to form coalescent masses of increasing size. Neoplastic lymphoid cells secondarily infiltrate the red pulp to a variable degree (*fig. 3*). Initial involvements of the spleen in B-cell NHL of the small-cell type (*fig. 2*) may be difficult to diagnose. Such lesions are characterized by an increased number of corpuscles, whose size and shape are not altered. A peripheral rim of normal lymphocytes may persist. Detailed cytological analysis of the affected corpuscles is necessary to ascertain the diagnosis of neoplastic lymphoid involvement. Such lesions must not be confused with reactive lymphoid hyperplasias of the spleen. Criteria for the differential diagnosis are identical to those used in the distinction between follicular lymphomas and follicular hyperplasias in lymph nodes. Three

additional signs are to be mentioned: (**a**) in reactive lymphoid hyperplasias of the spleen, all the corpuscles are usually involved, while in malignant involvements, normal corpuscles coexist with neoplastic ones (8) (*fig. 4*); (**b**) reactive hyperplasias of the spleen are generally associated with red pulp plasmacytosis; and (**c**) malignant involvements are generally associated with sub-endothelial vascular infiltration (*fig. 5*). Immunohistochemistry may be helpful in solving some diagnostic problems by showing a monotypic B-cell proliferation.

Secondary spleen involvement in **T-cell NHL** characteristically affects the periarteriolar sheath of the white pulp, which constitutes a thymo-dependent zone in the normal spleen. Involvement further progresses either through the entire corpuscle or towards the red pulp (9). It should be remembered that massive involvements of

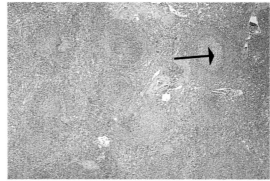

Fig. 4: **Small-cell lymphoma of spleen:** *coexistence of normal and tumorous corpuscules*

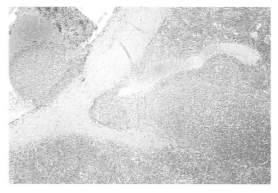

Fig. 5: **Small-cell lymphoma of spleen:** *infiltration of the white pulp with sub-endothelial infiltration*

the red pulp by B-cell lymphomas may be observed. In these cases, the characteristic lesions of the white pulp are difficult to identify. In consequence, immunohisto-chemistry is necessary to ascertain the diagnosis of T-cell lymphoma in the spleen. Splenic involvement by T-cell lymphomas raises specific diagnostic problems. Their polymorphic appearance together with the possible existence of pseudo-Reed-Stern-berg cells may lead to confusion with Hodgkin's disease of the spleen. The predominant involvement of the red pulp observed in some cases may lead to confusion with hairy-cell leukaemia. This diagnosis may be refuted using cytological criteria and because of the absence of the angiomatous lesions characteristic of hairy-cell leukaemia (11,12).

Primary splenic non-Hodgkin's lymphomas

So-called "primary" NHL of the spleen cor-reponds to cases of lymphomas with primary presentation in the spleen, i.e. clinically isolated splenomegaly, absence of superficial lymphadenopathy, and absence of blood involvement (13-15). However splenomegaly is rarely strictly isolated. Regional lymphadenopathies are often found simultaneously, especially in the splenic hilum, mesentery and retroperitoneum.

Splenomegaly may be discovered because of functional symptoms (abdominal pain) or of hypersplenism, or on routine examination. Constitutional symptoms are rare. Radiological investigations (sonography and computed tomography) may reveal two distinct patterns: (a) a multinodular involvement; or (b) the existence of a single large mass. Splenectomy may be used to ascertain the diagnosis. However, surgical resection is not always necessary. Indeed, at this stage, diagnosis of NHL may often be achieved by indirect examinations, such as biopsy of bone marrow or of liver, which are involved in 60 and 30% of cases, respectively (13).

Primary presentation in the spleen may be observed in all types of NHL. The following types are the most frequent:

- small lymphocytic lymphomas (50% of primary splenic lymphomas) and their various subtypes, falling into the so-called "B-cell leukaemias with splenomegaly" category (17). A particular entity, named splenic B-cell lymphoma with circulating villous lymphocytes, in which neoplastic B cells resembling hairy cells involve both the white and the red pulp, and are found in varying numbers in the blood, has recently been described (17) (see pp. 249-269);

- small cleaved-cell lymphomas (20% of the primary splenic lymphomas); and

- large-cell and immunoblastic NHL (15 to 25% and 10% of the primary splenic lymphomas, respectively). Large-cell lymphomas of the spleen are characterized by the existence of a large and rapidly growing single mass with regional dissemination. The few cases subjected to immunohisto-chemical examination proved to be of B-cell type (16).

Before splenectomy, primary spleen NHL has to be distinguished from other primary splenic tumours. These tumours are exceedingly rare and their frequency is even less than that of primary NHL (16,18). Another problem of differential diagnosis is raised by an entity of uncertain significance and behaviour: so-called idiopathic spleno-megaly (19,20). Cases grouped under this name clinically simulate splenic NHL. His-tologically, they are characterized by a florid lymphoid hyperplasia of the spleen, sometimes accompanied by reactive infiltrates in liver and bone marrow. Some of these cases have evolved towards typical lymphoma after a variable delay ranging between a few months and 6 years (21).

The prognosis of primary splenic lymphomas depends on their histological type. It is comparable to that of nodal lymphomas of the same type (13,14). Cases of prolonged survival have been reported (22). Most authors have proposed that splenecto-my be included in the therapeutic protocol.

A particular clinical entity is constituted by the association between primary splenic lymphoma and C1 esterase-inhibitor deficiency (23). Treatment of the NHL is accompanied by regression of the clinical symptoms of angioneurotic oedema, and by regression of the biological abnormalities of the complement system.

References

1. GOFFINET DR, WARNKE R, DUNNICK DR et al.
   Clinical and surgical (laparotomy) evaluation of patients with non-Hodgkin's lymphomas.
   Cancer Treat Rep, 1977; 61: 981-992.

2. RIBAS-MUNDO M, ROSENBERG SA
   The value of sequential bone-marrow biopsy and laparotomy and splenectomy in a series of 200 consecutive untreated patients with non-Hodgkin's lymphoma.
   Eur J Cancer, 1979; 15: 941-952.

3. AHMANN DL, KIELY JM, HARRISON EG, PAYNE WS
   Malignant lymphoma of the spleen: a review of 49 cases in which the diagnosis was made at splenectomy.
   Cancer, 1966; 19: 461-469.

4. BAUER TW, HASKINS GE, ARMITAGE JO
   Splenic rupture in patients with hematologic malignancies.
   Cancer, 1981; 48: 2729-2733.

5. The Kiel Lymphoma Study Group:
   Clinical and prognostic relevance of the Kiel Classification of non-Hodgkin's lymphomas: results of a prospective multicenter study by the Kiel Lymphoma Study Group.
   Hematol Oncol, 1984; 2: 269-306.

6. BREITFELD V, LEE RE
   Pathology of the spleen in hematologic disease.
   Surg Clin North Amer, 1975; 55: 233-251.

7. DIEBOLD J
   La splénectomie en hématologie. Considérations anatomopathologiques.
   Ann Gastroentérol Hépatol, 1974; 10: 413-429.

8. BUTLER JJ
   Pathology of the spleen in benign and malignant conditions.
   Histopathology, 1983; 7: 453-474.

9. BURKE JS
   The diagnosis of lymphoma and lymphoid proliferations in the spleen.
   In: Surgical pathology of lymph nodes and related organs, Saunders, Philadelphia, 1985: p. 249-281.

10. BURKE JS
    Surgical pathology of the spleen: an approach to the differential diagnosis of splenic lymphomas and leukemias. Part I. Diseases of the white pulp.
    Am J Surg Pathol, 1981; 5: 551-563.

11. BURKE JS
    Surgical pathology of the spleen: an approach to the differential diagnosis of splenic lymphomas and leukemias. Part II. Diseases of the red pulp.
    Am J Surg Pathol, 1981 ; 5 : 681-694.

12. NANBA K, SOBAN EJ, BOWLING MC, BERARD CW
    Splenic pseudosinuses and hepatic angiomatous lesions : distinctive features of hairy-cell leukemia.
    Am J Clin Pathol, 1977; 67: 415-426.

13. SPIER CM, KJELKSBERG SR, EYRE HJ, BEHM FG
    Malignant lymphoma with primary presentation in the spleen. A study of 20 patients.
    Arch Pathol Lab Med, 1985; 109: 1076-1080.

14. KRAEMER BB, OSBORNE BM, BUTLER JJ
    Primary splenic presentation of malignant lymphoma and related disorders. A study of 49 cases.
    Cancer, 1984, 54: 1606-1619.

15. DAVEY FR, SKARIN AT, MOLONEY WC
    Pathology of splenic lymphoma.
    Am J Clin Pathol, 1973; 59: 95-103.

16. HARRIS NL, AISENBERG AC, MEYER JE, ELLMAN L, ELMAN A
    Diffuse large-cell (histiocytic) lymphoma of the spleen. Clinical and pathologic characteristics of ten cases.
    Cancer, 1984; 54: 2460-2467.

17. MELO JV, HEGDE U, PARREIRA A, THOMPSON I, LAMPERT IA, CATOVSKY D
    Splenic B-cell lymphoma with circulating villous lymphocytes: differential diagnosis of B-cell leukaemias with large spleen.
    J Clin Pathol, 1987; 40: 642-651.

18. WICK MR, SMITH SL, SCHEITHAUER BW, BEART RW Jr
    Primary non-lymphoreticular malignant neoplasms of the spleen.
    Am J Surg Pathol, 1982; 6: 229-242.

19. LONG JC, AISENBERG AC
    Malignant lymphoma diagnosed at splenectomy and idiopathic splenomegaly: a clinicopathologic comparison.
    Cancer, 1974; 33: 1054-1061.

20. DACIE JV, BRAIN MC, HARRISON CV, LEWIS SM, WORLLEDGE SM
    Non-tropical idiopathic splenomegaly ("primary hypersplenism"): a review of ten cases and their relationship to malignant lymphomas
    Br J Haematol, 1969; 17: 317-333.

21. DACIE JV, GALTON DAG, GORDON-SMITH EC, HARRISON CV

Non-tropical idiopathic splenomegaly: a follow-up study of ten patients described in 1969.

Br J Haematol, 1978; 38: 185-193.

22. MONTANARO A, PATTON R

Primary splenic malignant lymphoma, histiocytic type, with sclerosis: report of a case with long-term survival.

Cancer, 1976; 38: 1625-1628.

23. DREYFUS B

Lymphomes spléniques.

In: Hématologie, Flammarion, Paris, 1984: pp. 700-702.

ADDENDUM

FALK S, STUTTE HJ

Primary malignant lymphomas of the spleen. A morphologic and immunohistocheminal analysis of 17 cases.

Cancer, 1990; 66: 2612-2619.

STROUP RM, BURKE JS, SHEIBANI K, BEN-EZRA J, BROWNELL M, WINBERG CD

Splenic involvement by aggressive malignant lymphomas of B-cell and T-cell types.

Cancer, 1992; 69: 413-420

Extra-cranial non-Hodgkin's lymphomas of the head and neck

PH. SOLAL-CÉLIGNY, N. BROUSSE

NHL of Waldeyer's ring

Waldeyer's ring is formed by the lymphoid aggregates located at the junction of the upper digestive and respiratory tracts. It includes the palatine and facial tonsils, the lymphoid tissue of the nasopharynx and the base of the tongue. Secondary involvement of Waldeyer's ring is found in 7% (1) to 10% (2) of NHL. Higher incidences have been reported in series from Europe (3-5) where Waldeyer's ring involvement was systematically sought (*see pp. 101-105*). Apart from NHL, which frequently involve Waldeyer's ring in patients with HIV-1 infection, a non-malignant tumoral nasopharyngeal lymphoid hyperplasia has recently been described in HIV-infected patients (6). These patients complain of nasal twang, dyspnoea, otalgia and/or hypoacousia. Histological examination shows an intense follicular hyperplasia of the nasopharyngeal lymphoid tissue with prominent germinal centres but no monoclonal B-cell proliferation (6).

Primary non-Hodgkin's lymphomas of Waldeyer's ring represent 5 to 10% of all NHL (7,8). Palatine tonsils are the most frequent site of involvement [51% (7)] followed by nasopharynx [35% (7)] and the base of the tongue [9% (7)]. Several sites may be simultaneously involved. Symptoms at presentation depend upon the main site of involvement: sore throat and dysphagia with tonsil involvement, nasal obstruction and/or auditory symptoms in patients with nasopharynx involvement. In some patients, Waldeyer's ring involvement is revealed by cervical lymphadenopathy.

The architecture of most primary NHL of Waldeyer's ring is diffuse [from 70% (7) to 90% (8)] with a predominance of large-cell NHL *(fig. 1)* (1,7,8). Primary NHL of the

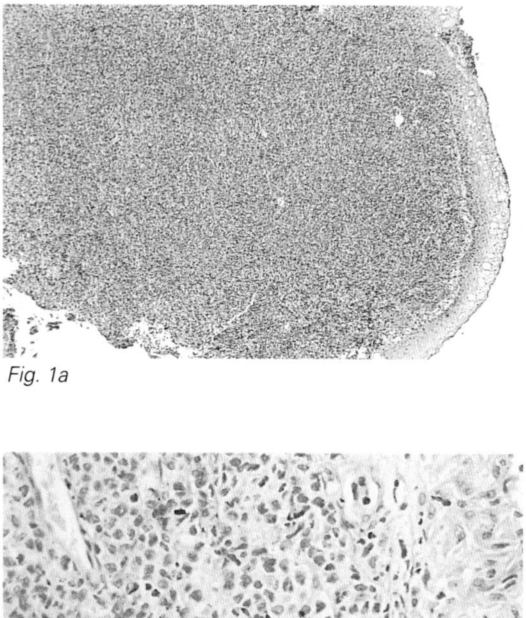

Fig. 1a

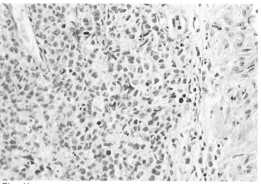

Fig. 1b

Fig. 1: Waldeyer's ring: diffuse lymphoma (fig. 1a), large-cell type (fig. 1b)

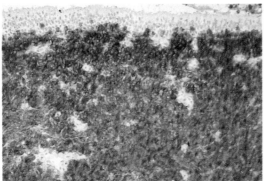

Fig. 2a

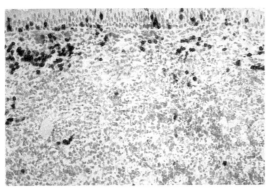

Fig. 2b

Fig. 2: Lymphoma of the tonsils, B-cell phenotype. Immunohistochemical analysis: immunoperoxidase technique on frozen tissue. 2a: staining with an anti-pan-B (CD22) antibody; tumoral cells express CD22 2b: with an anti-pan-T (CD3) antibody: reactional T cells express CD3

tonsils have a follicular pattern more often than those of the nasopharynx. Immunohistochemical studies show a B-cell phenotype (fig. 2) in most cases, even in Japan, where T-cell NHL are predominant (9).

Staging results show predominantly localized NHL [stages I and II in 59 to 88% of cases (1,7,8,9)]. Nevertheless, several authors have reported the high incidence of associated gastric involvement (10) [observed in 18% of patients in whom it was systematically sought (8)]. Gastric endoscopy must be routinely performed in the staging of head-and-neck extra-cranial NHL.

The optimal treatment of primary NHL of Waldeyer's ring is unknown. Most patients have been treated with radiotherapy alone or with combined radiotherapy and chemotherapy. In patients treated with radiotherapy alone, relapses outside Waldeyer's ring were frequent [75% in a series of 68 patients (7)]. Most authors therefore agree that patients with primary NHL of Waldeyer's ring must be treated with combined chemotherapy and radiotherapy (11-13).

Primary lymphoma of the nasal cavity and paranasal sinuses and lethal midline granuloma

Primary lymphomas of the nasal cavity and/or paranasal sinuses are rare (9,14-16). They are usually revealed by rhinorrhea and/or epistaxis and/or nasal congestion. They are almost all aggressive NHL, predominantly diffuse large-cell (14,15).

Lethal midline granuloma (LMG) is a clinical term generally used to describe ulcerative and destructive lesions occurring in the midface, nasal cavity, paranasal sinuses and other portions of the upper respiratory and digestive tract (17). LMG is composed of a non-malignant disorder, Wegener's granulomatosis, and malignant lymphomas. Cases initially reported under the names of "polymorphic reticulosis" (18) or "midline malignant reticulosis" (19,20), are now thought to be malignant lymphomas (21,22). As in lymphomatoid granulomatosis, most cases exhibit an angiocentric and angio-destructive infiltration of atypical lymphoid cells and areas of necrotic change (fig. 3). Phenotypic and genotypic studies (22,26) have shown that these entities were T-cell NHL and could be included in the group of peripheral T-cell NHL. As recently described in other T-cell lymphomas, five Japanese patients with lethal midline granuloma had serological signs of active EBV infection with high VCA-IgG antibody levels, EA-IgG positivity and low EBNA antibody titres. EBV was detected in tumour cells using EBV-DNA hybridization and immunofluorescence. Tumour cells lacked expression of CD21 antigen, regarded as the EBV receptor on B cells (27).

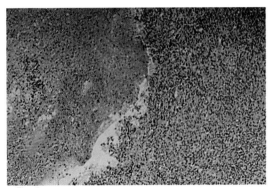

Fig. 3a

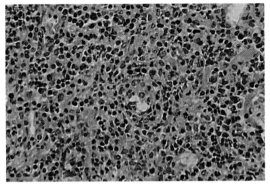

Fig. 3b

Fig. 3: Lethal midline granuloma. Low magnification: diffuse massive infiltration with large areas of necrosis (fig. 3a). High magnification: angiocentric infiltration with large atypical lymphoid cells (fig. 3b)

Primary lymphoma of the thyroid gland

Primary lymphomas of the thyroid gland, although rare, represent approximately 5 to 10% of thyroid neoplasias (28). Most of these lymphomas develop upon an underlying or preexistent thyroid disease, especially Hashimoto's thyroiditis. Recently, the prevalence of primary lymphoma of the thyroid increased simultaneously with that of autoimmune thyroiditis (28,29). The relative risk of thyroid lymphoma in patients with thyroiditis has been estimated to be approximately 70 times greater than in controls (30).

Most patients with primary lymphoma of the thyroid are elderly women. In one series of 76 patients, the median age was 63.3 years (range 27-84) (31). Female predominance is reported in all series (male-to-female ratio of 1: 8 in the group of Anscombe et al.) and more pronounced in patients over 60 years (28).

Most patients present with symptoms suggestive of a malignant tumour of the thyroid gland: rapid enlargement of one lateral lobe or both, often associated with obstructive symptoms (28-36): dysphagia, dyspnoea or stridor, hoarseness and, more rarely, vocal-cord paralysis or superior vena caval syndrome. Thyroid may be grossly enlarged, firm, fixed to adjacent tissues or, more rarely, the site of one nodule (28,31,32,34). Approximately 20 % of patients have enlarged cervical lymph nodes (37). Scintigraphic scan results vary: no isotope uptake, multinodular goitre, one or several cold nodules (28,29,33,34). Patients are either euthyroid or, in a ratio varying from one series to another, have impaired thyroid function (28,38) [12 of 30 patients in one series (28)]. Hyperthyroidism is exceedingly rare. Circulating antibodies to thyroid constituents (thyroglobulin and/or thyroid microsomes) were found in most of the patients tested [19 out of 29 (28), 39 out of 47 (39)], reflecting the incidence of underlying autoimmune thyroiditis.

Most patients have a localized lymphoma at presentation. But associated gastro-intestinal involvement has been reported prior to death (40) or at autopsy (31,33). Because of the morbidity possibly related to GI involvement at the initiation of chemotherapy (haemorrhage, perforation), stomach and intestine involvement should probably be sought in most patients.

Diagnosis can be performed either by needle or surgical biopsy. In the patients reported by Hamburger et al. (28), multiple needle biopsies allowed an accurate diagnosis in 24 of 30 cases. But distinction between severe autoimmune thyroiditis and lymphoma may be difficult and may require immunohistochemical studies (39,40) more easily performed upon surgical specimens. Accordingly, in a patient with a rapidly enlarging thyroid gland or obstructive symptoms, surgi-

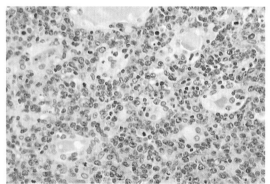

Fig. 4: Primary lymphoma of the thyroid gland, large-cell type

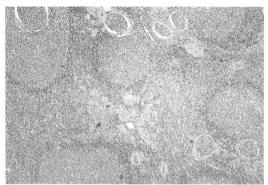

Fig. 5: Primary lymphoma of the thyroid gland, small-cell type: lymphoid follicular hyperplasia and lymphoid proliferation infiltrating thyroid vesicles

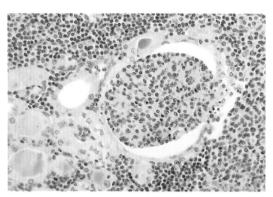

Fig. 6: Primary lymphoma of the thyroid glan, small-cell type: infiltration of thyroid vesicles by "centrocyte-like" cells forming lymphoepithelial lesions

cal biopsy must be performed if needle biopsies do not demonstrate thyroid neoplasia.

Almost all primary NHL of the thyroid are derived from B-lymphoid cells (28, 30, 31,33, 40, 41). In high-grade thyroid NHL (fig.4), the most frequent type, the infiltrate is formed of large cells, often associated with smaller centrocyte-like cells suggesting transformation of low-grade NHL (42). Low-grade primary NHL of the thyroid are diffuse small-cell lymphomas. Their histological aspects can be very similar to those of "florid" Hashimoto's thyroiditis (41,42).

Primary lymphoma of the thyroid gland is currently included in the group of malignant lymphomas of the Mucosa-Associated Lymphoid Tissue (MALT) (see pp. 171-178) (30,33,41,42) since typical features of lymphomas of the MALT can be observed:

- follicular hyperplasia (fig. 5);

- development of lymphoma from the parafollicular ("centrocyte-like") B cells;

- lymphoepithelial lesions (compression and infiltration of thyroid vesicles by lymphoma cells) (fig. 6);

- plasma-cell differentiation of tumour cells in some cases; and

- associated involvement of other MALT sites, especially in the digestive tract (31).

Low-grade primary NHL of the thyroid must be distinguished from Hashimoto's thyroiditis. In Hashimoto's thyroiditis, pathological lesions include diffuse lymphoid infiltration, sometimes polymorphic, with prominent follicles and an oncocytic metaplasia of the epithelium of thyroid vesicles (Hürthle cells). Lymphoepithelial lesions may be observed. Immunohistochemical studies of Hashimoto's thyroiditis have shown, in a significant number of cases, a light-chain restriction leading to amendment of the diagnosis and to consideration of these cases as low-grade primary NHL (42). These studies suggest that low-grade primary NHL of the thyroid arise from parafollicular B cells. The demonstration of lymphoepithelial lesions in

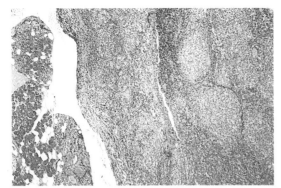

Fig. 7: lymphoma of the parotid: follicular lymphoma of an intra-parotid lymph node

Hashimoto's thyroiditis as well as in low-grade NHL suggest that there is a continuum between these two diseases. Such a continuum also exists from low-grade to high-grade primary NHL of the thyroid.

The prognosis of primary lymphoma of the thyroid gland depends upon the histological type, the age of the patient, the duration of goitre before therapy, and the extent of the disease [5-year survival of 80% of patients with disease limited to the thyroid gland vs 40% of patients with extensive disease (28)] (28,34,38,43-47).

The role of surgery remains to be determined. In some series, patients who had total removal of the tumour had the longest survival period (45,46). Surgical removal may be proposed to patients with limited disease, if parathyroid glands, recurrent laryngeal nerves or post-operative appearance will not be compromised. Most patients have been treated with radiotherapy or combined radiotherapy and chemotherapy. Extended field radiotherapy, including the neck, axillae and mediastinum, has been advocated as better than local radiotherapy in terms of recurrence rate (47). Patients with low-grade NHL may be treated by thyroidectomy.

NHL of the salivary glands

Non-Hodgkin's lymphomas of the salivary-glands were previously considered as rare [4.7% of extranodal NHL for Freeman et al. (48)]. Recently Colby and Dorfman (49) reported a series of 59 cases. The mean age of their patients was 56 years with an unusual female predominance, also mentioned in other series (50,52).

As with all tumours of salivary-glands, parotid localizations are the most frequent; bilateral or multiple salivary-gland involvements are exceedingly rare.

In most cases, the distinction between true parotid involvement or intra- or periparotid lymph node involvement is very difficult (*fig*.7) (52). Schmid et al. (59) found a strictly glandular involvement in 7 out of 25 cases, nodal-only involvement in 8 cases, and mixed glandular and nodal involvements in 10 cases. An associated lymph node involvement is described in 41 of 42 cases by Colby and Dorfman (49).

Salivary-gland NHL may arise either in normal glands, or in glands previously involved by myoepithelial sialadenitis (49,53,54) sometimes associated with Sjögren's syndrome. The relative risk of NHL in patients with Sjögren's syndrome is significantly increased [approximately 44 times higher than in controls (55)]. In myoepithelial sialadenitis, pathological aspects include clustering of lymphoid B cells around acini, with secondary involvement of these acini forming lympho-myo-epithelial lesions. Numerous follicles with large germinal centres are often associated. Lymphoepithelial lesions are not specific to salivary-gland NHL. In salivary gland NHL, a "centrocyte-like cell" proliferation is associated with lymphoepithelial lesions.

Immunohistochemical studies have shown a continuum from "benign" lymphoepithelial lesions to primary salivary-gland NHL. For instance, light-chain restriction may be observed in some cases of "benign" lymphoepithelial lesions (56,57).

Immunohistochemical studies help solve most of the problems in the diagnosis of salivary-gland lymphoid infiltrates: in Sjögren's syndrome, the lymphoid infiltrate is

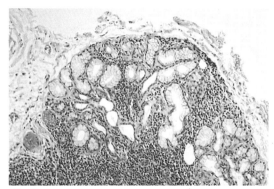

Fig. 8a

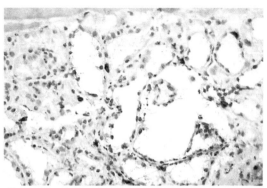

Fig. 8b

Fig. 8: Sjögren's syndrome: lymphoid infiltrate in the salivary gland

composed of T cells, with predominantly CD4+ cells *(fig. 8)* and polyclonal B cells (58). Lymphoepithelial lesions consist of B cells. In contrast, primary NHL of salivary glands are proliferations of monotypic B cells. Molecular studies have also added data to demonstrate that myoepithelial sialadenitis can be considered as a "prelymphomatous" disorder. They have shown a limited number of immunoglobulin gene rearrangements typical of oligoclonal B-cell proliferations (59).

Primary salivary-gland NHL are B-cell NHL (53), often with an IgM κ phenotype (53). With the exception of nodal intraglandular NHL, most primary salivary-gland NHL are of low grade. They were previously considered as follicular NHL (16,51,52).

In fact they are MALT-derived low-grade NHL with an associated follicular hyperplasia. High-grade NHL are rare and often associated with a low-grade component *(fig. 9)*.

NHL of the eye and ocular adnexa

In decreasing order of frequency, NHL of the ocular region involve the orbit, the conjunctiva, the eyelids and, more rarely, the eye itself.

Lymphoid tumours of the orbit represent 10 to 15% of orbit tumours (60,61). In a series of 60 cases (61) they were revealed by a

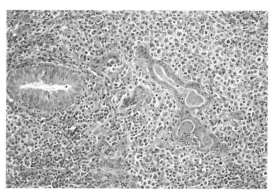

Fig. 9a

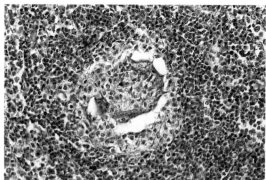

Fig. 9b

Fig. 9: Primary lymphoma of the maxillary gland, large-cell type with a small-cell type component: numerous lymphoepithelial lesions (fig. 9a); lympho-myoepithelial lesion (fig. 9b)

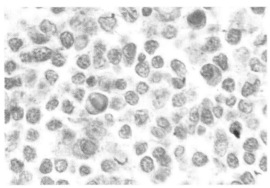

Fig. 10: Primary lymphoma of the orbit, low-grade, small-cell type with plasma cell differentiation: intra-nuclear vacuoles (acknowledgements to Dr. P. Dhermy)

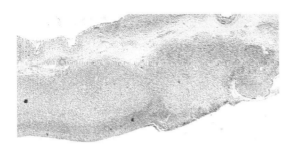

Fig. 11: Benign lymphoid follicular hyperplasia of the orbit: numerous lymphoid follicles with germinal centres (acknowledgements to Dr. P. Dhermy)

mass in 57% of cases, exophthalmia in 27% or, less often, ptosis, ocular pain or visual disorders.

Lesions are most often unilateral. CT scan is mandatory to look for posterior extension or contiguous bone involvement. Most orbital NHL are primarily retrobulbar (60). Diagnosis of orbit NHL is difficult since biopsies are often small and "crushed" and NHL must be distinguished from benign lymphoid hyperplasias. Orbital NHL are low-grade (59-62), small lymphocytic, sometimes with plasma-cell differentiation, (fig. 10) diffuse small-cleaved or, less often, follicular.

Small lymphocytic NHL with plasma-cell differentiation are the ones most often encountered [7 out of 8 cases in the series of Lazzarino et al. (62)] and are often asso-

ciated with type-II cryoglobulinaemia (62). All immunohistochemical studies have shown a B-cell phenotype (62-66). As previously mentioned, low-grade NHL are often difficult to distinguish from benign lymphoid hyperplasias (fig. 11). These infiltrates develop in the orbit either in isolation or in association with other lymphoid infiltrates in patients with immune disorders such as Sjögren's syndrome (68). Knowles and Jakobiec (65) have distinguished 4 histological types of lymphoid infiltration (Table I): inflammatory pseudotumours, reactive lymphoid hyperplasia, atypical lymphoid infiltrate and lymphocytic lymphoma. For other authors (69), well-defined limits, cellular polymorphism and the presence of germinal centres are suggestive of benign lymphoid infiltration. Even before immunohistochemical studies were available, these morphological criteria were considered as non-specific since some proliferations which were described as benign were either associated, at presentation or during the course of the disease, with extraorbital lymphoid infiltrations or they evolved towards malignant lymphomas (70).

Immunohistochemical studies have greatly modified the importance of these morphological criteria. For instance, cases described as "inflammatory pseudotumours" or "atypical lymphocytic infiltrations" were B-cell monotypic proliferations (60,64,66). Like all low-grade NHL, orbital lymphomas are associated with other involvement sites, especially bone marrow (62).

Patients with conjunctival lymphomas present with one or several small, firm, regular, dark pink tumours. As orbital lymphomas, they are low-grade NHL which must be distinguished from benign lymphoid hyperplasias possibly arising from normal lymphoid aggregates of the conjunctiva. Morphological criteria similar to those described for orbital NHL have been proposed, but immunohistochemical studies have greatly decreased their usefulness (66).

Intraocular lymphomas (71) are most often simultaneously or subsequently associated with primary brain NHL. These lymphomas extend to the choroid and are often revealed by serious, steroid-resistant,

TABLE I:

Histological classification of ocular lymphoid infiltrates [from Knowles and Jakobiec (65)]

Diagnosis	Description
Inflammatory pseudotumour	Variable cellularity, polymorphic (small lymphocytes, rare immunoblasts, polymorphonuclears, eosinophils), hyalinisation, oedema, large endothelial cells, rare germinal centres
Reactive lymphoid hyperplasia (follicular or diffuse)	Small-lymphocyte infiltration, vessel proliferation, large endothelial cells Numerous and large germinal centres in the follicular type
Atypical lymphoid infiltrate	Admixture of small lymphocytes and atypical and larger lymphoid cells Frequent extension to fat and muscles
Lymphocytic lymphoma	Monomorphic proliferation of small, diffuse or follicular lymphocytes

uveitis. If no other site is involved, diagnosis may be confirmed only by pathological examination of the surgically removed ocular globe. Lymphoid proliferations of the choroid are more often reactive than malignant. They are revealed by a rapidly worsening amblyopia, unilateral in most cases. When they are one site of a multifocal NHL, they involve anterior and posterior uvea. When isolated or associated with CNS lymphoma, they involve, usually on one side, the retina, the retineal epithelium and the root of the optic nerve. All intraocular lymphomas are high-grade.

References

1. HOPPE RT, BURKE JS, GLATSTEIN E, KAPLAN HS
   Non-Hodgkin's lymphomas: involvement of Waldeyer's ring.
   Cancer, 1978; 42: 1096-1104.
2. ROSENBERG SA, DIAMOND HD, JASLOWITZ B, CRAVER LF
   Lymphosarcoma: a review of 1 269 cases.
   Medicine, 1961; 40: 381-385.
3. BANFI A, BONADONNA G, CARNEVALI G et al.
   Lymphoreticular sarcomas with primary involvement of Waldeyer's ring. Clinical evaluation of 225 cases.
   Cancer, 1970; 26: 341-351.
4. BAJETTA E, BUZZONI R, RILKE F et al.
   Non-Hodgkin's lymphomas of Waldeyer's ring.
   Tumori, 1983; 69: 129-136.
5. ALBADA J, HORKIJK GJ, VAN UNNIK JAM, DEKKER AW
   Non-Hodgkin's lymphoma of Waldeyer's ring.
   Cancer, 1985; 56: 2911-2913.
6. OKSENDHENDLER E, LIDA H, D'AGAY MF et al.
   Tumoral nasopharyngeal lymphoid hyperplasia in human immunodeficiency virus-infected patients.
   Arch Intern Med, 1989; 149: 2359-2361.
7. SAUL SH, KAPADIA SB
   Primary lymphoma of Waldeyer's ring. Clinicopathologic study of 68 cases.
   Cancer, 1985; 56: 157-166.
8. BANFI A, BONADONNA G, RICCI SB et al.
   Malignant lymphomas of Waldeyer's ring: natural history and survival after radiotherapy.
   Br Med J, 1972; 3: 140-143.

9. YAMANAKA N, HARABUCHI Y, SAMBE S et al.

Non-Hodgkin's lymphoma of Waldeyer's ring and nasal cavity. Clinical and immunologic aspects.

Cancer, 1985; 56: 768-776.

10. REE HJ, REGE VB, KINSLEY RE et al.

Malignant lymphoma of Waldeyer's ring following gastrointestinal lymphoma.

Cancer, 1980; 46: 1528-1535.

11. OSSENKOPPELE GJ, MOL JJ, SNOW GB et al.

Radiotherapy versus radiotherapy plus chemotherapy in stages I and II non-Hodgkin's lymphoma of the upper digestive and respiratory tract.

Cancer, 1987; 60: 1505-1509.

12. SHIRATO H, TSUTII H, ARIMOTO T et al.

Early stage head and neck non-Hodgkin's lymphoma. The effect of tumor burden on prognosis.

Cancer, 1986; 58: 2312-2319.

13. NASH JR, ROTHERY GA, WILLATT DJ, RUGMAN F, STELL PM

Non-Hodgkin's lymphoma of the head and neck. Prognostic factors.

Clin Otolaryngol, 1987; 12: 203-210.

14. ROBBINS KT, FULLER LM, VLASAK M et al.

Primary lymphomas of the nasal cavity and paranasal sinuses.

Cancer, 1985; 56: 814-819.

15. WONG DS, FULLER LM, BUTLER JJ, CHULLENBERGER CC

Extra-nodal non-Hodgkin's lymphomas of the head and neck.

Am J Radiol, 1975; 123: 471-481.

16. DUNCAVAGE JA, CAMBELL BH, HANSON GA et al.

Diagnosis of malignant lymphomas of the nasal cavity, paranasal sinuses and nasopharynx.

Laryngoscope, 1983; 93: 1276-1280.

17. STEWART JP

Progressive lethal granulomatosis ulceration of the nose.

J Laryngol, 1933; 48: 657-701.

18. EICHEL BS, MAYBERY TE

The enigma of lethal midline granuloma.

Laryngoscope, 1968; 78: 1367-1386.

19. KASSEL SH, ECHVARRIA RA, GUZZO FP

Midline malignant reticulosis (so-called lethal midline granuloma).

Cancer, 1969; 23: 920-935.

20. FECHNER RE, LAMPPIN DW

Midline malignant reticulosis, a clinicopathologic entity.

Arch Otolaryngol, 1972; 95: 467-476.

21. ISHII Y, YAMANAKA N, OGAWA K et al.

Nasal T-cell lymphoma as a type of so-called "lethal midline granuloma".

Cancer, 1982; 50: 2336-2344.

22. CHOTT A, RAPPERSBERGER K, SCHLOSSAREK W, RADASZKIEWICZ T

Peripheral T-cell lymphoma presenting primarily as lethal midline granuloma.

Hum Pathol, 1988; 19: 1093-1101.

23. GAULARD P, HENNI T, MAROLLEAU JP et al.

Lethal midline granuloma (polymorphic reticulosis) and lymphomatoid granulomatosis. Evidence for a monoclonal T-cell lymphoproliferative disorder.

Cancer, 1988; 62: 705-710.

24. DUBOIS A, ROSSI JF, MARTY-DOUBLE C et al.

Le granulome malin centro-facial de Stewart est-il un lymphome T périphérique?

Rev Laryngol, 1989; 110: 151-155.

25. CHAN JKC, NG CS, LAU WH et al.

Most nasal/nasopharyngeal lymphomas are peripheral T-cell neoplasms.

Am J Surg Pathol, 1987; 11: 418-423.

26. LIPPMAN SM, GROGAN TM, SPIER CM et al.

Lethal midline granuloma with a novel T-cell phenotype as found in peripheral T-cell lymphoma.

Cancer, 1987; 59: 936-939.

27. HARABUCHI Y, YAMANAKA N, KATAURA A et al.

Epstein-Barr virus in nasal T-cell lymphomas in patients with lethal midline granuloma.

Lancet, 1990; 1: 128-130.

28. HAMBURGER JI, MILLER JM, KINI SR

Lymphoma of the thyroid.

Ann Intern Med, 1983; 99: 685-693.

29. CHAK LY, HOPPER RT, BURKE JS, KAPLAN HS

Non-Hodgkin's lymphoma presenting as thyroid enlargement.

Cancer, 1981; 48: 2712-2716.

30. HOLM LEW, BLOMGREN H, LOWHAGEN T

Cancer risk in patients with chronic lymphocytic thyroiditis.

N Engl J Med, 1985; 312: 601-604.

31. ANSCOMBE AM, WRIGHT DH

Primary malignant lymphoma of the thyroid: a tumour of mucosa-associated lymphoid tissue. Review of seventy-six cases.

Histopathology, 1985; 9: 81-97.

32. RIGAUD C, BOGOMOLETS WV, DELISLE MJ

Lymphomes malins (primitifs et secondaires) de la thyroïde. Description de 9 observations et revue de la littérature.

Bull Cancer (Paris), 1985; 72: 210-219.

33. COMPAGNO J, OERTEL JE

Malignant lymphoma and other lymphoprolifera-tive disorders of the thyroid gland. A clinicopatho-logic study of 245 cases.

Am J Clin Pathol, 1980; 74: 1-11.

34. OERTEL JE, HEFFESS CS

Lymphoma of the thyroid and related disorders.

Sem Oncol, 1987; 14: 33-342.

35. VAN RUISWYK J, CUNNINGHAM C, CERLETTY J

Obstructive manifestations of thyroid lymphoma.

Arch Intern Med, 1989; 149: 1575-1577.

36. BURKE JS, BUTLER JJ, FULLER LM

Malignant lymphomas of the thyroid: a clinical pathologic study of 35 patients including ultrastuc-tural observations.

Cancer 1977; 39: 1587-1602.

37. DEVINE RM, EDIS AH, BANKS PM

Primary lymphoma of the thyroid: a review of the Mayo Clinic experience through 1978.

World J Surg, 1981; 5: 33-38.

38. AOZASA K, INOUE A, TAJIMA K, MIYAUCHI A, MATSUZUKA F, KUMA K

Malignant lymphomas of the thyroid gland. Analy-sis of 79 patients with emphasis on histologic prog-nostic factors.

Cancer, 1986; 58: 100-104.

39. STONE CW, SLEASE RB, BRUBAKER D, FABIAN C, GROZEA PN

Thyroid lymphoma with gastrointestinal involve-ment. Report of 3 cases.

Am J Hematol, 1986; 21: 357-365.

40. FAURE P, CHITTAL S, WOODMAN-MENETEAU F et al.

Diagnostic features of primary malignant lym-phomas of the thyroid with monoclonal antibodies.

Cancer, 1988; 61: 1852-1861.

41. ISAACSON P, WRIGHT DH

Extranodal malignant lymphoma from Mucosa-Associated Lymphoid Tissue.

Cancer, 1979; 44: 576-589.

42. HYJEK E, ISAACSON P

Primary B-cell lymphoma of the thyroid and its relationship to Hashimoto's thyroiditis.

Hum Pathol, 1988; 19: 1315-1326.

43. TUPCHONG G, HUGHES F, HARMER CL

Primary lymphoma of the thyroid : clinical fea-tures, prognostic factors and results of treatment.

Int J Radiat Oncol Biol Phys, 1986; 12: 1813-1821.

44. ROSEN IB, SUTCLIFFE SB, GOSPODAROWICZ MK, CHUA T, SIMPSON WJ

The role of surgery in the management of thyroid lymphoma.

Surgery, 1988; 104: 1095-1099.

45. IFRAH N, ROHMER V, SAINT-ANDRE JP, JARDEJ H, BOASSON M, BIGORGNE JC

Lymphome primitif du corps thyroïde. Discussion diagnostique et thérapeutique à propos de 4 obser-vations.

Ann Med Interne, 1988; 139: 344-348.

46. MAKEPEACE AR, FERMONT DC, BENNETT MH

Non-Hodgkin's lymphoma of the thyroid.

Clin Radiol, 1987; 38: 277-281.

47. BLAIR TJ, EVANS RG, BUSKIRK SJ, BANKS PM, EARLE JD

Radiotherapeutic management of primary thyroid lymphoma.

Int J Radiat Oncol Biol Phys, 1985; 11: 365-370.

48. FREEMAN C, BERG JW, CUTLER SJ

Occurrence and prognosis of extranodal lym-phomas.

Cancer, 1972; 29: 252-260.

49. COLBY TV, DORFMAN RF

Malignant lymphomas involving the salivary glands.

In: Sommers SC and Rosen PP Eds: Pathology Annual, Part 2, New York, Appleton-Century, Crofts, 1979; 14: 307-324.

50. NIME FA, COOPER HS, EGGLESTON JC

Primary malignant lymphomas of the salivary glands.

Cancer, 1976; 37: 906-912.

51. HYMAN GA, WOLFF M

Malignant lymphomas of the salivary glands: review of the literature and report of 33 new cases, including four cases associated with the lymphoep-ithelial lesion.

Am J Clin Pathol, 1976; 65: 421-438.

52. SCHMID U, HELBRON K, LENNERT K

Primary malignant lymphomas localized in salivary glands.

Histopathology, 1982; 6: 673-687.

53. SCHMID U, HELBRON K, LENNERT K

Development of malignant lymphoma in myoepithe-lial sialadenitis (Sjögren's syndrome).

Virchows Arch (Pathol Anat), 1982; 395: 11-43.

54. HYJEK E, SMITH WJ, ISAACSON PG

Primary B-cell lymphoma of salivary glands and its relationship to myoepithelial sialadenitis.

Hum Pathol, 1988; 19: 766-776.

55. KASSAN SS, THOMAS TL, MOUTSOPOULOS HM et al.

Increased risk of lymphoma in sicca syndrome.

Ann Intern Med, 1978; 89: 888-892.

56. ISAACSON PG, SPENCER J

Malignant lymphoma of Mucosa-Associated Lym-phoid Tissue.

Histopathology, 1987; 11: 445-462.

57. FALZON M, ISAACSON PG

The natural history of benign lymphoepithelial lesion of the salivary gland in which there is a monoclonal population of B cells.

Am J Surg Pathol, 1991; 15: 59-65.

58. ADAMSON TC, FOX RI, FRISMAN DM, HOWELL FV

Immunohistologic analysis of lymphoid infiltrates in primary Sjögren's syndrome using monoclonal antibodies.

J Immunol, 1983; 130: 203-208.

59. FISHLEDER A, TUBBS R, HESSE B et al.

Uniform detection of immunoglobulin-gene rearrangements in benign lymphoepithelial lesions.

N Engl J Med, 1987; 316: 1118-1125.

60. TEWFIK HH, PLATZ CE, CORDER MP, PANTHER SK, BLODI FC

A clinicopathologic study of orbital and adnexal non-Hodgkin's lymphoma.

Cancer, 1979; 44: 1022-1028.

61. KNOWLES DM, JAKOBIEC FA

Orbital lymphoid neoplasms. A clinicopathologic study of 60 patients.

Cancer, 1980; 46: 576-589.

62. LAZZARINO M, MORRA E, ROSSO R et al.

Clinicopathologic and immunologic characteristics of non-Hodgkin's lymphomas presenting in the orbit. A report of eight cases.

Cancer, 1985; 55: 1907-1912.

63. MEDEIROS LJ, HARRIS NL

Immunohistologic analysis of small lymphocytic infiltrates of the orbit and conjunctiva.

Hum Pathol, 1990; 21: 1126-1131.

64. HARRIS NL, PILCH BZ, BHAN AK, HARMON DC, GOODMAN ML

Immunohistologic diagnosis of orbital lymphoid infiltrates.

Am J Surg Pathol, 1984; 8: 83-91.

65. KNOWLES DM, JAKOBIEC FA

Ocular adnexal lymphoid neoplasms. Clinical, histopathologic electron microscopic and immunologic characteristics.

Hum Pathol, 1982; 13: 148-162.

66. TURNER RR, EGBERT P, WARNKE RA

Lymphocytic infiltrates of the conjunctiva and orbit: immunohistochemical staining of 16 cases.

Am J Clin Pathol, 1984; 81: 447-452.

67. DHERMY P

Les lymphomes des annexes de l'oeil.

Bull Mem SFO, 1986; 97: 77-89.

68. JAKOBIEC FA, McLEAN I, FONT R

Clinicopathologic characteristics of orbital lymphoid hyperplasia.

Ophtalmology, 1979; 86: 948-966.

69. ASTARITA RW, MINCKLER D, TAYLOR CR, LEVINE A, LUKES RJ

Orbital and adnexal lymphomas. A multiparameter approach.

Am J Clin Pathol, 1980; 73: 615-662.

70. MORGAN G, HARRY J

Lymphocytic tumors of indeterminate nature: a 5 years follow-up of 98 conjunctival and orbital lesions.

Br J Ophtalmol, 1978; 62: 381-383.

71. QUALMAN SJ, MENDELSOHN G, MANN RB, GREEN WR

Intraocular lymphomas. Natural history based on a clinicopathologic study of eight cases and review of the literature.

Cancer, 1983; 58: 878-886.

Central nervous system involvement in non-Hodgkin's lymphomas

P. SOLAL-CÉLIGNY, G. GANEM, N. BROUSSE

Secondary central nervous system (CNS) involvement in NHL

The overall frequency of secondary CNS involvement in patients with NHL ranges from 5 to 11% [5%, n = 1039 (1); 6.3%, n = 602 (2); 8.4%, n = 347 (3); 8.5%, n = 445 (4); 11%, n = 292 (5)].

Histological type of NHL is the most significant risk factor for secondary CNS involvement. The highest incidence is observed in patients with lymphoblastic NHL [23% in a series of 66 patients (2)] or small non-cleaved cell NHL [23% in a series of 64 patients with non-endemic Burkitt's lymphoma (6)]. CNS involvement is extremely rare in low-grade NHL (1-5).

In addition to the histological type, the presence of an underlying immune deficiency greatly increases the risk of secondary CNS involvement. Among 238 patients with NHL occurring after a kidney transplantation (7), 93 (39%) had CNS involvement. Such a high incidence has also been observed in patients with NHL and HIV infection: 30 out of 88 (34%) homosexual men with NHL presented with CNS involvement (8).

Other factors may slightly increase the risk of CNS involvement: other extranodal sites [especially involving bone marrow, bone, the digestive tract, or testis (1,2,4,5,9-13)] and youth (below 40 years), regardless of the histological type (1,2,5).

Unlike lymphoblastic leukaemias, CNS prophylaxis in NHL is not a major issue since most relapsing patients do not have isolated CNS relapse.

In general, prophylaxis by "elective" CNS therapy was considered separately because CNS has usually been considered as a "sanctuary" for chemotherapeutic agents included in the first-and most of the second-generation protocols. There is no clear consensus as to the most efficient prophylactic treatment (14). The classical RT scheme delivered 24 Gy with conventional fractionation to the midplane of the skull, including all meningeal surfaces of the brain and below the inferior level of the second cervical vertebra (15). The rationale for the use of this scheme was the poor diffusion of intrathecal chemotherapy in the upper meningeal structures. When the two modalities are combined, it is now well-demonstrated that RT must be delivered after intrathecal chemotherapy in order to reduce the risk of neurological sequelae. Although this combined "elective" prophylactic therapy has been recommended for certain patients with diffuse large-cell NHL (4,10), it remains questionable whether it was beneficial. The development of more intensive chemotherapy regimens, including high or intermediate doses of Methotrexate and Cytarabine, should probably reduce the risk of CNS relapse to less than 5% and prophylactic RT is no longer included in most

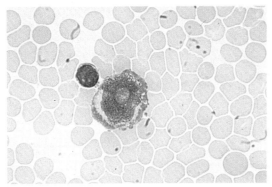

Fig.1: Cerebro-spinal fluid. Large immunoblastic cells

recent programmes (16-18). In childhood NHL, RT is also no longer used for CNS prophylaxis (19,20).

Secondary CNS involvement is rarely observed at presentation [10 to 20% of patients with CNS involvement (1,2,11)] but more often occurs during the course of the disease. In some patients, CNS is the first site of relapse, preceding an overt relapse by weeks or months (11). In rare cases, CNS is the only site of relapse. The pattern of CNS involvement varies according to the immune status. Most patients without an underlying immune deficiency have diffuse leptomeningeal involvement [from 61% (5) to 78% (1)] even at autopsy [69% (10)]. In patients with post-transplant or HIV-associated NHL, isolated brain- or associated leptomeningeal- and-brain involvements are the most usual pattern (7,8). Symptoms of CNS involvement include one or more of the following: headache, sight disorders, weakness of legs and/or arms, disturbed consciousness, nausea and vomiting (2,4). In some patients, CNS involvement is asymptomatic and diagnosis is performed by routine lumbar puncture. Cranial-nerve (oculomotor) palsies, spinalroot or nerve deficiency and papillary oedema are the most usual signs (1,2,5,10,11).

Diagnosis of CNS involvement is usually performed by cerebrospinal fluid (CSF) analysis. Most patients have increased protein and beta-2-microglobulin (21) CSF levels. Lymphoma cells are found in the CSF of 58 to 100% of patients (1,2,10,11) *(fig. 1)*. If lymphoma cells are rare or have a normal appearance, immunocytochemistry may help diagnosis if it shows a monotypic lymphoid-cell population (22-24) *(fig. 2)*. Except for patients with an underlying immune deficiency, brain CT scan is usually normal.

Except for patients with CNS disease at presentation, one-year survival of patients with CNS involvement by NHL is less than 20% in almost all series (10,14). However, only 10 to 20% of the patients ultimately died from CNS disease. Thus, even for patients with apparently isolated CNS relapse, systemic therapy in addition to "elective" CNS treatment is indicated. In this setting, RT is delivered to the whole brain or to the total neuraxis. Although there is no dose-control relationship, a dose of 30 to 35 Gy is recommended and delivered with conventional fractionation (10); in this study, multivariate analysis has shown that, in addition to the status of systemic NHL, three factors were associated with a better survival after CNS involvement; age under 30, the use of CNS irradiation and a good symptom response.

More recent studies suggest that chemotherapy alone (systemic or intraventricular) is highly effective (14). Thus, the role of RT has become still more difficult to define. The use of total neuraxis irradiation is limited, partly because of its bone-marrow toxicity; its role may be advocated if cerebrospinal fluid contains lymphoma cells (17) and/or if nerve roots are involved, and/or for patients who do not rapidly respond to chemotherapy. In other settings, classical whole-brain irradiation alone may be indicated particularly if there is evidence of major brain involvement by NHL and if a response to chemotherapy is not rapidly achieved. If long-term survival is anticipated, a low dose-per-fraction, long-term schedule should probably be used in order to reduce the risk of long-term neurological sequelae (25).

NHL and spinal-cord compression

Lymphoma may cause spinal-cord compression in a number of ways (26-30):

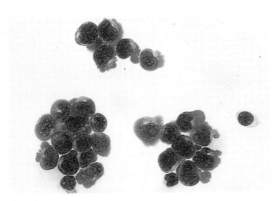

Fig. 2a

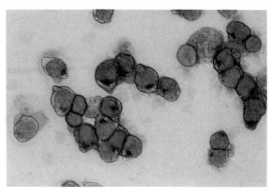

Fig. 2c

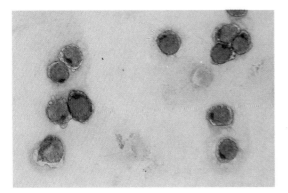

Fig. 2b

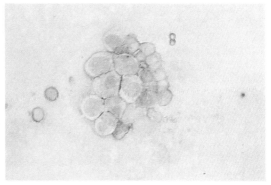

Fig. 2d

Fig. 2: Cerebrospinal fluid. Presence of lympho-plasma-cytic cells (fig.2a). Immunocytochemical studies confirm their tumoral origin: staining of lymphoid cells by anti-μ antibodies (fig.2b) and anti-κ (fig.2c), and absence of staining with anti-λ antibodies (fig.2d)

- spreading from paraspinal lymph nodes into the epidural space;

- compression of involved vertebral bodies with rupture of the posterior wall; or

- expansion from involved vertebral bodies into the epidural space.

However, the development of *de novo* NHL in the epidural space has not been proved (30).

Most patients with NHL spinal-cord compression complain of chronic back pain and recent leg weakness, dysesthesiae or paresthesiae in the lower limbs.

Computed tomography scan and/or magnetic resonance imaging and/or myelography usually show a posterolateral extradural mass which produces a block, in most cases at the thoracic level [10 of 15 cases (30)]. Fewer than a third of patients with lym-

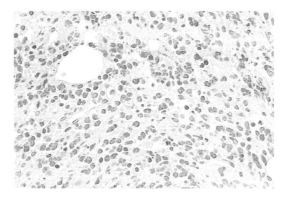

Fig. 3: Epidural involvement by a large-cell NHL

phomatous epidural compression of the cord have evidence of vertebral bone changes (28). CSF analysis only shows increased protein level without lymphoma cells.

Most patients with spinal-cord compression have high-grade diffuse large-cell NHL. Other histological types are rarer; particularly lymphoblastic or follicular lymphomas (26-30).

Unlike Hodgkin's disease, spinal-cord compression is most often seen at presentation and the diagnosis of NHL is performed on a laminectomy specimen.

RT classically has a major role in the treatment of this severe complication (26,31,32). The radiation portal upper and lower limits are usually defined to one or two vertebral bodies from the occlusion of the spinal canal as determined by myelography, magnetic resonance imaging and/or computed tomography. Clinical response is achieved in 70 to 90% of patients. In general, there is no difference in improvement of neurological signs between patients undergoing laminectomy compared with patients receiving RT only. Failures in irradiated areas occur in 0 to 24% of cases. In the series published by Friedman et al. (26), a dose higher than 25 Gy appears to be optimal for local control. Steroids are usually given during the RT session. Chemotherapy is also highly effective (34,35). However, the majority of authors still recommend the use of RT as part of the treatment for this complication (36).

Primary central nervous system NHL

Epidemiology

Until recently, primary CNS non-Hodgkin's lymphoma, also called "microglioma", was a rare tumour accounting for only 0.85 to 1.5% of malignant brain tumours (37,38) and 0.5 to 0.9% of NHL (39,40). The frequency has greatly increased in the last decade (41). The high incidence of primary brain NHL in AIDS patients (42,43) only partly explains this rising incidence.

Prior to 1980, primary CNS lymphoma had the same epidemiological characteristics as other nodal or extranodal NHL: slight male predominance, median age of about 55 years. Since the endemic spread of AIDS, male predominance has increased and patients are younger.

At present, more than half of patients with CNS-NHL are at increased risk, i.e. have an underlying immune deficiency. Among constitutional immune deficiencies, Wiskott-Aldrich syndrome and severe combined immune deficiency predispose to CNS-NHL (44). For instance, 75% of the cancers reported in patients with Wiskott-Aldrich syndrome were NHL and, among them, 24% were primary CNS-NHL (44). Primary CNS-NHL is rare among patients with the X-linked lymphoproliferative syndrome (1 out of 17 patients) (45).

Among transplant recipients - either kidney (46), heart (47) or bone marrow (48) - the risk of NHL is greatly increased [about 100- to 350-fold greater than for the population at large (46-48)]. Approximately half of these patients have primary CNS-NHL (7).

About 3% of patients with AIDS develop NHL during the course of the disease and 30% of them present with brain lymphoma (8,42,43,49) even if staging discloses other involvement sites. Some of these patients have typical histological features of lymphomatoid granulomatosis (50).

Other diseases may predispose to primary CNS-NHL such as systemic lupus erythematosus (51), rheumatoid arthritis (52) and IgA deficiency (53).

In patients with an immunodeficiency, Epstein-Barr virus could play a key role in the development of CNS-NHL (54). In most - but not all - cases of CNS-NHL associated with immunodeficiency, lymphoma cells contain EBV genome (55-57). The brain could be a sanctuary for EBV and CNS-NHL may be the result of EBV reactivation related to immune deficiency and followed by B proliferation.

Diagnosis

Symptoms of primary CNS-NHL are non-specific (39,40,58-60): seizures, focal neurological deficit, symptoms related to increased intracranial pressure, progressive

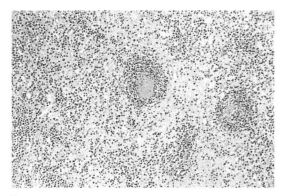

Fig. 4a

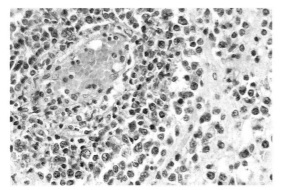

Fig. 4b

Fig. 4: Large-cell lymphoma of the brain: lymphoid infiltration of the white subsistance (fig.4a) with a predominant perivascular localization (photograph Prof. D. Hennin)

dementia or visual changes. A few patients complained of an unexplained dysphagia (39,62). Blurred vision often points to vitreous, choroid and/or retina involvement by NHL (41,63,64). Vitreous or uveal lymphoma deposits may precede clinically evident primary CNS-NHL by weeks or months (63).

Precontrast scans typically show one or several uniform, most often homogeneous, lesions that are isodense to, or hyperdense to normal brain tissue (64-68). In approximately 75 % of primary CNS-NHL, lesions are supratentorial; lesions are infratentorial or both supratentorial and infratentorial in the remaining cases (41,58). Following contrast administration, intense, homogeneous and well-circumscribed enhancement is usual. Tumour nodules are surrounded by varying degrees of white-matter oedema. In one series of 32 cases, nodules had an average size of 39 mm (68). The most usual

angiographic finding, suggestive of primary CNS-NHL, is a diffuse, homogeneous, cloud-like tumour stain at capillary and venous phases (68).

Diagnosis of primary CNS-NHL may be made by surgery, CT-guided stereotaxic or needle biopsy depending upon lesion location. If there is vitreous involvement, vitrectomy is an easy way to obtain accurate diagnostic material, thus obviating an intracranial approach (66).

Primary CNS-NHL always have a diffuse architecture and are predominantly large-cell (fig.4) or immunoblastic, less often small non-cleaved NHL (41,69-71). The cellular infiltrate in primary NHL of the brain is angiocentric with multiple foci of perivascular malignant cells. Immunophenotyping suggests a B-cell origin in most cases studied (60,70-72), although a few cases of primary T-cell brain NHL have been described (72,73). In approximately 30% of patients, CSF examination discloses lymphoma cells (58).

Treatment

Until recently, the treatment of primary CNS-NHL was disappointing. The median survival period in one series of 61 patients was 13.5 months (41) and other series gave similar results (37,40,58,60,64-66,74,75). Radical surgical excision is not warranted (61,64). Radiation therapy has been the primary therapeutic procedure (74,76-80). As cerebral involvement is often multifocal, most patients have been treated with whole-brain RT. Although there is no clear dose-efficacy relationship above 30 Gy, the majority of patients received 40 Gy under whole-brain treatment, often followed by a 15-20 Gy boost in the tumour mass. With increasing doses, there is a major risk of radiation encephalopathy (81). Craniospinal-axis RT has been proposed by some investigators because seeding of the spinal axis occurred in 5 to 25% of the patients (58,74); spinal RT delivered 18 to 30 Gy, but there is no clear advantage of craniospinal-axis RT over whole-brain RT alone. Except for AIDS-related CNS-NHL (82), the survival rates at 1 and 5 years following exclusive RT are respectively 60 and 5%: around 90% of relapses occurred within the brain.

Few studies addressed the role of chemotherapy (83,84). Using high-dose methotrexate, Abelson et al. obtained in 11 patients a CR rate of 45% and a PR rate of 36% (83). Other similar results have been reported (85). Encouraging results using high-dose dexamethasone and high-dose cytosine-arabinoside with cisplatin have also been observed (86). Neuwelt et al. have used intra-arterial chemotherapy in conjunction with blood-brain barrier modification by hyperventilation with 100% O_2 and mannitol infusion (61). They obtained 13 CR out of 17 patients and the median survival for the whole group is 44.7 months. At present, combined whole-brain radiotherapy and chemotherapy using drugs known to cross the blood-brain barrier (high-dose methotrexate, high-dose cytosine-arabinoside, teniposide, nitrosoureas) is the treatment likely to yield the best results. These procedures may improve the prognosis of primary CNS lymphoma, at least in patients without any underlying immune deficiency as suggested by the most recent studies (87-89).

References

1. HERMAN TS, HAMMOND J, JONES SE, BUTLER JJ, BYRNE GE, McKELVEY EM
   Involvement of the central nervous system by non-Hodgkin's lymphoma. The Southwest Oncology Group Experience.
   Cancer, 1979; 43: 390-397.

2. ERSBOLL J, SCHULTZ HB, THOMSEN BLR, KEIDING N, NISSEN NI
   Meningeal involvement in non-Hodgkin's lymphoma: symptoms, incidence, risk factors and treatment.
   Scand J Haematol, 1985; 35: 487-496.

3. JOHNSON CJ, OKEN MM, ANDERSON JR, O'CONNELL MJ, GLICK JH
   Central nervous system relapse in unfavourable histology non-Hodgkin's lymphoma: is prophylaxis indicated ?
   Lancet, 1984; 2: 685-687.

4. YOUNG RC, HOWSER DM, ANDERSON T, FISHER RI, JAFFE E, DE VITA VT
   Central nervous system complications of non-Hodgkin's lymphomas. The potential role for prophylatic therapy.
   Am J Med, 1979; 66: 435-443.

5. LITAM JP, CABANILLAS F, SMITH LT, BODEY GL, FREIREICH EJ
   Central nervous system relapse in malignant lymphomas: risk factors and implications for prophylaxis.
   Blood, 1979; 54: 1249-1257.

6. SARIBAN E, EDWARDS B, JANUS C, MAGRATH J
   Central nervous system involvement in American Burkitt's lymphoma.
   J Clin Oncol, 1983; 1: 677-681.

7. PENN I
   Lymphomas complicating organ transplantation.
   Transplant Proc, 1983; 15: 718-722.

8- ZIEGLER JL, BECKSTEAD JA, VOLDERDING PA et al.
   Non-Hodgkin's lymphoma in 90 homosexual men. Relation to generalized lymphadenopathy and the Acquired Immunodeficiency Syndrome.
   N Engl J Med, 1984; 311: 565-570.

9. HAROUSSEAU JL, VALLANTIN X, TRICOT G, GISSELBRECHT C, JACQUILLAT C
   Les localisations neuro-méningées au cours des lymphomes non hodgkiniens de l'adulte.
   Sem Hop Paris, 1983; 59: 221-225.

10. McKINTOSH FR, COLBY TV, PODOLSKY WJ et al.
    Central nervous system involvement in non-Hodgkin's lymphoma: an analysis of 105 cases.
    Cancer, 1982; 49: 586-595.

11. BUNN PA, SCHEIN PS, BANKS PM, DE VITA VT
    Central nervous system complications in patients with diffuse histiocytic and undifferentiated lymphoma.
    Blood, 1976; 47: 3-10.

12. DOLL DC, WEISS RB
    Malignant lymphoma of the testis.
    Am J Med, 1986; 81: 515-524.

13. MARTENSON JA, BUSKIRK SJ, ILSTRUP DM et al.
    Patterns of failure in primary testicular non-Hodgkin's lymphoma.
    J Clin Oncol, 1988; 6: 297-302.

14. RECHT L, STRAUS DJ, CIRRINCIONE C et al.
    Central nervous system metastases from non-Hodgkin's lymphoma: treatment and prophylaxis.
    Am J Med, 1988; 84: 425-435.

15. HUSTU HO, AUR RJA, VERZOSA MS et al.
    Prevention of central nervous system leukemia.
    Cancer, 1973; 32: 585-597.

16. COIFFIER B, GISSELBRECHT C, HERBRECHT R et al.
    LNH-84 regimen: A multicenter study of intensive chemotherapy in 737 patients with aggressive malignant lymphoma.
    J Clin Oncol, 1979; 7: 1018-1026.

17. SHIPP MA, YEAP BY, HARRINGTON DP et al.

    The m-BACOD combination chemotherapy regimen in large-cell lymphoma: analysis of the completed trial and comparison with the M-BACOD regimen.

    J Clin Oncol, 1990; 8: 84-93.

18. SCHNEIDER AM, STRAUS DJ, SCHLUGER AE et al.

    Treatment results with an aggressive chemotherapeutic regimen (MACOP-B) for intermediate - and some high-grade non-Hodgkin's lymphomas.

    J Clin Oncol, 1990; 8: 94-102.

19. MURPHY SB, BLEYER WA

    Cranial irradiation is not necessary for central-nervous system prophylaxis in pediatric non-Hodgkin's lymphoma.

    Int J Radiation Oncology Biol Phys, 1987; 13: 467-468.

20. MANDEL LR, WOLLNER N, FUKS Z

    Is cranial radiation necessary for CNS prophylaxis in pediatric NHL?

    Int J Radiation Oncology, 1987; 13: 359 363.

21. MAVLIGIT GM, STUCKEY SE, CABANILLAS FF et al.

    Diagnosis of leukemia or lymphoma in the central nervous system by beta-2-microglobulin determination.

    N Engl J Med, 1980; 303: 718-722.

22. EZRIN-WATERS C, KLEIN M, DECK J, LANG AE

    Diagnostic importance of immunological markers in lymphoma involving the central nervous system.

    Ann Neurol, 1984; 16: 668-672.

23. GOODSON J, STRAUSS GM

    Diagnosis of lymphomatous leptomeningitis by cerebrospinal fluid lymphocyte cell surface markers.

    Am J Med, 1979; 66: 1057-1059.

24. CHIN-YANG LI, WITZIG TE, PHYLIKY RL, ZIESMER SC, YAM LT

    Diagnosic of B-cell non Hodgkin's lymphomas of the central nervous system by immunocytochemical analysis of cerebrospinal fluid lymphocytes.

    Cancer, 1986; 57: 737-744.

25. FOWLER JF

    Principles of fractionation in radiotherapy.

    In: Radiobiology in radiotherapy.

    BLEEHEN NM (Ed.) New-York, Springer, 1988: pp. 53-58.

26. FRIEDMAN M, KIM TH, PANAHON AM

    Spinal cord compression in malignant lymphoma. Treatment and results.

    Cancer, 1976; 37: 1485-1491.

27. SICHEZ JP, RAPHAEL M, LE PORRIER M et coll.

    Compressions médullaires tumorales dans les hémopathies malignes. A propos de 28 observations.

    Ann Méd Int, 1982; 33: 251-255.

28. HADDAD P, THAELL JF, KIELY JM, HARRISON EG, MILLER RH

    Lymphoma of the spinal extradural space.

    Cancer, 1976; 38: 1862-1866.

29. MULLINS GM, GLYNN J, EL-MAHDI AM, McQUEEN JD, OWENS AH

    Malignant lymphoma of the spinal epidural space.

    Ann Inter Med, 1971; 74: 416.

30. GRANT JW, KAECH D, JONES DB

    Spinal cord compression as the first presentation of lymphoma. A review of 15 cases.

    Histopathology, 1986; 10: 1191-1202.

31. AABO K, WALBOM-JORGENSEN S

    Central nervous system complications by malignant lymphomas: radiation schedule and treatment results.

    Int J Radiation Oncology Biol Phys, 1986; 12: 197-202.

32. EPELBAUM R, HAIM N, BEN-SHAHAR M et al.

    Non-Hodgkin's lymphoma presenting with spinal epidural involvement.

    Cancer, 1986; 58: 2120-2124.

33. VASUDEV RAO T, NARAYANA SWAMY KS, SHANKAR SK, DESHPANDE DH

    "Primary" spinal epidural lymphomas. A clinico-pathological study.

    Acta Neurochirurgica, 1982; 62: 307-317.

34. OVIATT DL, KIRSHNER HS, STEIN RS

    Successful chemotherapeutic treatment of epidural compression in non-Hodgkin's lymphoma.

    Cancer, 1982; 49: 2446-2448.

35. BURCH PA, GROSSMAN SA

    Treatment of epidural cord compression from Hodgkin's disease with chemotherapy.

    Am J Med, 1988; 84: 555-558.

36. DE VITA VT, JAFFE ES, MAUCH P, LONGO DL

    Lymphocytic lymphomas.

    In: Principles & Practice of Oncology.

    DE VITA VT, HELLMAN S and ROSENBERG SA Eds., Philadelphia, Lippincott, 1989: pp. 1741-1798.

37. JELLINGER K

    Primary lymphomas of the CNS.

    Arch Neurol, 1982; 39: 458-464.

38. ZIMMERMAN HM

Malignant lymphomas of the nervous system.

Acta Neuropathol suppl, 1975; 6: 69-74.

39. WOODMAN R, CHIN K, PINEO G

Primary non-Hodgkin's lymphoma of the brain. A review.

Medicine, 1985; 64: 425-430.

40. HENRY M, HEFFNER RR, DILLARD SH, EARLE KM, DAVIS RL

Primary malignant lymphomas of the central nervous system.

Cencer, 1974; 34: 1293-1302.

41. HOCHBERG FH, MILLER DC

Primary central nervous system lymphoma.

J Neurosurg, 1988; 68: 835-853.

42. SNIDER WD, SIMPSON DM, ARONYK KE, NIELSEN SL

Primary lymphoma of the nervous system associated with acquired immuno-deficiency syndrome.

N Engl J Med, 1983; 308: 45.

43. GILL PS, LEVINE AM, MYER PR et al.

Primary central nervous system lymphoma in homosexual men. Clinical, immunologic and pathologic features.

Am J Med, 1985; 78: 742-748.

44. FILOPOVICH AH, HEINITZ KJ, ROBISON LL et al.

The immunodeficiency cancer registry. A research resource.

Am J Pediatr Hematol Oncol, 1987; 9: 183-184.

45. HARRINGTON DS, WEISENBURGER DD, PURTILO DT

Malignant lymphoma in the X-linked lymphoproliferative syndrome.

Cancer, 1987; 59: 1419-1429.

46. HOOVER R, FRAUMENI JF

Risk of cancer in renal transplant recipients.

Lancet, 1973; 2: 55-57.

47. WEINTRAUB J, WARNCKE RA

Lymphoma in cardiac allotransplant recipients. Clinical and histological features and immunological phenotypes.

Transplantation, 1982; 33: 347-351.

48. SHAPIRO RS, Mc CLAIN K, FRIZZERA G et al.

Epstein-Barr virus associated B-cell lymphoproliferative disorders following bone-marrow transplantation.

Blood, 1988; 71: 1234-1243.

49. SO YT, BECKSTEAD JM, DAVIS RL

Primary central nervous system lymphoma in acquired immune deficiency syndrome: a clinical and pathological study.

Ann Neurol, 1986; 20: 566-572.

50. ANDERS KH, LATTA H, CHANG BS, TOMIYASU U, OUDOUSI AS, VINTERS HV

Lymphomatoid granulomatosis and malignant lymphoma of the Central Nervous System in the Acquired Immuno-Deficiency Syndrome.

Hum Pathol, 1989; 20: 326-334.

51. LIPSMEYER EA

Development of malignant lymphoma in a patient with systemic lupus erythematosus treated with immunosuppression.

Arth Rheum, 1972; 15: 183-186.

52. GOOD AE, RUSSO RH, SCHNITZER B, WEATHERBEE L

Intracranial histiocytic lymphoma with rheumatoid arthritis.

J Rheumatol, 1978; 5: 75-78.

53. GREGORY MC, HUGUES JT

Intracranial reticulum cell sarcoma associated with immunoglobulin A deficiency.

J Neurol Neurosurg Psych, 1973; 36: 769-776.

54. SOLLIVAN JL

Epstein-Barr virus and lymphoproliferative disorders.

Semin Hematol, 1988; 25: 269-279.

55. HOCHBERG FH, MILLER G, SCHOOLEY RT et al.

Central nervous system lymphoma related to Epstein-Barr virus.

N Engl J Med, 1983; 309: 745-748.

56. ROSENBERG NL, HOCHBERG FH, MILLER G et al.

Primary central nervous system lymphoma related to Epstein-Barr virus in a patient with acquired immune deficiency syndrome.

Ann Neurol, 1986; 20: 98-102.

57. KATZ BZ, ANDIMAN WA, EASTMAN R et al.

Infection with two genotypes of Epstein-Barr virus in an infant with AIDS and lymphoma of the central nervous system.

J Infect Dis, 1986; 153: 601-604.

58. HELLE TL, BRITT RH, COLBY TV

Primary lymphoma of the central nervous system. Clinicopathological study of experience at Stanford.

J Neurosurg, 1984; 60: 94-103.

59. KAWAKAMI Y, TABUCHI K, OHNISHI R, ASARI S, NISHIMOTO A

Primary central nervous system lymphoma.

J Neurosurg, 1985; 62: 522-527.

60. de MASCAREL A, VITAL C, RIVEL J et al.

Lymphomes malins non hodgkiniens primitifs du cerveau. Etude anatomo-clinique et immunopathologique de 21 cas.

Sem Hop Paris, 1983; 59: 179-184.

61. NEUWELT EA, GOLDMAN DL, DAHLBORG SA et al.

Primary CNS lymphoma treated with osmotic Blood-Brain Barrier disruption: prolonged survival and preservation of cognitive function.

J Clin Oncol, 1991; 9: 1580-1590.

62. BENJAMIN SB, EISOLD J, GERHARDT DC, CASTELL DO

Central nervous system lymphoma presenting as dysphagia.

Dig Dis Sci, 1982; 27: 155-158.

63. KATTAH JC, JENKINS RB, PILKERTON AR et al.

Multifocal primary ocular and central nervous system malignant lymphoma.

Ann Ophtalmol, 1982; 13: 589-593.

64. MENDENHALL NP, THAR JL, AGEE OF, HARTY-GOLDER F, BALLINGER WE, MILLION RE

Primary lymphoma of the central nervous system. Computerized tomography scan characteristics and treatment results in 12 cases.

Cancer, 1983; 52: 1993-2000.

65. ENZMANN DR, KRIKORIAN J, NORMAN D et coll.

Computed tomography in primary reticulum cell sarcoma of the brain.

Radiology, 1979; 130: 165-170.

66. LETENDRE L, BANKS PM, REESE DF, MILLER RH, SCANLON PW, KIELY JM

Primary lymphoma of the central nervous system.

Cancer, 1982; 49: 939-943.

67. WEINGARTEN K, ZIMMERMAN RD

CT of intracranial lymphoma.

Sem Ultrasoud, CR, and MR, 1986; 7: 9-17.

68. JACK CR, REESE DF, SCHEITAUER BW

Radiographic findings in 32 cases of primary CNS lymphoma.

AJR, 1986; 146: 271-276.

69. CASADEI GP, GAMBACORTA M

A clinicopathological study of seven cases of primary high-grade malignant non-Hodgkin's lymphoma of the central nervous system.

Tumori, 1985; 71: 501-507.

70. ALLEGRANZA A, MARIANI C, GIARDINI R, BRAMBILLA MC, BOERI R

Primary malignant lymphomas of the central nervous system: a histological and immunohistological study of 12 cases.

Histopathology, 1984; 8: 781-791.

71. SIMON J, JONES EL, TRUMPER MM, SALMON MV

Malignant lymphomas involving the central nervous system. A morphological and immunohistochemical study of 32 cases.

Histopathology, 1987; 11: 335-349.

72. GRANT JW, GALLAGHER PJ, JONES DB

Primary cerebral lymphoma. A histologic and immunohistochemical study of 6 cases.

Arch Pathol Lab Med, 1986; 110: 897-901.

73. MARSH WL, STEVENSON DR, LONG HJ

Primary leptomeningeal presentation of T-cell lymphoma.

Cancer, 1983; 51: 1125-1133.

74. LOEFFLER JS, ERVIN TJ, MAUCH P et coll.

Primary lymphomas of the central nervous system: patterns of failure and factors that influence survival.

J Clin Oncol, 1985; 3: 490-494.

75. POLLACK IF, LUNSFORD LD, FLICKINGER JC, DAMESHEK HL

Prognostic factors in the diagnosis and treatment of primary central nervous system lymphoma.

Cancer, 1989; 63: 939-947.

76. BERRY MP, SIMPSON WJ

Radiation therapy in the management of primary malignant lymphoma of the brain.

Int J Radiat Oncol Biol Phys, 1980; 7: 55-59.

77. RAMPEN FHJ, VAN ADEL JG, SIZOO W et al.

Radiation therapy in primary non-Hodgkin's lymphoma of the CNS.

Eur J Cancer, 1967; 88: 552-554.

78. GONZALEZ-GONZALEZ D, SCHUSTER-VITTERHOEVE ALJ

Primary non-Hodgkin's lymphomas of the central nervous system. Results of radiotherapy in 15 cases.

Cancer, 1983; 51: 2048-2052.

79. AMENDOLA BE, McCLATCHEY KD, AMENDOLA MA et al.

Primary large-cell lymphoma of the central nervous system.

Amer J Clin Oncol, 1986; 9: 204-208.

80. LEIBEL SA, SHELINE GE

Radiation therapy for neoplasms of the brain.

J Neurosurg, 1987; 66: 1-22.

81. ASAI A, MATSUTANI M, KOHNO T et al.

Subacute brain atrophy after radiation therapy for malignant brain tumor.

Cancer, 1989; 63: 1962-1974.

82. FORMENTI SC, GILL PS, LEAN E et al.

Primary central nervous system lymphoma in AIDS: results of radiation therapy.

Cancer, 1989; 63: 1101-1107.

83. ABELSON HT, KUFE DW, SKARIN AT et al.

Treatment of central nervous system tumors with methotrexate.

Cancer Treat Rep, 1981; 65: 137-140.

84. COHEN IJ, VOGEL R, MATZ S et al.
Successful non-neurotoxic therapy (without radiation) of a multifocal primary brain lymphomas with a methotrexate, vincristine and BCNU protocol (DEMOB).
Cancer, 1986; 57: 6-11.

85. ERVIN T, CANELLOS GP
Successful treatment of recurrent primary central nervous system lymphoma with high-dose methotrexate.
Cancer, 1980; 45: 1556-1557.

86. McLAUGHLIN P, VELASQUEZ WJ, REDMAN JR et al.
Chemotherapy with dexamethasone, high-dose cytarabine and cisplatin for parenchymal brain lymphoma.
J Natl Cancer Inst, 1988; 80: 1408-1412.

87. SOCIE G, PIPROT-CHAUFFAT C, SCHLIENGER M et al.
Primary lymphoma of the central nervous system: an unresolved therapeutic problem.
Cancer, 1990; 65: 322-326.

88. SHIBAMOTO Y, TSUTSUI K, DODO Y et al.
Improved survival rate in primary intracranial lymphoma treated by high-dose radiation and systemic vincristine-doxorubicin-cyclophosphamide-prednisolone chemotherapy.
Cancer, 1990; 65: 1907-1912.

89. YAHALOM J, M de ANGELIS L
Primary CNS lymphoma-improved survival with an intensive combined modality treatment approach.
Int J Radiation Oncology Biol Phys, 1990; 19 (suppl 1): 135 A39.

Non-Hodgkin's lymphomas of bone

J.-L. LE BAIL, M. PEUCHMAUR

Lymphomas of bone can be divided into:

– primary lymphomas of bone [previously called "Parker and Jackson's reticulum cell sarcoma" (1)]. This lymphoma comprises a single tumour, limited to bone, without nodal or extranodal extension;

– secondary lymphomas characterized by bone involvement from a nodal or extranodal lymphoma by contiguous or haematogenic spread.

Clinically, it is simpler to distinguish a lymphoma which presents as a solitary bone tumour (primary lymphoma) from disseminated lymphoma associated with sites of bone involvement which are often numerous, either at the onset or during development.

Primary lymphomas of bone

Lymphomas represent only 5% of all primary bone tumours (2). Diagnosis is never made before the histological study is complete. Primary lymphoma of bone occurs in any age group, but the majority of patients are usually younger than 15 years. Clinical manifestations are not specific: fixative bone pain, spontaneous fracture.

Primary lymphomas of bone involve preferentially metaphysis of long bones (femur, and in order of decreasing frequency, tibia, fibula, humerus and radius), and, rarely, flat bones (2-6).

Radiological features of bone lesions (lysis, condensation, or periosteal reaction) observed in bone tumours are more or less associated in lymphomas of bone. Lesions were monomorphous in one patient. Osteolysis is described as either "moth-eaten" or as a permeative pattern. "Moth-eaten" osteolysis is characterised by multiple holes, more or less confluent, of varying diameter. When the tumour originates from the medullary, osseous trabeculae are sometimes thickened by osseous apposition. When the tumour originates from the medulla, it destroys first the endosteum, followed by the cortex, with deep geodes parallel to the large axis of the diaphysis. Permeative osteolysis occurs only in the cortex, and comprises multiple tiny holes parallel to the long axis of the bone, with subperiosteal new bone.

Intra-tumour osteocondensation is either secondary to lysis, with increased osseous density around the lysis, or tumoral, forming the classical "ivory bone" pattern.

Periosteal reaction may be prominent and mimic Ewing's sarcoma and it may be associated with cortical destruction (3-6). In about 40% of patients with primary bone lymphoma, the most frequent radiological change comprises areas of increased transparence with a moth-eaten appearance, occurring in the metaphysis of long bone, sometimes associated with sclerotic rim, cortical destruction with soft-tissue invasion, and periosteal reaction. Magnetic resonance imaging accurately pinpoints the topography and extent of the lesions.

Histological diagnosis requires either a needle- or an open biopsy. Primary bone lymphomas are always high-grade (7), being diffuse large-cell or immunoblastic, or more rarely, Burkitt-type.

Immunohistochemical techniques demonstrate that primary bone lymphomas are more often of B phenotype, with tumour cells expressing CD20. In 60 to 70% of cases a light-chain restriction involving kappa chain was demonstrated (8). In Japan, rare primary T-cell lymphomas of bone have been described (9).

In lymphomas revealed by bone tumour, other involved sites can be demonstrated in most cases (3,4,7).

The treatment of primary bone lymphoma relies on chemotherapy (4) combined with limited-field radiotherapy (10).

Secondary bone involvement

Secondary bone involvement in lymphomas is rarely observed at presentation (1 to 2% of cases in adults, 20% in children). It is more frequent during the course of the disease (15% in adults and 25% in children).

It is discovered either because of specific symptoms or during systematic staging; ^{99}Tc scintigraphy is the most sensitive examination, but true negative results are possible. All abnormalities must be confirmed by radiological examination, possibly by computed tomography or magnetic resonance imaging. Secondary involvement mostly concern axial skeleton and presents as permeative or moth-eaten lysis of the rachis or sacrum, less often as mixed lytic and condensant lesions, and rarely as a purely condensant lesion. Radiological aspects can be evocative, but they are not characteristic.

Secondary bone involvement is observed in high-grade lymphoma. In the African endemic form of Burkitt's lymphoma, facial involvement occurs in more than 50% of cases.

These secondary sites can induce complications: spontaneous fractures (20% of cases), medullary or radicular compression from a spinal lesion, as well as hypercalcaemia.

References

1. PARKER FJR, JACKSON H JR
   Primary reticulum cell sarcoma of bone.
   Surg Gynecol Obstet, 1939; 68: 45-53.
2. PARKER BR, MARGLIN S, CASTELLINO RA
   Skeletal manifestations of leukemia, Hodgkin's disease, and non-Hodgkin's lymphoma.
   Sem Oncol, 1980; 15: 302-315.
3. REIMER RR, CHABNER BA, YOUNG RC, REDDICK R, JOHNSON RE
   Lymphoma presenting in bone. Results of histopathology, staging and therapy.
   Ann Intern Med, 1977; 80: 50-55.
4. BACCI G, JAFFE N, EMILIANI E et al.
   Therapy for primary non-Hodgkin's lymphoma of bone and a comparison of results with Ewing's sarcoma.
   Cancer, 1986; 57: 1468-1472.
5. NGAN H, PRESTON BJ
   Non-Hodgkin's lymphoma presenting with osseous lesions.
   Clin Radiol, 1975; 26: 351-356.
6. BRAUSTEIN EM, WHITE SJ
   Non-Hodgkin's lymphoma of bone.
   Radiology, 1980; 135: 59-63.
7. DUMONT J, MAZABRAUD A
   Primary lymphomas of bone (so-called "Parker and Jackson's reticulum cell sarcoma"): histological review of 75 cases according to the new classifications of non-Hodgkin's lymphomas.
   Biomedicine, 1979; 31: 271-275.
8. PETTIT CK, ZUKERBERG LR, GRAY MH et al.
   Primary lymphoma of bone. A B-cell neoplasm with a high frequency of multilobated cells.
   Am J Surg Pathol, 1990; 14: 329-334.

9. UEDA T, AOZASA K, OHSAWA M,
YOSHIKAWA H, UCHIDA A, ONO K,
MATSUMOTO K

Malignant lymphomas of bone in Japan.

Cancer, 1989; 64: 2387-2392.

10. DOSERETZ DE, MURPHY GF,
RAYMOND AK et al.

Radiation therapy for primary lymphoma of bone.

Cancer, 1983; 51: 44-46.

Urogenital involvement in non-Hodgkin's lymphomas

P. SOLAL-CÉLIGNY, N. BROUSSE

Renal involvement

Renal involvement is often found at autopsy, with a frequency ranging from 42 to 57% (1,2), but clinical manifestations are very rare ranging from 0.5 (3) to 5.8% (4) of patients.

Most often, renal involvement is asymptomatic and found at ultrasonographic (5-8) or CT scan examination (9) during staging procedures. In rare cases, lymphoma involvement is responsible for kidney failure, generally mild [but bilateral ureteral compression by retroperitoneal lymph nodes is the most frequent cause of kidney failure in patients with NHL] (8-13).

Unilateral or bilateral kidney enlargement, homogeneous or nodular, is the most frequent manifestation of lymphoma involvement (7,8). Among 48 patients, there was a single nodule in 22% of patients, multiple nodules in 33%, diffuse enlargement in 17% and contiguous spreading from retroperitoneal lymph nodes in 28%. The involvement was bilateral in 44% of cases (8). In most cases NHL has been previously diagnosed and the diagnosis of renal involvement relies on radiographic abnormalities (7,8). More rarely, kidney involvement is the first manifestation of NHL and the diagnosis is established by transcutaneous or surgical kidney biopsy (14).

Almost all cases of kidney involvement have been described in aggressive NHL (large-cell or immunoblastic) (3,7,10-15). A high frequency has been observed, particularly at relapse, in female patients with diffuse large B-cell NHL of the mediastinum.

Several cases of glomerulonephritis - especially extramembranous or proliferative - associated with NHL have been reported. The relationship between these two disorders is unknown (16).

Testicular involvement

Primary NHL of the testis is defined by a presentation as a testicular tumour, even if the staging discloses other involvement sites, especially retroperitoneal lymph-node involvement. A denomination of secondary testis involvement is reserved for relapsing patients or those presenting with disseminated disease.

Primary NHL of the testis are very rare, accounting for less than 1% of all NHL (18-22). They are observed in patients older than 50 years. In this group of patients, primary NHL accounts for more than 30% of testicular tumours (18). It is the most common type of testicular tumour in men over the age of 60 (22). Patients present with unilateral testis enlargement, very uncommonly bilateral. Except in rare cases, primary NHL of the testis are of intermediate- or high-grade malignancy; and are diffuse large-cell or immunoblastic (17,20). They often spread to retroperitoneal lymph nodes. In several series, a high frequency of associated head-and-neck (17,22) and/or cerebromeningeal involvement (18,22) has been reported, especially as site(s) of relapse.

Prostate involvement

Primary or secondary involvement of the prostate is very rare (25) and is observed only in elderly patients. Dysuria and/or pollakiuria with prostate enlargement are the usual mode of presentation. All histological types of NHL have been described in the prostate (25).

Ovarian, uterine and vulvo-vaginal involvement

Ovarian involvement is very rare, except in African endemic forms of Burkitt's lymphoma (26). Limited series of ovary NHL have been reported (27,28). The diagnosis relies on pathological examination of unilateral or bilateral cyst(s) of the surgically removed ovary (28). Bilateral involvement is found in more than 50% of cases (27,28).

Uterine and vulvo-vaginal involvements have been reported in patients with highly disseminated disease. Very few cases of primary uterine or vulvo-vaginal NHL have been reported (29,30). They were high grade in two-thirds of cases, and follicular in the others.

Malignant lymphomas of the breast

Non-Hodgkin's lymphomas represent less than 1% of all breast malignancies [estimated incidence of 0.14% (31)]. Most of them are intermediate- or high-grade NHL [50 out of 53 cases (32)]. A right-sided predominance has been reported in several series (31-34). Primary NHL of the breast must be distinguished from anaplastic carcinoma and granulocytic sarcomas. In contrast with carcinomas, lymphomas most often surround but spare lobules and ducts, although cases have been reported with a lymphomatous infiltration in the mammary ductules and acini (32). Two cases of synchronous occurrence of axillary NHL and ipsilateral breast carcinoma have been reported (36).

References

1. RICHMOND J, SHERMAN RS, DIAMOND HD et al.
   Renal lesions associated with malignant lymphomas.
   Am J Med, 1962; 32: 184-207.

2. MARTINEZ-MALDONADO M, RAMIREZ DE ARELLANO GA
   Renal involvement in malignant lymphomas: a survey of 49 cases.
   J Urol, 1966; 95: 485-488.

3. STRAUSS DJ, FILIPPA DA, LIEBERMAN PH et al.
   The non-Hodgkin's lymphomas: I. A retrospective clinical and pathologic analysis of 499 cases diagnosed between 1958 and 1969.
   Cancer, 1983; 51: 101-109.

4. GOFFINET DR, WARNKE R, DUNNICK NR et al.
   Clinical and surgical (laparotomy) evaluation of patients with non-Hodgkin's lymphomas.
   Cancer Treat Rep, 1977; 61: 981-992.

5. KAUDE JV, LACY GD
   Ultrasonography in renal lymphoma.
   J Clin Ultrasound, 1978; 6: 321-323.

6. SHIRKHODA A, STAAB EV, MITTELSTAEDT CA
   Renal lymphoma imaged by ultrasound and gallium-67.
   Radiology, 1980; 137: 175-180.

7. HARTMAN DS, DAVIS CJ, GOLDMAN SM et al.
   Renal lymphoma: radiologic-pathologic correlation of 21 cases.
   Radiology, 1982; 144: 759-766.

8 DUPRIEZ B, MOREL P, COIFFIER B et al.
   Renal involvement in aggressive non-Hodgkin's lymphomas included in the LNH-84 and LNH-87 protocols. A report of 48 patients.
   Personal communication.

9. KANFER A, VANDERWALLE A, MOREL-MAROGER L et al.
   Acute renal insufficiency due to lymphomatous infiltration of the kidneys.
   Cancer 1976; 38: 2588-2599

10. ALEDORT LM, HODGES M, BROWN JA
    Irreversible renal failure due to malignant lymphoma.
    Ann Intern Med, 1966; 65: 117-122

11. GLIKLICH D, SUNG HW, FREY M
    Renal failure due to lymphomatous infiltration of the kidney. Report of 3 new cases and review of the literature.
    Cancer, 1986; 58: 745-7583.

12. GEFFEN DB, FISHER RI, LONGO DL, YOUNG RD, DE VITA VT

Renal involvement in diffuse aggressive lymphomas: results of treatment with combination chemotherapy.

J Clin Oncol, 1985; 3: 646-653.

13. RANDOLPH VL, HALL W, BRAMSON W

Renal failure due to lymphomatous infiltration of the kidneys.

Cancer, 1983; 52: 1120-1126.

14 SILBER SJ, CHANG CY

Primary lymphoma of kidney.

J Urol, 1973; 110: 282-284.

15. D'AGATI V, SABLAY LB, KNOWLES DM, WALTER L

Angiotropic large-cell lymphoma (intravascular malignant lymphomatosis) of the kidney: presentation as minimal change disease.

Hum Pathol, 1989; 20: 263-268.

16. PERRONE T, FRIZZERA G, ROSAI J

Mediastinal diffuse large-cell lymphomas with sclerosis, A clinicopathologic study of 60 cases.

Am J Surg Pathol, 1986; 10: 176-191.

17. DABBS DJ, MOREL-MAROGER-STRIKER L, MIGNON F, STRIKER G

Glomerular lesions in lymphomas and leukemias.

Am J Med, 1986; 80: 63-70.

18. GANEM G, GISSELBRECHT C, JOUAULT H, TRICOT G, MARTIN M, BOIRON M

Lymphomes malins du testicule.

Presse Med, 1985; 14: 1739-1742

19. TALERMAN A

Primary malignant lymphoma of the testis.

J Urol, 1977; 118: 783-786.

20. TURNER RR, COLBY TV, MACKINTOSH FR

Testicular lymphomas: a clinicopathologic study of 35 cases.

Cancer, 1981; 48: 2095-2102.

21. DUNCAN PR, CHECA F, GOWING NPC, McELWAIN TJ, PECKHAM MJ

Extranodal non-Hodgkin's lymphoma presenting in the testicle: a clinicopathologic study of 24 cases.

Cancer, 1880; 45: 1578-1584.

22 DOLL DC, WEISS RB

Malignant lymphoma of the testis.

Am J Med, 1986; 81: 515-524.

23. HAMLIN JA, KAGAN R, FRIEDMAN NB

Lymphomas of the testicle.

Cancer, 1972; 29: 1352-1356.

24. WOOLEY PU, OSBORNE CK, LEVI JA, WIERNIK PH, CANELLOS GP

Extranodal presentation of non-Hodgkin's lymphomas in the testis.

Cancer, 1976; 38: 1026-1035.

25. BOSTWICK DG, MANN RB

Malignant lymphomas involving the prostate. A study of 13 cases.

Cancer, 1985; 56: 2932-2938.

26. BERARD CW, O'CONOR GT, THOMAS LB, TORLONI H

Histopathological definition of Burkitt's tumor.

Bull WHO, 1969; 40: 601-607.

27. PALADUGU RR, BEARMAN RM, RAPPAPORT H

Malignant lymphoma with primary manifestation in the gonad; a clinicopathologic study of 38 patients.

Cancer, 1980; 45: 561-571.

28. OSBORNE BM, ROBBOY SJ

Lymphomas or leukemia presenting as ovarian tumors. An analysis of 42 cases.

Cancer, 1983; 52: 1933-1943.

29. KOMAKI R, COX JD, HANSEN RM, GUNN WG, GREENBERG M

Malignant lymphoma of the uterine cervix.

Cancer, 1984; 54: 1699-1704.

30 HARRIS NL, SCULLY RE

Malignant lymphoma and granulocytic sarcoma of the uterus and vagina. A clinicopathologic analysis of 27 cases.

Cancer, 1984; 53: 2530-2545.

31. FISHER MG, CHIDECKER NJ

Primary lymphoma of the breast.

Breast, 1984; 10: 9-12.

32. BRUSTEIN S, KIMMEL M, LIEBERMAN PH, FILIPPA DA, ROSEN PP

Malignant lymphoma of the breast. A study of 53 patients.

Ann Surg, 1987; 205: 144-150.

33 MAMBO NC, BURKE JS, BUTLER JJ

Primary malignant lymphoma of the breast.

Cancer, 1977; 39: 2033-2040.

34. HUGH JC, JACKSON FI, HANSON J, POPPEMA S

Primary breast lymphoma. An immunohistologic study of 20 new cases.

Cancer, 1990; 66: 2602-2611.

35. TELESINGHE PU, ANTHONY PP

Primary malignant lymphoma of the breast.

Histopathology, 1985; 9: 297-307.

36. STIERER M, ROSEN HR, HEINZ R, HANAK H

Synchrony of malignant lymphoma and breast cancer.

JAMA, 1990; 263: 2922-2923.

5.

TREATMENT OF NON-HODGKIN'S LYMPHOMAS

edited by

C. GISSELBRECHT, B. COIFFIER

Methodology and problems in the comparison of treatment results in non-Hodgkin's lymphomas

B. COIFFIER

As stated earlier in this book, lymphomas are very heterogeneous in presentation, prognosis and evolution. Interpretation of results from published trials should be cautious and should take into account this heterogeneity. The first problem arises from the difficulty of diagnosing the subtype of the lymphoma. The most popular classification schemes used around the world (Rappaport's, Lukes-Collins' and Kiel's nomenclatures, the Working Formulation) are not truly reproducible. Totally accurate diagnosis is essential if therapeutic trials are to be comparable. Unfortunately, there is a high degree of discordance between pathologists. A prospective therapeutic trial should comprise the reappraisal of all slides for the accuracy of diagnosis of the lymphoma subtype and the expression of this reappraisal in at least two of the currently used classifications (the Working Formulation and another) in order to be comparable with other trials. As mentioned earlier, the Working Formulation is not the best classification owing to inadequacies in the classification of T-cell NHL and other rare subtypes but it is currently the most useful for clinical purposes.

The second difficulty is due to the fact that most reported trials have mixed together several types of lymphoma with no homogeneous prognosis and no stratification on the basis of the major prognostic factors: stage, tumoral mass, performance status, LDH level and so on. Very few prospective randomized trials exist where this problem is properly addressed.

Armitage and Cheson have presented guidelines for the analysis of published data and comparison of different regimens for large-cell NHL (1). These guidelines could be applied to all the lymphomas and are summarized below:

- Long-term follow-up is necessary. Results from newer regimens are usually reported with median follow-up of 2 to 3 years. Median follow-up of 5 years should be required for definitive results.

- Percentages of CR patients at 2 years do not imply cure. Late relapses do occur up to 7 years afterwards in the CHOP series and in updated newer regimens. The likelihood of cure for patients in CR at 2 years is approximately 70 to 90%.

- Results obtained with newer regimens require confirmation. Newer regimens are usually reported with results of the first 70 or 100 patients treated in one institution. To reflect the heterogeneity of NHL, results should at least be reproduced with more patients in the original group and in a multicentre trial: reproducibility and "exportability" of the results must be demonstrated before such a regimen may be recommended as a standard treatment.

- Variability of percentage of patients with major prognostic factors. Due to the low number of patients, certain factors with prognostic value in one series do not predict the outcome in another series. Nevertheless, major prognostic factors have been described in large patient groups and the breakdown of patients according to these factors should always be stated. Prognostic indexes have been described and will be summarized in the following pages. Prospective studies should be stratified using one of these indexes.

- Recent regimens should be evaluated prospectively in comparison with older, widely recognized regimens.

Reference

1. ARMITAGE JO, CHESON BD
   Interpretation of clinical trials in diffuse large-cell lymphomas.
   J Clin Oncol, 1988; 6: 1335-1347.

Treatment of low-grade non-Hodgkin's lymphomas

C. GISSELBRECHT, J.-M. COSSET

The therapeutic approach to low-grade NHL (i.e. small lymphocytic, follicular small cleaved-cell and follicular mixed) remains controversial. The major controversy is whether any treatment can induce long-term disease-free survival and alter the natural course of the disease. The debate is more directed towards disseminated disease, which accounts for 80 to 90% of low-grade lymphomas, since there is evidence that radiation therapy for early-stage disease is potentially curative.

Treatment of early stage I, II, low-grade lymphomas

The efficacy of radiation therapy has been demonstrated in the treatment of clinically staged patients with localized disease. Most of the studies reported (1-10) are composed of patients with follicular small-cleaved-cell or follicular mixed lymphomas since small lymphocytic lymphoma is rarely localized at presentation. However, these studies also included follicular large-cell lymphomas, which have a different behaviour from other follicular lymphomas (11). Their prognosis is the same as for intermediate-grade NHL.

Doses of radiation therapy usually range from 30 to 50 Gy depending in part on the extent of the field (5,6,9). The cure rate does not appear to be any different whether the dose is 20 Gy or 40 Gy (12).

The main results for disease-free survival are given in *Table I*.

At least 54% of patients are disease-free at 10 years (9). A higher freedom from relapse of up to 80% is reported in stage I disease (2) and only 10% of the patients who were treated with total lymphoid radiation relapsed (3,4,9). The absence of relapse after 6 years (13) in studies with long follow-up may indicate that a subset of patients can be cured. For stage II patients, localized irradiation produces a 61% disease-free survival rate at 5 years (2,14), whereas an 83% disease-free survival has been reported in patients treated with total nodal irradiation (3,4).

The contiguous and non-contiguous nodal relapses seen in patients who received limited-field radiation in all studies suggest that stage II patients should receive total nodal irradiation. However, in non-laparotomy staged patients with disease above the diaphragm, no significant difference in either survival or freedom from relapse has been observed between limited and extended total nodal irradiation (2,9). Whether or not total nodal irradiation should be routinely used in carefully staged stage I disease remains unclear. Staging laparotomy may be of interest in such patients as overall survival is better in surgically staged stage I patients than in clinically staged ones (9). In an analysis of various prognostic factors (5,9,12) age, stage and B symptoms were found to be independently significant in Cox regression analysis (5,15). The bulk of the tumour mass, if greater than 5 cm, was found to be of value in at

TABLE I

**Radiation therapy: stage I-II
follicular lymphoma (including some follicular large-cell lymphomas)**

Authors	Stage		Number	Treatment modality		Disease-free survival
Chen (2)	I	II	28	IF EF	I II	88% at 10 yr 61%
Gallagher (3)	I	II	22	IF TLI		83% at 10 yr
Gomez (4)	I	II	29	IF EF		83% at 10 yr
Gospodarowicz (5)	I	II	252	IF		53% at 10 yr
Paryani (9)	I	II	124	IF EF TLI		54% at 10 yr
Reddy (10)	I	II	24	EF		70% at 10 yr
Carde (1)	I		55	IF IF + CVP EF TLI + CVP		67% 92% 39% 54
McLaughlin (7)	I	II	76	IF + CHOP or COP BLEO		37% 64%
Monfardini (8)	I	II	26	IF IF + CVP		54 % at 5 yr
Lawrence (6)	I	II	54	IF EF ± chemo.		48 % at 10 yr

IF: involved field.
EF: extended field.
TLI: total lymphoid irradiation.

least two studies (5,12). Three main groups can be defined. In the first, which includes patients less than 70 years old, with limited stage I or II non-bulky NHL, there is a 10-year disease-free survival rate of 75%; in the second, which includes patients with extensive stage II and bulky disease, a disease-free survival rate of 45% and a survival rate at 10 years of 58% have been observed; the last group, of very unfavourable prognosis, includes patients older than 70, whatever the other parameters, with a survival and disease-free survival rate at ten years of less than 20% (5,12).

The role of combination chemotherapy in the treatment of early-stage follicular lymphoma has been studied in randomized trials where Cyclophosphamide, Vincristine and Prednisone (CVP) were used in association with localized radiotherapy (8). No clear superiority was seen in the combined modality arm when compared to radiation therapy alone. However, when using a combination of Cyclophosphamide, Doxorubicin, Vincristine and Prednisone (CHOP) (7), McLaughlin reported a higher relapse-free survival rate at 5 years (64%) than for those treated with radiation alone (37%).

TABLE II

**Radiation therapy: stage III-IV
low-grade lymphomas**

Authors	Stage	Number	Treatment modality	CR	Disease-free survival
Glastein (19)	III	51	TLI	100%	35% at 10 yr
Cox (20)	III	29	TLI + abdomen	97%	61% at 5 yr
Thar (21-22)	II III IV	28	TBI f + b	83%	35% at 5 yr
Choi (23)	III IV	31	TBI f	84%	26% at 4 yr
Carabell (24)	III IV	43	TBI + b	-	15% at 8 yr
Hoppe (25)	III IV	17	TBI + b	71%	25% at 4 yr
Chaffey (26)	III IV	36	TBI	-	20% at 5 yr
Paryani (27)	III	66	TBI + b TLI + CVP	100%	39% at 10 yr
Johnson (28)	III	13	TBI	100%	70% at 5 yr
Mendenhall (29)	II III IV	27	TBI	74%	10% at 10 yr

TLI: total lymphoid irradiation
TBI: total body irradiation (100-200 Gy)
f: fractionated
b: boost

The low relapse-free survival reported in these series underlines the need for adding other prognostic factors such as age, tumour bulk, LDH and B symptoms to the Ann Arbor Classification.

Thus, it is possible that the use of chemotherapy might improve the results obtained with radiation alone in stage II disease with adverse prognostic factors, i.e. bulky abdominal disease, number of node areas involved > 2, B symptoms or increased LDH level. Repeat biopsy in these cases should be recommended as the propensity of the disease to evolve to more aggressive lymphoma is well known and will modify the therapeutic approach in favour of chemotherapy (1).

It is unlikely that there will be a definitive answer in the near future as to the best approach for early-stage indolent lym-phomas, since this would require a randomized multicentre trial spanning decades for such a low number of patients.

Treatment of advanced stages III and IV

The optimal treatment approach to patients with advanced-stage low-grade lymphoma is one of the most controversial topics despite more than 20 years of clinical investigation (16,17). This type of lymphoma is, in fact, an unusualy slow-growing advanced malignancy and despite the absence of durable complete remission, patients develop a capacity to live with their disease. However, all patients ultimately die of their disease. The paradox of this indolent lymphoma is that more patients survive after

TABLE III

Single-agent chemotherapy in low-grade lymphomas

Authors	Number	Chemotherapy	CR	Median survival
Kennedy (33)	13	Cyclophosphamide 150 mg/d	46%	30 m
Hoppe (25)	17	Cyclophosphamide 1.5 - 2.5 mg/kg/d Chlorambucil 0.1 - 0.2 mg/kg/d	64%	> 48 m
Rosenberg (17)	37	Cyclophosphamide 1.5 - 2.5 mg/kg/d Chlorambucil 0.1 - 0.2 mg/kg/d	65%	133 m
Lister (34)	31	Chlorambucil 10 mg/d X 6 wk then 15 d/m X 5 m	13%	> 48 m
Portlock (31)	26	Chlorambucil 16 mg/m^2 X 5 d/m	42%	> 60 m
Cavallin-Stahl (32)	106	Prednimustine 150-200 mg X 5 d/m	63%	42 m

15 years with higher grade non-Hodgkin's lymphomas than with low-grade subtypes. There is no evidence that the rarer forms of indolent lymphomas, diffuse small lymphocytic or mantle-zone lymphomas, require a distinct therapeutic approach as most of the information about these entities is hidden in large series of the more common follicular small-cleaved and follicular mixed types. Proof of the perplexity of oncologists is evident in the numerous therapeutic approaches that have been developed: single-agent, combination chemotherapy, whole-body irradiation, chemotherapy and radiotherapy, local-field irradiation, autologous bone-marrow transplantation or no initial therapy (16-18).

Radiation therapy at stages III and IV

Total lymphoid irradiation (TLI) has been proposed mostly in stage III follicular lymphomas. Recommended doses are 25 to 35 Gy. The frequent involvement of mesenteric nodes and relapses occurring in non-irradiated epitrochlear nodes argue in favour of extending the field to those areas. Results are given in *Table II*. CR is achieved in almost all patients (19,20,27) with probability of survival of 65 to 78% and a 5-year relapse-free survival rate of 43 to 61% (19,20). Approximately 40% of patients remain disease-free. Adverse prognostic factors are B symptoms, tumour burden and number of sites involved. Selection of patients for radiotherapy alone is necessary and unfortunately only 12% of stage III patients fall into this favourable subset (27).

Low-dose total-body irradiation with 150 to 200 cGy delivered in fractions of 10 to 15 cGy, often with boost irradiation delivered to initially-involved sites has been widely used. Complete remission is achieved easily (22-28). However 60 to 75% of patients experienced relapses. The haematological toxicity with delayed thrombocytopenia is generally transient and in most cases does not prohibit the subsequent use of chemotherapy (29).

Low-dose limited-field radiation therapy (4 Gy in 2 fractions over 3 days) has recently

TABLE IV

Combination chemotherapy in low-grade lymphomas: CVP regimen

Authors	Number	CR	Median survival
Portlock (36)	32	41%	> 24 m
Hoppe (25)	17	88%	> 60 m
Bagley (37)	75	57%	–
Young (38)	29	65%	> 60 m
Parlier (39)	31	65%	> 60 m
Anderson (40)	49	67%	83 m
Jones (41)	74	48%	48 m
Steward (42)	162	56%	64 m
Kennedy (33)	28	68%	> 60 m
Lister (34)	35	37%	> 48 m
Kalter (35)	40	67%	48 m
C: Cyclophosphamide per os or intravenously with different dosage. V: Vincristine P: Prednisone			

been reported to achieve an 89% response rate (38% CR and 51% PR) in irradiated volumes and could have several clinical applications in the general management of low-grade NHL (30)

Single agent chemotherapy

Chlorambucil and Cyclophosphamide have been widely used for decades *(Table III)*. Complete remission can be achieved in 13 to 65% of patients, depending on the time of evaluation and the extent of restaging procedures. Median time to reach complete remission is 12 months (25), with some patients requiring 24 months of therapy. Chlorambucil was generally administered orally on a daily basis. More recently, high-dose pulses of Chlorambucil or Prednimustine (31,32) have been proposed with a similar or superior response-rate, depending on the application of careful restaging crite-

ria. For patients treated with a single agent, the median duration of remission is close to 30 months in reported series (12 months to 36 months) but only 20 to 30% of the patients are disease-free at 10 years, with a median survival period of about 8 years (17,25,31-35).

Combination chemotherapy

Regimens without anthracycline

CVP regimen

The most widely used association of chemotherapy in follicular lymphomas has been Cyclophosphamide, Vincristine and Prednisone (CVP). Cycles are repeated every 3 to 4 weeks. Different schedules and dosages of moderate intensity have been proposed. Results are shown in *Table IV*.

TABLE V

Combination chemotherapy in low-grade lymphomas without anthracycline

Authors	Number	Regimen	CR	Median survival
Oken (47)	89	BCVP	70%	> 42 m
Glick (46)	14	BCVP	50%	> 48 m
Ezdinli (43)	53	BCVP	53%	> 50 m
Ezdinli (43)	27	COPrP	56%	> 50 m
Glick (46)	18	COPrP	61%	41 m
Bitran (45)	29	COPrP	48%	> 48 m
Anderson (44)	31	COPrP	77%	> 101 m
Lepage (48)	57	COPrP	43%	> 48 m
Longo (13)	24	CMOPrP	79%	114 m
C: Cyclophosphamide B: BCNU V: O: Vincristine Pr: Procarbazine P: Prednisone				

TABLE VI

Combination chemotherapy in low-grade lymphomas with anthracycline

Authors	Number	Regimen	CR	Median survival
Rodriguez (49)	16	CHOP - BLEO	61%	NP
McKelvey (50)	20	CHOP or HOP	70%	NP
Jones (51)	92	CHOP	69%	NP
Kalter (35)	45	CHOP - BLEO HOP	79%	> 96 m
Peterson (52)	14	CHOP - BLEO	56%	> 36 m
Sullivan (15)	16	CHOP	69%	54 m
Anderson (53)	18	M.BACOD	55%	> 60 m
Lepage (48)	56	PACOP	47%	> 38 m

Complete remission is observed in 65 to 85% of cases. In a randomized trial (36), patients were assigned to receive either Chlorambucil or CVP combined or not with total lymphoid irradiation. Although the CR rate after the first 6 months was higher in the CVP arm, over time the CR rate with Chlorambucil was equivalent and no difference in survival could be observed in any group. Median time to achieve remission is generally 12 months with single-agent chemotherapy and 6 months with polychemotherapy. Several other studies comparing CVP with single-agent chemotherapy have also failed to demonstrate significant advantages in more aggressive therapy (33,34). Median duration of remission ranges from 18 months to 36 months, with a median survival period of between 6 and 8 years. Less than 30% of the patients are expected to be disease-free after 7 years.

Other regimens without anthracycline

Several attempts have been made to improve the CVP regimen (Table V). The COPP regimen, with added Procarbazine, (43) achieved CR in 56% of patients with advaced follicular small-cleaved lymphoma, and 57% of the CR lasted more than 5 years (43). Similar experiences have been shared by others, with regimens containing Procarbazine (13,44-46) or BCNU (46,47).

Regimens with anthracycline

Attempts at improving the chemotherapy treatment results of low-grade lymphomas started by using mainly active regimens in diffuse large-cell lymphoma (Table VI). In the initial comparison between CVP and CHOP (Cyclophosphamide, Adriamycin, Vincristine, Prednisone) (51), the CR rate with CHOP was 60% and was not significantly different from CVP. The introduction of Bleomycin (CHOP-BLEO) did not improve the CR rate (27,49) and a prolongation of the disease-free survival period has not been reported. With regimens such as M-BACOD (Methotrexate, Bleomycin, Doxorubicin, Cyclophosphamide, Vincristine and Dexamethasone), the complete response rate is 55% and the 5-year disease-free survival rate 40% (36). Comparison of regimens including or not including anthra-cyclines, PACOP- PCOP [Procarbazine (Doxorubi-cin), Cyclophosphamide, Vincri-stine, Prednisone] in randomized trials (48) did not exhibit superiority of anthracycline-containing regimens, either in terms of remission (43% vs 47%) or of disease-free survival (61% at 3 years in both arms).

However, several authors have reported in non-randomized studies a better disease-free survival in patients treated with an anthracycline-containing regimen (35,54).

Duration of treatment

Duration of treatment oncc complete remission is obtained is not well-established.

In most reported series, at least one year of maintenance was used (31,42,43,48). The impact of maintenance therapy is difficult to assess. Prolonged survival without progression is observed in patients treated with BCVP (26) or with Chlorambucil. Although no impact on survival has been described clearly, a study which is of interest is that by Jones (55), where chemotherapy was stopped after complete remission and patients were randomly assigned to BCG or no therapy. A similar increase in disease-free survival was observed in the BCG arm. In any case, it must be pointed out that patients who do not achieve complete remission are generally treated for months or years and survival is poor for these patients (35,48).

Combined-modality therapy

Relapses occur in nodal areas in most patients treated with chemotherapy and outside irradiated areas in patients treated with radiation alone. Radiation is only suitable in patients without bone-marrow involvement, non-bulky disease or B symptoms.

Consequently, although the aim of treatment should be a curative one, combined chemotherapy and irradiation may provide another approach in reducing tumour burden, B symptoms and bone-marrow involvement, allowing radiation to play a role in a consolidation phase in order to prevent relapse.

TABLE VII

Combined modality in advanced-stage low-grade lymphomas

Authors	Stage	Number	Treatment	CR	Survival % (year)
Sullivan (15)	II-III-IV	16	CHOP X 5	69%	33% (6yr)
McLaughlin (56)	III	74	CHOP Bléo + IF	81%	75% (5yr)
Portlock (36)	IV	63	Single-agent vs CVP vs CVP + TLI	65% 83% 70%	no difference
Hoppe (25)	III-IV	51	Single-agent vs CVP vs CVP + TLI	64% 88% 71%	84% no difference
Young (38)	III-IV	75	TLI + boost vs CVP vs C-MOPP	84% 65% 53%	no difference
Hancock (57)	III-IV	100	Systemic RT vs chemo.	- -	no difference at 10 yr
Johnson (28)	III-IV	72	TBI+CVP/MOPP vs CVP	-	no difference at 5 yr
Brereton (58)	II-III-IV	39	TBI+CVP/MOPP vs CVP/MOPP	70%	no difference at 5 yr

TBI: low-dose total-body irradiation
IF: involved field irradiation
TLI: total lymphoid irradiation

Several pilot studies reported in *Table VII*, have addressed this question. As expected, CR rate was over 80% and disease-free survival at five years ranged from 33 to 75% (56).

Durable remission is only observed in stage III disease (55) with a decreasing risk of relapse after 4 to 5 years. Disappointing results with combined modality therapy in randomized trials *(Table VII)* may be due to the inclusion of stage IV patients or to problems of treatment design. Secondary leukaemia might be a risk, especially when using Procarbazine in combination chemotherapy (38).

At present there is no clear evidence that combined modality therapy is better than chemotherapy alone as regards long-term disease-free survival except for a subset of limited stage III patients. Whether or not this approach is better than conservative treatment in all stage III and IV patients remains in debate. In a prospective randomized study (13,38) comparing conservative treatment with aggressive combined-modality therapy with Pro MACE/MOPP flexitherapy followed by low-dose total lymphoid-radiation therapy for those achieving CR with chemotherapy, 78% achieved CR and 86% of those achieving CR remained in their initial remission with a median follow-up of more than 4 years. There is no significant impact on overall survival as yet (13).

No initial therapy

The apparent incurability of patients whose disease is at an advanced stage has often led to deferral of treatment until overt clinical manifestations (18,59). This attitude was supported by the experience of Rosenberg (17) at Stanford who selected for no initial therapy patients asymptomatic for at least 2 months after their initial evaluation. Often they were of advanced age or had concurrent medical problems that made intensive treatment somewhat riskier, or a history of several months of gradually enlarging non-tender adenopathy. Criteria for initiating therapy were rapid progression, development of a site of disease that threatened the function of an organ or B symptoms. Eighty-three patients with stage III or IV were managed in this way (17,60). In 51 patients (61%) the median time for requiring treatment was 3 years with for differences follicular mixed (16.5 months), follicular small cleaved (48 months) and small lymphocytic (72 months). The median survival was 11 years. The actuarial survival curves did not differ significantly from those of two prospective randomized studies being carried out at the same time (17). Of interest is the report of spontaneous regression in patients managed without initial therapy (61). The overall rate was 23%, the highest occurring in patients with follicular small cleaved subtype (30%). The duration was usually longer than one year and 7% experienced complete remission.

It is a unique characteristic of the low-grade lymphoma that there is an increasing probability with time of histological change to a higher grade. Such a transition occurs at a rate of about 8% per year. The actuarial probability of histological transformation was the same for patients who had had no initial therapy, as compared in a series of 131 patients assigned to therapeutic protocols (17).

Thus the data from conservatively treated patients make it difficult to discern the effect of aggressive treatment. However, many centres have found that their patients with follicular lymphoma do not fare as well as the Stanford patients (62). The percentage of true indolent disease was estimated at 56% in the Stanford series, but seems lower in others groups (34%, GELF protocol). Straus (62) found that patients with advanced stage had a median survival of less than 5 years with conservative treatment. Patients with follicular mixed lymphoma will in any case require therapy in the year following diagnosis.

Moreover, follicular mixed lymphomas are more likely to respond to combination chemotherapy with durable CR (13,63). The potential benefit of withholding initial therapy is mainly a prolonged treatment-free interval without exposure to drugs. However, there are certain disadvantages associated with the conservative approach. Many patients are adversely affected by the constant and visible enlargement of lymph nodes and need close follow-up to detect any unexpected rapid progression. Several series (35,48,51) reported that patients who achieve complete remission have better prognosis and survival.

Before choosing the option of no initial therapy the first question to be answered is whether any initial therapy is indicated (18). Factors which should be considered include:

(1) histopathology: patients with follicular small cleaved or small lymphocytic NHL appear to derive the greatest benefit from the deferred approach;

(2) stage: only patients who have stage III or IV should be considered; stage I and II should be treated with curative intent;

(3) sites of disease: if it is locally bulky or in a threatening site it may require therapy;

(4) pace of disease: rapid progression would be inappropriate for deferment of therapy;

(5) systemic symptoms require palliation with systemic therapy;

(6) general medical condition and psychological behaviour; and

(7) age: although young patients have a better prognosis, deferment therapy might be difficult to justify as they are candidates for new approaches.

In any case, even if the criteria for no initial therapy are well-defined and rely upon prognostic factors, the experience of Stanford was not randomized, which makes it difficult to assess the reproducibility of the results. Randomized trials are mandatory and are in progress in France and in the U.S.

Although the concept of a "favourable" indolent disease has been widely accepted, acceptance of low-grade lymphoma as incurable is clearly counterproductive. What may be adequate therapy for clinical practice is not necessarily optimal clinical investigation. The large body of evidence which fails to demonstrate any advantage for combination therapy only serves to reinforce the need for new approaches to the management of these patients.

Prognostic factors

Prognostic factors which have been reported to adversely influence the results of therapy include the following:

(1) age greater than 50 years (5,14,64);

(2) sex, generally with a poorer survival among male patients (65-69);

(3) systemic symptoms (3,14);

(4) extranodal involvement, other than bone marrow and liver (36) in some reports, while bone-marrow involvement is characterized as the main factor in others (48,68,69);

(5) stage, if disseminated stage IV (14,69);

(6) bulk of the disease in localized stage (3,12,68,69);

(7) LDH level (7,13,69);

(8) prior chemotherapy (65);

(9) absence of response to initial treatment (44,48,65,69); and

(10) histological subtype (14,69,70) and degree of nodularity.

Histological subtype

Although not statistically significant, diffuse small lymphocytic lymphoma patients survive longer than those with follicular subtypes (17,48). However, treatment studies have generally included relatively few patients, and complete response rates have been slightly lower.

Reports suggesting superior disease-free survival in patients with follicular mixed lymphoma (13,34,71) have not been confirmed by others (18,48,68,69).

On the basis of the experience of the National Cancer Institute, it has been proposed that all advanced follicular mixed lymphomas should be treated aggressively with curative intent (14). However, proper multivariate analysis failed to demonstrate any advantage in disease-free survival for follicular mixed lymphoma when treated with COPP regimen (46,48).The coexistence of nodular and diffuse patterns in follicular lymphomas does not influence survival rate (14,70). The clinical approach to such patients should be similar to that in those with a "nodular-only" pattern. However, a pure nodular pattern involving 75% or more of the cross-sectional area was found to be an important favourable prognostic indicator (71). The presence of interfollicular fibrosis is associated with a longer survival period (69) Clinicopathological studies of non-Hodgkin's lymphomas have demonstrated histological variation in examination of sequential biopsies from patients who presented with follicular lymphomas (72). This histological variation was apparent as a change from a nodular to a diffuse pattern or an increased proportion of large cells or both. With time, there is an increasing probability of histological change to a non-Hodgkin's lymphoma of a higher grade and more aggressive subtype (68,73). By five to ten years after diagnosis, as many as 50% of patients who have required and undergone a second biopsy procedure have transformed to a more progressed aggressive histological subtype (63,74,75), especially diffuse large-cell lymphomas.

Multiple recurrent chromosomal alterations in follicular lymphomas may be integrated into the development of the disease (75). Type or amount of chromosomal defects could serve as objective markers to assist in histopathological classification and as prognostic indicators.

Histological conversion is highly likely in patients who fail to achieve remission with initial therapy or relapse after achieving complete initial response (68,74).The actuarial probability of histological conversion seems the same for patients who have had no initial therapy (74). Such a transition occurs at a rate of about 8% per year, by evolving through follicular mixed- and follicular large-cell stages first (74). However, the probability of transformation may decrease after 6 years (68). When the histology changes, the natural course accelerates, with a median survival period of 5 months (68). Few series have enough patients to be able to speculate on the efficacy of therapy once histological conversion has taken place. However, there is some indication that complete response may be durable (40,44,74). Such patients should be candidates for new approaches with bone-marrow transplantation (76).

Response to therapy

Pathologically documented complete remission can be achieved in approximately 40 to 80% of patients using one of the previously described treatments. Prompt responses are observed with all approaches except daily alkylating agent, where the time to achieve CR may be as long as 1 to 2 years (25). No significant differences among treatments have been observed.

It remains controversial whether or not achieving a complete remission of disease with any form of therapy confers a survival advantage to patients (17). Several studies found a significant advantage in survival in patients who achieved complete remission (3,40,42,51,68,76-78). However, patients who achieve complete remission may have better prognostic factors and cannot be compared with more unfavourable patients. In a multivariate analysis, Lepage et al. (47) identified 3 main prognostic factors for survival: achievement of complete remission, bone-marrow involvement and age. However, in other multiparametric studies, complete remission was not identified as an independent parameter (68).The notion that emerges from these studies is that complete remission prolongs disease-free survival and is more likely to be seen in young patients with stage III disease of follicular mixed histology. Once a systemic treatment has been initiated, the goal must be to obtain a pathologically documented complete remission and then to discontinue all therapy.

Prior chemotherapy

Exposure to prior therapy has been described as affecting survival (11) in multi-

varia,te analysis. The reason probably has to do with its influence on complete remission rate. Possible mechanisms might include a decrease in bone-marrow tolerance and the induction of resistance in the tumour cells. Few data are available on the efficacy of salvage therapy at relapse. Nevertheless, shorter survival has been observed in patients who are unable to achieve complete remission or who relapse after CR (35,48,65,68).

LDH level and other biological markers

Increased LDH level is associated with poor survival in follicular mixed lymphoma (13) or among patients staged I, II or III (7,56). LDH level also affects relapse-free survival (13,42,56,69). Low haemoglobin level was found to be significant (3,65) in univariate analysis, as well as a low platelet count. Beta-2 microglobulin was found to be correlated with bulky disease (78), which itself affects survival (69). However, covariability exists among prognostic factors and the assessment of the relative impact of each factor is difficult to determine because of the limited number of patients covered in each report.

Tumour bulk

Bulky disease is associated with a lower survival (3,5,42,48,56,67,68,79) and relapse-free survival. The importance of this parameter will depend upon the type of therapy used. Patients with a tumour treated with radiotherapy alone will experience a poor prognosis (5,15) but this factor will remain significant in patients treated with chemotherapy alone or combined-modality therapy (56,65). Even so, survival is better than with radiation alone. The number of sites involved, a factor which affects the bulk of the disease, adversely influences survival (42,48,67).

Stage

As reported above, survival of patients with stage I or stage II non-bulky desease is significantly superior to that of stage III and IV and more than 50% of patients with localized stage can expect to be cured of their disease (2,3,5,7). Data regarding the prognostic importance of stage III versus stage IV are scarce. Nevertheless stage III patients generally have a longer survival period than stage IV patients (3,14), especially in limited stage III without bulky disease, with normal LDH and without systemic symptoms.

Extranodal involvement

Among stage IV patients, bone-marrow involvement was not associated with a less favourable prognosis in several studies (3,18,65,67,68,77,81). It has recently been characterized as an independent adverse prognostic factor for both complete remission and survival in a randomized prospective study (48) and a non-randomized study (67).

In fact, by using immunological techniques and probes or molecular biology it has been found that circulating abnormal clone is readily detectable in nearly 70% of patients with advanced stage disease (82,83). Thus, bone-marrow involvement is likely to be present in most advanced-stage patients, with the rate clearly depending on the extent of the staging procedures. A degree of bone-marrow involvement of > 20% adversely affects survival and relapse-free survival (67,68), and massive involvement is a clear indicator of unfavourable prognosis. Other extranodal involvement sites have been generally associated with more unfavourable prognosis (81,84) although the prognostic significance of liver involvement is not clear (14,18). Overall, a number of extranodal sites involved of ≥ 2 is an independent adverse prognostic factor (67,68).

Systemic symtoms

The presence of systemic symptoms is linked with more agressive disease (3,14,48,65,68) but their prognostic value does not reach a significant level in most studies (65,67).

Sex

A more favourable prognosis is described among women patients (42,65-67) whereas it is not found significant in other reported studies (3,40,48,85).

Age

Age greater than 60-65 years is one of the most important determinant factors adversely affecting survival in the localized and disseminated stages (5,14,40,43,48,67,79-82). Though 45% of patients are still alive after ten years and 29% after 20 years, this proportion, which might be acceptable for older patients, is dramatically low for younger patients, who may be candidates for new investigational approaches despite their better prognosis.

The selection of patients for new programmes is difficult since models of prognostic factors which have been established have not been validated in other studies (5,48,65,67,68). Nevertheless, patients with bulky disease, massive bone-marrow involvement, extensive stage with extranodal site ≥ 2, represent a subset of patients with poor prognosis. Intensive treatment should be restricted to younger patients with adverse prognostic factors with the goal of achieving durable and complete remission.

Only two new approaches are currently under development:

- intensification of treatment with autologous or allogenic bone-marrow transplantation and

- use of biological response modifiers.

Unless dramatic improvements emerge from pilot studies, it will take at least 8 years before the impact of these new strategies can be evaluated.

Interferon therapy

In a disorder where the clinical course of the disease is slow, the rate of proliferation of tumour cells is low, and numerous immunological defects occur, molecules such as Interferon (IFN) that modulate growth and interact extensively with the immune system are an attractive proposition for clinical and experimental development.

TABLE VIII

Single-agent chemotherapy in low-grade lymphomas

Authors	Type IFN	Dose	Patient Numbers	CR+PR	Follicular	Small lymphocytic
Louie (87)	HuI	5MU X 2d X 30 d	8	4	4/8	-
Gutterman (88)	HuI	3MU/d X 28 d	10	5	3/6	2/4
Horning (89)	HuI	9MU/d X 28 d	18	6	6/18	0/10
Siegert (85)	Hurβ	4.5-9MU X 43 d	10	2	2/10	-
Leavitt (90)	Hurα	10MU X 2/wk	21	10	10/15	0/6
Wagstaff (91)	Hurα	2MU X 2/wk	34	17	13/23	4/11
Foon (92)	Hurα	50MU X 3/wk	24	13	-	-
O'Connell (93)	Hurα	12MU/m² X 3/wk	16	7	7/16	-
Chiesi (94)	Hurα ι CB	3MU/m² X 3/wk 10 mg/d	10	8	8/10	-
Rohatiner (95)	Hurα	2MU/m² X 3/wk + CB 10 mg/d	11	8	8/11	-
Ozer (96)	Hurα + CP	2MU/m² X 3/wk 100 mg/d	60	31	-	-

HuI: Human leucocyte interferon
Hur: Human recombinant interferon
MU: Million units
CB: Chlorambucil
CP: Cyclophosphamide

A summary of published findings with various IFN preparations is given in *Table VIII*.

Patients with follicular histology responded more frequently than those with diffuse small lymphocytic histology, with a response rate of about 40% versus 20% (87-94). However, documented CR does not exceed 20%. There is no clear evidence in favour of a dose/response relationship, but patients who have never received chemotherapy may respond more frequently to IFN than those who have received prior treatment (90).

Synergie, or additive effects, between interferon alpha and several cytotoxic drugs has been demonstrated *in vitro* (reviewed in reference 97) especially with certain drugs which are active in non-Hodgkin's lymphoma, such as cyclophosphamide, doxorubicin and vinca-alkaloids.

Several trials based on these data have tested the potential interferon therapeutic benefits of alpha combined with chemotherapy in an historical comparison, the MD-Anderson group has shown that patients treated with interferon alpha after responding to a CHOP-Bleomycin induction therapy have a longer-disease-free survival than those who received no maintenance treatment (98). In a prospective randomized trial, the EORTC is currently testing interferon alpha as a maintenance treatment after a response to chemotherapy. Patients are first treated with a CVP regimen and irradiation of bulky tumours. Responding patients are then randomly assigned to receive either interferon alpha-2a ($3 \times 10^6/m^2$ IU three times per week by subcutaneous injection for 12 months) or no treatment. A first analysis of this trial has recently been reported (99). There was a significantly longer time-to-treatment failure in patients treated with interferon alfa during maintenance (136 weeks vs. 85 weeks, p = 0.02). There was no difference in overall survival between the two groups.

Recently two prospective and randomized trials have tested the efficacy of recombinant interferon alpha combined with chemotherapy. In the ECOG trial, patients with clinically aggressive follicular non-Hodgkin's lymphoma or intermediate-grade non-Hodgkin's lymphoma were treated with a COPA regimen (cyclophosphamide 750 mg/m^2 D$_1$, doxorubicin 50 mg/m^2 D$_1$, vincristine 1.4 mg/m^2 D$_1$, prednisone 100mg/m^2 D$_1$-D$_5$, 1 cycle every 4 weeks, 8 cycles) with or without interferon alfa-2a. Interferon was given by intramuscular injection for 5 days at a dose of 6 MU/m^2 every 4 weeks, just before a course of COPA. 249 patients were randomized and analyzed, 127 in the COPA-only group, and 122 in the COPA + interferon alpha-2a group. Patients treated with COPA + interferon alpha-2a had a significantly longer time-to-treatment failure compared to those treated with COPA only (30 months vs. 19.2 months, p < 10^{-3}). Although there was no significant difference in overall survival using a log-rank test for comparison, the use of interferon alpha in combination with COPA was a significant favourable prognostic factor for survival in a multivariate analysis (100).

Finally, in 1986 the GELF group from France and Belgium began a prospective trial of concomitant administration of interferon alfa-2b with a CHOP-like regimen in follicular lymphoma patients with a high tumor burden. Two hundred and forty two patients were treated with either a CHVP regimen (cyclophosphamide 600mg/m^2, doxorubicin 25mg/m^2, teniposide 60 mg/m^2 all on Day 1, prednisone 40 mg/m^2 D$_1$ to D$_5$, 1 cycle every 4 weeks for 6 months then 1 cycle every 8 weeks for 12 months) (119 patients), or with the same chemotherapy regimen associated with interferon alfa-2 b (5 MU three times per week subcutaneously) for 18 months from the onset of chemotherapy (123 patients). Compared to patients treated with CHVP only, those treated with CHVP + interferon alpha-2b had a higher overall response rate (86 % vs. 70 %, p = 0.002), a longer median event-free survival (34.5 months vs. 18.5 months, p < 10^{-4}) and a higher 3-year survival (86 % vs. 69 %, p = 0.02) (101). These trials clearly demonstrate the benefits of a combinaison of a doxorubicin-containing chemotherapy regimen and interferon alpha in low-grade follicular non-Hodgkin's lymphoma.

Another trial testing a combination of interferon alfa-2b and chlorambucil vs. chlorambucil alone in low-grade follicular lymphoma is currently in progress (102).

Monoclonal antibody therapy studies

Virtually all the therapeutic trials with monoclonal antibodies (MAbs) have been phase I studies designed mainly to evaluate dose and toxicity. Nevertheless, they have indicated clinical responses that are reasonably consistent with the results seen in animal models (103). Several features have limited the efficacy of monoclonal antibodies in man. The duration of response was generally short, the target antigen was modulated on the surface of the malignant cells and the patients developed an antibody response to the murine antibody used for therapy.

An attractive approach is the use of anti-idiotype MAbs, which are reactive with the idiotype of the immunoglobulins on the malignant B-cells. An initial report (104) in a patient with refractory low-grade lymphoma was encouraging since a complete remission was observed lasting 6 years. Of 10 other lymphoma patients, five attained partial remission. Circulating idiotypes are common. This protein, if present in large amounts, can block the antibody, antagonizing the therapeutic action of the monoclonal anti-idiotype. Moreover, patients may develop an anti-mouse antibody which limits the anti-tumour effect of the mouse hybridoma. Other workers using anti-idiotype antibodies have not been successful in producing anti-tumour response (105,106).

Of great interest has been the demonstration of more than one idiotype in immunophenotyping of tumour sections. Antigenic heterogeneity will lead to the use of MAb "cocktails"' (107) to overwhelm or dampen the immunogenicity of murine MAbs. The use of human or near-human antibodies produced by genetic engineering opens the way for new therapies. However, it is possible that human MAbs can still generate an immune response against the antigen-binding region, a so-called anti-idiotype response.

Radio-immunotherapy

Despite dramatic advances in curative combination chemotherapy, few patients with low-grade lymphomas or relapsed aggressive lymphomas can be cured with conventional therapy.

One approach involves the use of monoclonal antibodies which recognize tumour-associated antigens as a mean of targeting drugs or radio-isotopes to tumour cells. Several groups have used radiolabelled antibodies.

Most human studies have employed modest individual doses of radio-iodine in order to avoid myelosuppression (86,108). Most tumour regressions have been partial in small numbers of patients.

The use of a large single dose of antibody and radio-iodine in conjunction with autologous marrow transplantation has recently been developed (105). In 10 patients with refractory non-Hodgkin's lymphomas, 7 follicular and 3 diffuse, complete response was observed in 9 patients. Myelosuppression was the only significant toxicity and two patients required autologous marrow rescue. However, only two patients remain in continous CR 11 + and 8 + months after therapy.

Interleukin-2

Trials of cytokines other than Interferon in lymphomas are just beginning. Anecdotal responses to high-dose IL-2 (109) or low-dose IL-2 (110) or IL-2 with LAK cells (111,112) have been described in low-grade or high-grade non-Hodgkin's lymphomas. In a recent ongoing phase II study in 14 pretreated patients only one complete remission was observed (Gisselbrecht et al.). The number of patients who at the present time have received such therapy is too small to allow valid conclusions to be drawn.

Fludarabine phosphate

Fludarabine is a fluorinated adenine nucleoside which is effective in chronic lymphocytic leukemia. Thirthy-four patients with follicular lymphoma have been included in a recent phase II trial (113) with Fludarabine which was given at a dose of 25 to 30 mg/m^2/day, IV, for 5 days every 3-4 weeks. 42% of the patients received $\geq$ 3 prior chemotherapy regimens. Response rate was 74% for the 27 patients with follicular small cleaved cell lymphoma; 10 complete remissions were observed; partial response was observed in all 7 patients with follicular mixed lymphoma. Fludarabine is an active drug in low-grade lymphoma and future investigations will assist in determining its optimal role.

References

1. CARDE P, BURGERS JMV, VAN GLABBEKE M et al.
   Combined radiotherapy-chemotherapy for early stages in non-Hodgkin's lymphoma: the EORTC controlled lymphoma trial.
   Radiotherapy and Oncology, 1984; 2: 301-312.
2. CHEN MG, PROSNITZ LR, GONZALES-SERVA A et al.
   Results of radiotherapy in control of stage I and II non-Hodgkin's lymphoma.
   Cancer, 1979; 43: 1245-1254.
3. GALLAGHER CJ, GREGORY WM, JONES AE et al.
   Follicular lymphoma: prognostic factors for response and survival.
   J Clin Oncol, 1986; 4: 1470-1480.
4. GOMEZ GA, BARLOS M, KRISHNAMSETTY RM et al.
   Treatment of early - stage I and II - nodular poorly differentiated lymphocytic lymphoma.
   Am J Clin Oncol, 1986; 9: 40.
5. GOSPODAROWICZ MG, BUSH RS, BROWN TC et al.
   Prognostic factors in nodular lymphomas: a multivariate analysis based on the Princess Margaret Hospital experience.
   Int J Radiat Oncol Biol Phys, 1984; 10: 489-497.
6. LAWRENCE TS, URBA WJ, STEINBERG SM, et al.
   Retrospective analysis of stage I and II indolent lymphomas at the National Cancer Institute.
   Int J Radiat Oncol Biol Phys, 1988; 14: 417-424.

7. MCLAUGHLIN P, FULLER LM, VELASQUEZ WS et al.
Stage I-II follicular lymphoma: treatment results of 76 patients.
Cancer, 1986; 58: 1596-1602.

8. MONFARDINI S, BANFI A, BONADONNA G et al.
Improved five-year survival after combined radiotherapy-chemotherapy for stage I and II non-Hodgkin's lymphoma.
Int J Radiat Oncol Biol Phys, 1980; 6: 125-134.

9. PARYANI SB, HOPPE RT, COX RS
Analysis of non-Hodgkin's lymphomas with nodular and favourable histologies, stages I and II.
Cancer, 1983; 52: 2300-2307.

10. REDDY S, SAXEMA VS, PELLETIERE EV, HENDRICKSON FR
Stage I and II non-Hodgkin's lymphomas: long term results of radiation therapy.
Int J Radiat Oncol Biol Phys, 1989; 16: 687-692.

11. STEIN RS, MAGEE MJ, LENOX RK et al.
Malignant lymphomas of follicular center cell origin in man. Large cleaved cell lymphoma.
Cancer, 1987; 60: 2704-2711.

12. SUTCLIFFE SB, GOSPODAROWICZ MK, BUSH RS et al.
Role of radiation therapy in localized non-Hodgkin's lymphoma.
Radiotherapy and Oncology, 1985; 4: 211-223.

13. LONGO DL, YOUNG RC, HUBBARD SM et al.
Prolonged initial remission in patients with nodular mixed lymphomas.
Ann Intern Med, 1984; 100: 651.

14. RUDDERS RA, KADDIS M, DE LELLIS RA et al.
Nodular non-Hodgkin's lymphoma. Factors influencing prognosis and indications for aggressive treatment.
Cancer, 1979; 43: 1643-1651.

15. SULLIVAN M, NETMAN PR, KADIN ME
Combined modality therapy of advanced non-Hodgkin's lymphoma: an analysis of remission duration and survival in 95 patients.
Blood, 1983; 62: 51-61.

16. LONGO DL
Lymphocytic lymphoma Cancer: Principles and Practice of Oncology.
De Vita VT, Hellman S, Rosenberg SA editors. J.B. Lippincott Company Philadelphia, Toronto, 1989.

17. ROSENBERG SA
The low grade non-Hodgkin's lymphomas: challenges and opportunities.
J Clin Oncol, 1985; 3: 299-310.

18. PORTLOCK CS
The role of treatment deferral in the management of patients with advanced indolent non-Hodgkin's lymphomas.
Semin Hematol, 1983; 20: 25-34.

19. GLATSTEIN E, FUKS Z, GOFFINET DR et al.
Non-Hodgkin's lymphoma of stage III extent. Is total lymphoid irradiation appropriate treatment?
Cancer, 1976; 37: 2806-2812.

20. COX JD, HOMAKI R, KUN LE et al.
Stage III nodular lymphoreticular tumours (non-Hodgkin's lymphoma): results of central lymphatic irradiation.
Cancer, 1981; 47: 2247-2251.

21. THAR TL, MILLIAN RR, NOYES WD et al.
Total body irradiation in non-Hodgkin's lymphoma.
Int J Radiat Oncol Biol Phys, 1979; 5: 171-176.

22. THAR TL, MILLIAN RR
Total body irradiation in non-Hodgkin's lymphoma.
Cancer, 1978; 42: 926-931.

23. CHOI NC, TIMOTHY AR, KAUFMAN SD et al.
Low dose fractionated whole body irradiation in the treatment of advanced non-Hodgkin's lymphoma.
Cancer, 1979; 43: 1636-1642.

24. CARABELL SC, CHAFFEY JT, ROSENTHAL DS et al.
Results of total body irradiation in the treatment of advanced non-Hodgkin's lymphomas.
Cancer, 1979; 43: 994-1000.

25. HOPPE RT, KUSHLAN P, KAPLAN HS et al.
The treatment of advanced stage favorable histology non-Hodgkin's lymphoma: a preliminary report of a randomized trial comparing single agent chemotherapy, combination chemotherapy and whole body irradiation.
Blood, 1981; 58: 592-598.

26. CHAFFEY JT, HELLMAN S, ROSENTHAL DS et al.
Total body irradiation in the treatment of lymphocytic lymphoma.
Cancer Treat Rep, 1977; 61: 1149.

27. PARYANI SB, HOPPE RT, COX RS et al.
The role of radiation therapy in the management of stage III follicular lymphomas.
J Clin Oncol, 1984; 2: 841-848.

28. JOHNSON RE, CANELLOS GP, YOUNG RC et al.
Chemotherapy (cyclophosphamide, vincristine and prednisone) vs radiotherapy (Total Body Irradiation) for stages III-IV poorly differentiated lymphocytic lymphoma.
Cancer Treat Rep, 1978; 62: 321-325.

29. MENDENHALL NP, NOIGES WD, MILLION RR
Total body irradiation for stage II-IV Non-Hodgkin's Lymphoma: Ten-year follow up.
J Clin Oncol, 1989; 7: 67-74.

30. GANEM G, LAMBIN P, SOCIE G et al.
    Low dose limited-field radiation therapy (2 x 2 Gy) in the management of low-grade non-Hodgkin's lymphomas.
    J Clin Oncol, (submitted for publication)

31. PORTLOCK CS, FISCHER D, CADMAN E et al.
    High-pulse chlorambucil in advanced, low-grade non-Hodgkin's lymphomas.
    Cancer Treat Rep, 1987; 71: 1029-1031.

32. CAVALLIN-STAHL E, MOLLER TR with the Swedish lymphoma group.
    Prednimustines, Cyclophosphamide-Vincristine-Prednisolone in the treatment of non-Hodgkin's lymphoma with favorable histopathology: results of a national cancer care program in Sweden.
    Seminars in Oncology, 1986; 13: 19-22.

33. KENNEDY B, BLOOMFIELD CD, KIANG DT et al.
    Combination versus successive single agent chemotherapy in lymphocytic lymphoma.
    Cancer, 1978; 41: 23-28.

34. LISTER TA, CULLEN MH, BEARD MEJ et al.
    Comparison of combined and single agent chemotherapy in non-Hodgkin's lymphoma of favorable histological type.
    Br Med J, 1978; 4: 523-537.

35. KALTER S, HOLMES L, CABANILLAS F
    Long-term results of treatment of patients with follicular lymphomas.
    Hematol Oncol, 1987; 5: 127-138.

36. PORTLOCK CS, ROSENBERG SA, GLATSTEIN E et al.
    Treatment of advanced non-Hodgkin's lymphomas with favorable histologies: preliminary results of a prospective trial.
    Blood, 1976; 47: 747-756.

37. BAGLEY CM, DE VITA VT, BERARD CW, CANELLOS GP
    Advanced lymphosarcoma: intensive cyclical combination chemotherapy with cyclophosphamide, vincristine and prednisone.
    Ann Intern Med, 1972; 76: 227-234.

38. YOUNG RC, LONGO DL, GLATSTEIN E et al.
    The treatment of indolent lymphomas: watchful waiting; an aggressive combined modality treatment.
    Semin Hematol, 1988; 25, Suppl. 2: 11-16.

39. PARLIER Y, GORIN NC, NAJMAN A et al.
    Combination chemotherapy with cyclophosphamide, vincristine, prednisone and the contribution of adriamycine in the treatment of adult non-Hodgkin's lymphomas. A report of 131 cases.
    Cancer, 1982; 50: 401-409.

40. ANDERSON T, DE VITA VT, SIMON RM et al.
    Malignant lymphoma II. Prognostic factors and response to treatment of 473 patients at the National Cancer Institute.
    Cancer, 1982; 50: 2708-2721.

41. JONES SE, FUKS Z, BULL M et al.
    Non-Hodgkin's lymphoma IV. Clinicopathologic correlation in 405 cases.
    Cancer, 1973; 31: 806-823.

42. STEWARD WP, CROWTHER D, McWILLIAM LJ et al.
    Maintenance Chlorambucil after CVP in the management of advanced stage, low-grade histologic type non-Hodgkin's lymphoma.
    Cancer, 1986; 61: 441-447.

43. EZDINLI EZ, ANDERSON JR, MELVIN F et al.
    Moderate versus aggressive chemotherapy of nodular lymphocytic poorly differentiated lymphoma.
    J Clin Oncol, 1985; 3: 769-75.

44. ANDERSON T, BENDER RA, FISHER RI et al.
    Combination chemotherapy in non-Hodgkin's lymphoma: results of long-term follow-up.
    Cancer Treat Rep, 1977; 61: 1057-1066.

45. BITRAN JC, GOLOMB HM, ULTMANN JE et al.
    Non-Hodgkin's lymphoma, poorly differentiated and mixed-cell types: results of sequential staging procedures, response to therapy and survey of 100 patients.
    Cancer, 1978; 42: 88-95.

46. GLICK JH, BARNES JM, EZDINLI EZ et al.
    Nodular mixed lymphoma: results of a randomized trial failing to confirm prolonged disease-free survival with COPP chemotherapy.
    Blood, 1981; 58: 920-925.

47. OKEN MM, COSTELLO WG, JOHNSON GJ et al.
    The influence of histologic subtype on toxicity and response to chemotherapy in non-Hodgkin's lymphoma.
    Cancer, 1983; 51: 1581-1586.

48. LEPAGE E, SEBBAN D, GISSELBRECHT C et al.
    Treatment of low grade non-Hodgkin's lymphomas: assessment of Doxorubicin in a controlled trial.
    Hematol Oncology, 1990; 8: 31-39.

49. RODRIGUEZ V, CABANILLAS F, BURGESS MA et al.
    Combination chemotherapy ("CHOP-Bleo") in advanced non-Hodgkin's lymphoma.
    Blood, 1977; 49: 325-333.

50. Mc KELVEY EM, GOTTLIEB JA, WILSON HE et al.
    Hydroxydaunomycin (Adriamycin) combination chemotherapy in malignant lymphoma.
    Cancer, 1976; 38: 1434.

51. JONES SE, GROZEA PN, METZ EN et al.
    Superiority of adriamycin-containing combination chemotherapy in the treatment of diffuse lymphoma. A Southwest Oncology Group Study.
    Cancer, 1979; 43: 417-425.

52. PETERSON BA, ANDERSON JR, FRIZZERA G et al.

Nodular mixed lymphoma: a comparative trial of cyclophosphamide and cyclophosphamide, adriamycin, vincristine, prednisone and bleomycin.

Blood, 1985; 66: 216a, abstr. 749.

53. ANDERSON KC, SKARIN AT, ROSENTHAL DS et al.

Combination chemotherapy for advanced non-Hodgkin's lymphomas other than diffuse histiocytic or undifferentiated histologies.

Cancer Treat Rep, 1984; 68: 1343-1350.

54. FAYOLLE M, COSSET JM

Le traitement des lymphomes non hodgkiniens de l'adulte stade III et IV d'histologie favorable: abstention ou aggressivité thérapeutique.

Bull Cancer, 1983; 70: 381-388.

55. JONES SE, GROZEA PN, MILLER TP et al.

Chemotherapy with cyclophosphamide, doxorubicin, vincristine and prednisone alone or with levamisole or with levamisole + BCG for malignant lymphoma: a Southwest Oncology Group Study.

J Clin Oncol, 1985; 3: 1318-1324.

56. McLAUGHLIN P, FULLER LM, VELASQUEZ WS et al.

Stage III follicular lymphoma: durable remissions with combined chemotherapy-radiotherapy regimen.

J Clin Oncol, 1987; 5: 867-874.

57. HANCOCK SL, YOUNG R, LONGO DL et al.

Advanced indolent lymphoma: update of a randomized comparison of chemotherapy and radiotherapy.

PROC ASCO, 1985; 4: Abstr 792.

58. BRERETON HD, YOUNG RC, LONGO DL et al.

A comparison between combination chemotherapy and total body irradiation + combination chemotherapy in non-Hodgkin's lymphoma.

Cancer, 1979; 43: 2227-2231.

59. PORTLOCK CS, ROSENBERG SA

No initial therapy for stage III and IV non-Hodgkin's lymphomas of favorable histologic types.

Ann Intern Med, 1979; 90: 10-13.

60. HORNING SJ, ROSENBERG SA

The natural history of initially untreated low-grade non-Hodgkin's lymphomas.

N Engl J Med, 1984; 311: 1471-1475.

61. KRIKORIAN JG, PORTLOCK CS, COONEY P, ROSENBERG SA

Spontaneous regression of non-Hodgkin's lymphomas: a report of nine cases.

Cancer, 1980; 46: 2093-2099.

62. STRAUS DJ, GAYNOR JJ, LEIBERMAN PH et al.

Non-Hodgkin's lymphomas: characteristics of long-term survivors following conservative treatment.

Am J Me, 1986; 82: 247.

63. HUBBARD JR, CHABNER BA, DE VITA VT et al.

Histologic progression in non-Hodgkin's lymphoma.

Blood, 1982; 59: 258-264.

64. QAZI R, AISENBERG AC, LONG CJ, et al.

The natural history of nodular lymphoma.

Cancer, 1976; 37: 1923.

65. CABANILLAS F, SMITH T, BODEY CP et al.

Nodular malignant lymphomas: factors affecting complete response and survival.

Cancer, 1979; 44: 1983-1989.

66. EZDINLI EZ, HARRINGTON DP, KUCUK O, et al.

The effect of intensive intermittent maintenance therapy in advanced low-grade non-Hodgkin's lymphoma.

Cancer, 1987; 60: 156-160.

67. LEONARD RCF, CUZICK J, McLENNAN ICF et al.

Prognostic factors in non-Hodgkin's lymphoma: the importance of symptomatic stage as an adjunct to the Kiel histopathological classification.

Br J Cancer, 1983; 47: 91-102

68. ROMAGUERA JE, McLAUGHLIN P, NORTHL et al.

Multivariate analysis of prognostic factors in stage IV follicular low-grade lymphomas: a risk model.

J Clin Oncol, 1991; 9: 762-769.

69. BASTION Y, BERGER F, BRYON PA, FELMAN P, FFRENCH M, COIFFIER B

Follicular lymphomas: assessment of prognostic factors in 127 patients followed for 10 years.

Ann Oncol, 1991; 2 (supp.2): 123-129.

70. WARNKE RA, KIM H, FUKS Z, DORFMAN RF

The coexistence of nodular and diffuse patterns in nodular non-Hodgkin's lymphomas: significance and clinicopathologic correlation.

Cancer, 1977; 40: 1229-1233.

71. EZDINLI EZ, COSTELLO WG, FIKRI I, et al.

Nodular mixed lymphocytic-histiocytic lymphoma. Response and survival.

Cancer, 1980; 45: 261-267.

72. EZDINLI EZ, COSTELLO WG, KUCUK O, et al.

Effect of the degree of nodularity on the survival of patients with nodular lymphomas.

J Clin Oncol, 1987; 5: 413-418.

73. FISHER RI, JONES RB, DE VITA VT et al.

Natural history of malignant lymphomas with divergent histologies at staging evaluation.

Cancer, 1981; 47: 2022-2025.

74. OVIATT DL, COUSAR JG, COLLINS RD et al.

Malignant lymphomas of follicular center-cell origin in human V. Incidence, clinical features and prognostic implications of transformation of small cleaved-cell nodular lymphoma.

Cancer, 1984; 53: 1109-1114.

75. ACKER B, HOPPE RT, COLBY TV et al.
Histological conversion in the non-Hodgkin's lymphomas.
J Clin Oncol, 1983; 1: 11-16.

76. YUNIS JJ, OKEN MM, KAPLAN ME et al.
Distinctive chromosomal abnormalities in histologic subtypes of non-Hodgkin's lymphoma.
N Engl J Med, 1982; 307: 1231-1236.

77. FREEDMAN AS, RITZ J, NEUBERG D et al.
Autologous bone-marrow transplantation in 69 patients with a history of low-grade B-cell non-Hodgkin's lymphoma.
Bllod, 1991; 77: 2524-2529.

78. DIGGS CH, WIERNIK PM, OSTROW SS et al.
Nodular lymphoma. Prolongation of survival by complete remission.
Cancer Clin Trials, 1981; 4: 107-114.

79. DUMONT J, ASSELAIN B, WEIL M, et al.
Evolution lointaine des lymphomes nodulaires. Devenir de 85 malades traités entre 1968 et 1975.
Nouv Presse Med, 1981; 10: 2261-2265.

80. HOERNI B, BONICHON F, COINDRE JM et al.
Pronostic des lymphomes folliculaires dans une série de 180 cas.
Bull Cancer, 1986; 73: 171-177.

81. CONSTANTINIDES IP, PATHOULI C, KARVOUNTSIS G et al.
Serum B2 microglobulin in malignant lymphoproliferative disorders.
Cancer, 1985; 55: 2384-2389.

82. BENNETT JM, CAIN KC, GLICK JH et al.
The significance of bone marrow involvement in non-Hodgkin's lymphoma: the Eastern Cooperative Oncology Group experience.
J Clin Oncol, 1986; 4: 1462-1469.

83. HU E, THOMPSON J, HORNING S et al.
Detection of B-cell lymphoma in peripheral blood by DNA hybridisation.
Lancet, 1985: 1092.

84. SMITH BR, WEINBERG DS, ROBERT NJ et al.
Circulating monoclonal B lymphocytes in non Hodgkin's lymphoma.
N Engl J Med, 1984; 311: 1476-1481.

85. SIEGERT W, THEML H, FINK U et al.
Treatment of non-Hodgkin's lymphoma of low-grade malignancy with human fibroblast interferon.
Anticancer Res, 1982; 2: 193-198.

86. DENARDO S, DENARDO G, O'GRADY L et al.
Pilot studies of radio-immunotherapy of B-cell lymphoma and leukemia using I - 131 Lym - 1 monoclonal antibody.
Antibod Immunoconjugates, Radiopharmaceu, 1988; 1: 17-33.

87. LOUIE AC, GALLAGHER JG, SIKORA K et al.
Follow-up observations on the effect of human leucocyte interferon in non-Hodgkin's lymphoma.
Blood, 1981; 58: 712-718.

88. GUTTERMAN JU, BLUMENSCHEIN GR, ALEXANIAN R et al.
Leucocyte interferon-induced tumor regression in human metastatic breast cancer, multiple myeloma and malignant lymphoma.
Ann Intern Med, 1980; 93: 399-406.

89. HORNING S, MERIGAN TC, KROWN SE et al.
Human interferon alpha in malignant lymphoma and Hodgkin's disease. Results of the American Cancer Society Trial.
Cancer, 1985; 56: 1305-1310.

90. LEAVITT RD, RATANATHARATHORN V, OZER H et al.
Alfa 2 b interferon in the treatment of Hodgkin's disease and non-Hodgkin's lymphoma.
Seminars in Oncology, 1987; 14: 18-23.

91. WAGSTAFF J, LOYNDS P, CROWTHER D
A phase II study of human rDNA alpha 2 - interferon in patients with low-grade non-Hodgkin's lymphoma.
Cancer Chemother Pharmacol, 1986; 18: 54-58.

92. FOON KA, SHERWIN SA, ABRAMS PG et al.
Treatment of advanced non-Hodgkin's lymphoma with recombinant leucocyte-A interferon.
N Engl J Med, 1984; 311: 1148-1152.

93. O CONNELL MJ, COLGAN JP, OKEN MM et al.
Clinical trial of recombinant leukocyte A interferon as initial therapy for favorable histology non-Hodgkin's lymphomas and chronic lymphocytic leukemia.
J Clin Oncol, 1986; 4: 128-136.

94. CHIESI T, CAPNIST G, VESPIGNANI M, DINI E
The role of interferon alpha-2b and chlorambucil in the treatment of non-Hodgkin's lymphoma.
Cancer Treat Rev, 1988; 15: 27-34.

95. ROHATINER AZS, RICHARDS MA, BARNETT MJ et al.
Chlorambucil and interferon for low-grade non-Hodgkin's lymphoma.
Br J Cancer, 1987; 55: 225-226.

96. OZER H, ANDERSON JR, PETERSON BA et al.
Combination trial of subcutaneous alpha-2 interferon and oral cyclophosphamide in favorable histology non-Hodgkin's lymphoma.
Investigational New Drugs. Martinus Nijhoff Publishers, Boston 1987; 27-33.

97. WALDER S, SCHWARTZ R.

    Antineoplastic activity of interferon and cytotoxic agents against experimental and human malignancies.

    A Review Cancer Res, 1990; 530: 3473-3486.

98. Mac LAUGHLIN P, CABANILLAS F, HAGEMEISTER F, et al.

    Alpha -interferon prolongs remission in stage IV lowgrade lymphoma.

    Ann.Oncol. (In press).

99. WAGENBEEK A, CARDE P, SOMMERS R, et al.

    Maintenance of remission with human recombinant alpha-2 interferon (Roferon A) in patients with stages III and IV low-grade malignant non-Hodgkin's lymphoma. Results from a prospective, randomised phase III clinical trial in 331 patients.

    Blood 1992, 80 (suppl. 1), 288 A.

100. SMALLEY RV, ANDERSEN JW, HAWKINS MJ, O'CONNELL MJ, OKEN MM, BORDEN EC.

    Interferon alfa combined with cytotoxic chemotherapy for patients with non-Hodgkin's lymphoma.

    N. Engl. J. Med. 1992 ; 327 : 1336-1341.

101. SOLAL-CELIGNY P, LEPAGE E, BROUSSE N. et al.

    Recombinant interferon-alfa 2b associated with a doxorubicin-containing regimen in advanced follicular lymphoma patients. Results of a randomized trial.

    Submitted for publication.

102. PRICE CGA, ROHATINER AZS, STEWARD W et al.

    Interferon a2b in the treatment of follicular lymphomas: preliminary results of a trial in progress.

    Ann Oncol, 1991; 2 (supp.2): 141-145.

103. NADLER LM, STASHENKO P, HARDY R et al.

    Serotherapy of a patient with a monoclonal antibody directed against a human lymphoma-associated antigen.

    Cancer Res, 1980; 40: 314-317.

104. MILLER RA, MALONEY DG, WARNKE R et al.

    Treatment of B-cell lymphoma with monoclonal anti-idiotype antibody.

    N Engl J Med, 1982; 306: 517-522.

105. LENHARD R, ORDER S, SPUNBERG J et al.

    Isotopic immunoglobulin: a new systemic therapy for advanced Hodgkin's disease.

    J Clin Oncol, 1985; 3: 1296-1300.

106. PRESS OW, EARY JF, BADGER CC et al.

    Treatment of refractory non-Hodgkin's lymphoma with radiolabelled MB-1 (anti-CD 37) antibody .

    J Clin Oncol, 1989; 7: 1027-1038.

107. RANKIN EM, HEKMAN A, SOMERS R et al.

    Treatment of two patients with B-cell lymphoma with monoclonal anti-idiotype antibodies.

    Blood, 1985; 65: 1373.

108. HAMBLIN TJ, CATTAN AR, GLENNIE MN et al.

    Initial experience in treating human lymphoma with a chimeric univalent derivative of monoclonal anti-idiotype antibody.

    Blood, 1987; 69: 790.

109. LOTZE MT, CHANG AE, SEIPP CA et al.

    High-dose recombinant Interleukin 2 in the treatment of patients with disseminated cancer: Responses, treatment-related morbidity and histologic findings.

    JAMA, 1986; 256: 3117-3124.

110. ALLISON MA, JONES SE, Mc GUFFEY P

    Phase II trial of out-patient Interleukin 2 in malignant lymphoma, chronic lymphocytic leukemia, and selected solid tumors.

    J Clin Oncol, 1989; 7: 75-80.

111. PACIUCCI PA, HOLLAND JF, GLIDEWELL O, ODCHIMAR R

    Recombinant Interleukin-2 by continous infusion and adoptive transfer of recombinant Interleukin-2. Activated cells in patients with advanced cancer.

    J Clin Oncol, 1989; 7: 869-878.

112. ROSENBERG SA, LOTZE MT, MUUL LM, et al.

    A progress report on the treatment of 157 patients with advanced cancer using lymphokine-activated killer cells and Interleukin-2 or high-dose Interleukin-2 alone.

    N Engl J Med, 1987; 316: 889-897.

113. REDMAN J, CABANILLAS F, McLAUGHLIN P, HOLMES L, HAGEMEISTER F, VELASQUEZ W, SWAN F, RODRIGUEZ M, KEATING M

    Fludarabine Phosphate (FAMP) treatment of low-grade lymphoma (LGL).

    Proc Am Soc Clin Onc, 1991; 283: 989.

The role of radiation therapy in the management of aggressive non-Hodgkin's lymphomas

G. GANEM

Combination chemotherapy has nowadays become the primary treatment of aggressive NHL and the place of radiation therapy (RT) - if any - in an optimal therapeutic strategy remains to be determined.

Management of localized disease

Radiation therapy alone

Historically, RT was recommended as the exclusive modality of treatment. Immediate local control was achieved in 90-95% of patients. Relapses occurred in 0 to 60% of stage I patients and in 35 to 90% of stage II patients *(Table I)* (1-13). Best results were reported in patients who had been pathologically staged and who had good prognostic features. Patients with pathological stage I and small-bulk tumour treated with radiation therapy alone have a 10-year disease-free survival rate (DFS) of around 90% (9,10,13). However, in the vast majority of clinically staged patients, a laparotomy is not justified simply to decide whether they are treatable with RT alone. Although the majority of the RT series are retrospective and not stratified for tumour bulk or other recently recognized prognostic features (11,14), and frequently include nodal and extranodal NHL, several remarks can be made.

Dose-control relationship (1,8,15)

A minimum tumour dose of 35 to 40 Gy must be delivered to achieve optimal local control. Higher doses may not increase local control but may increase the side-effects of RT. Thus, a tumour dose of 35 to 45 Gy delivered over 4 to 5 weeks with 4 to 5 fractions of 1.8 to 2 Gy per week is recommended. Adherence to a low dose per fraction appears essential to decrease the risks of late RT side-effects (16,17). Hypo-fractionated schemes may be used for emergencies and in patients with poor performance status.

Volumes

The Stanford Group (11) has reported a 67% 5-year disease-free survival rate in patients treated with "extensive" RT (i.e., subtotal or total lymphoid irradiation) compared with 25% for those receiving "limited" irradiation (i.e., treatment limited to one side of the diaphragm: involved-field or extended-field irradiation). However, for patients having 3 or more involvement sites or bulky disease, the most extensive irradiation achieved 55% five-year freedom-from-relapse, comparable to that observed with limited irradiation followed by a first-generation chemotherapy protocol in the same institution. The results are poorer in diffuse large-cell NHL than those with a nodular

TABLE I

Results of radiation therapy alone in localized aggressive NHL

Series (Ref.)	Staging[1]	Stage	N	Fields[2]	5 years	
					DFS	% survival
Jones[3] (1973) (1)	CS	I II	25 64	IF, EF, TLI	56 25	67 31
Tubiana[3] (1974) (2)	CS	I,II	69	IF	-	38
Peckman (1975) (3)	CS	I II	69 38		61 42	69 53
Hellman (1977) (4)	CS	I		IF	40	60
Chen[3] (1979) (5)	CS	I,II	58	IF, EF	37	59
Swett[3] (1979) (6)	PS	I II	58 14	IF, EF, TLI	100 43	
Hoppe[3] (1985) (7)	PS	I II	18 14	IF, EF	73 43	
Sutcliffe[4] (1985) (8)	CS	I-II Low-risk Intermediate-risk High-risk	 78 204 50	IF	 87 55 10	
Levitt (1985) (9)	PS	I-II	19	EF, TLI	75	83
Vokes[3] (1985) (10)	PS	I II	17 14	EF, TLI	94 56	94 62
Kaminski[3] (1986) (11)	CS, PS	I II			62 38	56 48
Reddy[4] (1989) (12)	CS, PS	I II	22	IF, EF	66 30	66 30
Hallahan[4] (1989) (13)	PS	I II	22 14	IF, EF, TLI	91 35	

1 Staging: PS pathological staging; CS clinical staging
2 Fields: IF - involved fields; EF = extended fields; TLI = total or subtotal lymphoid irradiation
3 Including extranodal NHL
4 Results with 10-year follow-up

component. Previous studies from Stanford and other series have not shown the superiority of extended-field over limited-field treatment, even for good-risk patients (*Table I*) and no prospective and randomized study has so far been reported. Moreover, the majority of relapses occurred in extranodal areas. Thus, extensive RT (i.e., subtotal or total lymphoid irradiation) is no longer recommended by most of the authors. For head-and-neck NHL, the irradiated volumes usually include Waldeyer's ring and cervical lymph nodes (18). Total abdominal irradiation has been used frequently for gastrointestinal NHL.

Patterns of relapse (9,12,13,19,20)

Approximately 70% of the relapses occurred in the 2 years following treatment. Infield recurrences occurred in less than 10% of patients with tumours of small bulk (maximal diameter < 5 cm) but increased to 60% in patients with large tumours. Overall, local control of RT-treated diffuse "histiocytic" localized NHL was achieved in 85% of patients. Most relapses (40 to 90%) occurred outside irradiated volumes, mostly in extranodal sites. Nodal recurrence in contiguous areas alone after involved-field irradiation was observed in less than 5% of patients.

In conclusion, patients with stage I disease only, particularly those under 65 years, without unfavourable prognostic factors can, if carefully staged, be treated with radiation therapy alone.

Radiation therapy combined with chemotherapy

At least two randomized studies have shown that chemotherapy following RT gives better disease-free survival and survival than RT alone (21,22).

Currently, when combined modality is used, RT always follows combination chemotherapy or is alternated with chemotherapy (23,24).

In this setting, the role of RT can be considered in two situations: (i) for the management of good-risk patients, does RT need to be included in the treatment programme? and (ii) for the management of bad-risk localized NHL (included in "advanced" NHL), is RT useful for patients with bulky masses or with "persistent" masses after induction chemotherapy?

To our knowledge, no randomized study allows any precise answer these questions.

In the former situation, short-term chemotherapy followed by involved-field chemotherapy is a highly successful treatment, resulting in a 5-year disease-free survival rate of 80 to 96% (25-28), without severe long-term side-effects.

Conversely, retrospective analysis, with chemotherapy-based treatment, has shown that "adjuvant" irradiation slightly improves 5-year disease-free survival and overall survival compared with the same chemotherapy administered over a generally longer period (i.e., 6 to 11 cycles) without RT. However, in all these studies the difference was not statistically significant (25,29,30), and interpretation of the data needs to take into account the selection of patients and the choice of treatment strategy (31).

There is no study of dose-control relationship of RT delivered after induction chemotherapy; lowering the total dose of RT in complete responders to chemotherapy has been used by the ECOG (32) in patients with clinical stages II and II_E; radiation therapy delivered at 25 to 30 Gy to involved fields after 8 cycles of a first-generation chemotherapy regimen. The 4-year disease-free survival rate for complete responders was 86%; two of five failures occurred within abdominal irradiated fields. The ECOG is currently studying prospectively the need for RT in selected patients with localized NHL.

A randomized study has recently been published in 129 eligible good-risk localized childhood NHL (33), comparing first- generation chemotherapy treatment regimens (total length: 33 weeks) with or without involved-field RT (27 Gy with conventional fractionation). The complete remission rate was 100% with a projected disease-free survival rate at 4 years in both arms of approximately 87%. The number of relapses in each group was too small for statistical comparisons (3 local relapses in the chemotherapy arm versus 1 in the combined arm).

Management of advanced disease

The potential role of RT in bad-risk localized NHL and in disseminated NHL (Stages III and IV) has not yet been defined. In these advanced cases, if RT is indicated, it should probably be limited to initially bulky areas and/or for patients not responding rapidly to chemotherapy.

In an earlier analysis of aggressive localized NHL treated with first generation adriamycin-containing regimens (29,34), the majority of first failures were observed in sites of prior disease (around 70%), raising the question whether adjuvant RT could increase long-term tumour control.

A retrospective series of 183 patients with stages III and IV NHL (35) treated with adjuvant "iceberg" irradiation for patients in whom the initial diameter of the tumour exceded 5 cm or when a complete remission was not achieved prior to the fourth course of chemotherapy showed that the benefit of irradiation was minimal and restricted to stage III patients.

More recent series using intensive chemotherapy regimens (36-39) in advanced aggressive NHL have suggested that "touch up" RT after completion of the chemotherapy program is not necessary because it does not affect the patterns of relapse. However, the lack of apparent benefit from RT in these series does not exclude its potential role, albeit minimal. Optimal scheduling of RT and chemotherapy probably needs an earlier introduction of RT into the treatment programme, especially for patients who do not rapidly respond to chemotherapy (40). Irradiation could be delivered either a using classical scheme or a modified one: an accelerated hyperfractionated regimen and/or concomitant with the administration of chemotherapy (with reduction of the total dose of RT) may be proposed to "selected" patients, in the hope of overcoming the development of tumour resistance (41-43).

References

1. JONES SE, FUKS Z, KAPLAN HS et al.
   Non-Hodgkin's lymphomas. V. Results of radiotherapy.
   Cancer, 1973; 32: 682-691.

2. TUBIANA M, POUILLART P, HAYAT M et coll.
   Résultats de la radiothérapie dans les stades I et II des lymphosarcomes et réticulosarcomes.
   Bull Cancer (Paris), 1974; 61: 93-110.

3. PECKAM MJ, GUAY JP, HAMLIN IME et al.
   Survival in localized nodal and extranodal non-Hodgkin's lymphomata.
   Br J Cancer, 1975; 31 (suppl II): 413-424.

4. HELLMAN S, CHAFFEY JT, ROSENTHAL DS et al.
   The place of radiation therapy in the treatment of non-Hodgkin's lymphomas.
   Cancer, 1977; 39: 843-851.

5. CHEN MG, PROSNITZ LR, GONZALES-SERVA A et al.
   Results of radiotherapy in control of stage I and II non-Hodgkin's lymphoma.
   Cancer, 1979; 43: 1245-1254.

6. SWEET DL, KINZIE J, GACKE MI et al.
   Survival of patients with localized diffuse histiocytic lymphoma.
   Blood, 1980; 58: 1218-1223.

7. HOPPE RT
   The role of radiation therapy in the management of the non-Hodgkin's lymphomas.
   Cancer, 1985; 55: 2176-2183.

8. SUTCLIFFE SB, GOSPODAROWICZ MK, BUSH RS et al.
   Role of radiation therapy in localized non-Hodgkin's lymphoma.
   Radiother Oncol, 1985; 4: 211-223.

9. LEVITT SH, LEE CKK, BLOOMFIELD CD et al.
   The role of radiation therapy in the treatment of early stage large-cell lymphoma.
   Hematol Oncol, 1985; 3: 33-37.

10. VOKES EE, ULTMANN JE, GOLOMB HM et al.
    Long-term survival of patients with localized diffuse histiocytic lymphoma.
    J Clin Oncol, 1985; 3: 1309-1317.

11. KAMINSKI MS, COLEMAN CN, COLBY TB et al.
    Factors predicting survival in adults with stage I and II large-cell lymphoma treated with primary radiation therapy.
    Ann Intern Med, 1986; 104: 747-756.

12. REDDY S, SAXENA VS, PELLETIERE EV et al.
    Stage I and II non-Hodgkin's lymphomas: long-term results of radiation therapy.
    Int J Radiation Oncology Biol Phys, 1989; 16: 687-692.

13. HALLAHAN DE, FARAH R, VOKES EE et al.
    The pattern of failure in patients with pathological stage I and II diffuse histiocytic lymphoma treated with radiation therapy alone.
    Int J Radiation Oncology Biol Phys, 1989; 17: 767-771.

14. SWAN F, VELASQUEZ WS, TUCKER S et al.

A new serologic staging system for large-cell lymphomas based on initial ß2-microglobulin and lactate dehydrogenase levels.

J Clin Oncol, 1989; 7: 1518-1527.

15. MUSHOFF K, LEOPOLD H

On the question of the tumoricidal dose in non-Hodgkin's lymphomas.

Rec Results Cancer Res, 1978: 203-206.

16. FOWLER JF

Principles of fractionation in radiotherapy?

In: Radiobiology in radiotherapy. Bleehen N.M. (Ed) New York, Springer, 1988: pp. 53-58.

17. COX JD

Presidential address: Fractionation: A paradigm for clinical research in radiation oncology.

Int J Radiation Oncology Biol Phys, 1987; 13: 1271-1281.

18. GLASTEIN E, WASSERMAN TH

Non-Hodgkin's lymphomas.

In Principles and Practice of radiation oncology. CA PEREZ and LW BRADY. Lippincott Ed, 1987: pp. 1073-1085.

19. HORWICH A, PECKHAM M

"Bad risk" non-Hodgkin's lymphomas.

Semin Hematol, 1983; 20: 35-56.

20. BUSH RS, GOSPODAROWICZ M, STURGEON J et al.

Radiation therapy of localized non-Hodgkin's lymphoma.

Cancer Treat Rep, 1977; 61: 1129-1136.

21. NISSEN NI, ERSBOLL J, HANSEN HS et al.

A randomized study of radiotherapy versus radiotherapy plus chemotherapy in stage I-II non-Hodgkin's lymphomas.

Cancer, 1983; 52: 1-7.

22. BONADONNA G, LATTUADA A, MONFARDINI S et al.

Combined radiotherapy-chemotherapy in localized non-Hodgkin's lymphomas: 5-year results of a randomized study.

In: Adjuvant therapy of Cancer II. JONES SE, SALMON SE, Eds New-York: Grune & Stratton, 1979: pp. 145-136.

23. COSSET JM, HENRY-AMAR M, VUONG T et al.

Alternating chemotherapy and radiotherapy combination for bulky stage I and II intermediate and high grade non-Hodgkin's lymphoma: an update.

Radiother Oncol, 1991; 20: 30-37.

24. BAJETTA E, VALAGUSSA P, BONADONNA G et al.

Combined modality treatment for stage I-II non-Hodgkin's lymphomas: CVP versus BACOP chemotherapy.

Int J Radiation Oncology Biol Phys, 1988; 15: 3-12.

25. MAUCH P, LEONARD R, SKARIN A et al.

Improved survival following combined radiation therapy and chemotherapy for unfavorable prognosis stage I-II non-Hodgkin's lymphomas.

J Clin Oncol, 1985; 3: 1301-1308.

26. CONNORS JM, KLIMO P, FAIREY RN et al.

Brief chemotherapy and involved-field radiation therapy for limited-stage, histologically aggressive lymphoma.

Ann Intern Med, 1987; 107: 25-30.

27. PRESTIDGE BR, HORNING SJ, HOPPE RT

Combined modality therapy for stage I-II large-cell lymphoma.

Int J Radiation Oncology Biol Phys, 1988; 15: 633-639.

28. LONGO DL, GLASTEIN E, DUFFEY PL et al.

Treatment of localized aggressive lymphomas with combination chemotherapy followed by involved-field radiation therapy.

J Clin Oncol, 1989; 7: 1295-1302.

29. MILLER TP, JONES SE

Initial chemotherapy for clinically localized lymphomas of unfavorable histology.

Blood, 1983; 62: 413-418.

30. JONES SE, MILLER TP, CONNORS JM

Long-term follow-up analysis for prognostic factors for patients with limited-stage diffuse large-cell lymphoma treated with initial chemotherapy with or without adjuvant radiotherapy.

J Clin Oncol, 1989; 7: 1186-1191.

31. LONGO DL

Combined modality therapy for localized aggressive lymphoma; enough or too much?

J Clin Oncol, 1989; 7: 1179-1181.

32. O'CONNEL MJ, HARRINGTON DP, EARLE JD et al.

Chemotherapy followed by consolidation radiation therapy for the treatment of clinical stage II aggressive histologic type non-Hodgkin's lymphoma.

Cancer, 1988; 61: 1754-1758.

33. LINK MP, DONALDSON SS, BERARD CW et al

Results of treatment of childhood localized non-Hodgkin's lymphoma with combination chemotherapy with or without radiotherapy.

N Engl J Med, 1990; 322: 1169-1174.

34. CABANILLAS F

Chemotherapy as definitive treatment of stage I-II large-cell and diffuse mixed lymphomas.

Hematol Oncol, 1985; 3: 25-31.

35. FRIEDMAN S, BURGERS M, CARDE P et al.

    Iceberg irradiation in advanced non-Hodgkin's lymphoma.

    Europ Soc Therapeutic Radiation Oncology, 5th meeting, Baden-Baden, 1986: abst 252.

36. SHIPP MA, HARRINGTON DP, KLATT MM et al.

    Identification of major prognostic subgroups of patients with large-cell lymphoma treated with m-BACOD or M-BACOD.

    Ann Int Med, 1986; 104: 757-765.

37. SHIPP MA, KLATT MM, YEAP B et al.

    Patterns of relapse in large-cell lymphoma patients with bulk-disease: implications for the use of adjuvant radiation therapy.

    J Clin Oncol, 1989; 7: 613-618.

38. COIFFIER B, GISSELBRECHT C, HERBRECHT R et al.

    LNH-84 Regimen : a multicenter study of intensive chemotherapy in 737 patients with aggressive malignant lymphoma.

    J Clin Oncol, 1989; 7: 1018-1026.

39. SURBONE A, LONGO DL, DE VITA VT et al.

    Residual abdominal masses in aggressive non-Hodgkin's lymphoma after combination chemotherapy : significance and management.

    J Clin Oncol, 1988; 6: 1832-1837.

40. ARMITAGE JO, WEISENBURGER DD, HUTCHINS M et al.

    Chemotherapy for diffuse large-cell lymphoma. Rapidly responding patients have more durable remissions.

    J Clin Oncol, 1986; 4: 160-164.

41. LOONEY WB, HOPKINS HA

    Rationale for different chemotherapeutic and radiation-therapy strategies in cancer management.

    Cancer, 1991; 67: 1471-1483.

42. TANNOCK IF

    Combined modality treatment with radiotherapy and chemotherapy.

    Radiother Oncol, 1989; 16: 83-101.

43. GOFFMAN TE, RAUBITSCHEK A, MITCHELL JB et al.

    The emerging biology of modern radiation oncology.

    Cancer Res, 1990; 50: 7735-7744.

Treatment of aggressive lymphomas (intermediate and high grade)

B. COIFFIER

Over the past 10 years durable remissions have been achieved in an increasing proportion of patients with aggressive malignant lymphomas and there is evidence that remission rates and survival rates may be improved by using intensive chemotherapy regimens (1-6). These more aggressive approaches to the treatment of malignant lymphomas are associated with increased toxicity (7). Thus, an accurate pretreatment prognostic assessment of patients is required to guide physicians in selecting the most appropriate therapeutic regimen. Currently, therapeutic policy is determined by histological subtype (8-10) and extent of disease as defined by the Ann Arbor staging system (11). This staging system was originally described for Hodgkin's disease and, although applied worldwide to malignant lymphoma, it is not always suited to NHL, 40% of which are of extranodal origin (12). Tumour burden and LDH levels were found to be the most important prognostic factors by univariate analyses (13-18) and multivariate analyses (19,20) but are not part of the Ann Arbor staging system. Many institutions treating large numbers of patients with aggressive malignant lymphomas have presented multivariate analyses of prognostic factors and prognostic models (21-26). The major prognostic factors will be briefly reviewed before describing a possible future staging system for aggressive NHL.

Prognostic factors

Age

Lymphomas tend to be more aggressive with increasing age, whatever the histological type, but this is far more obvious for aggressive NHL. The importance of age has been much debated in recent years and it has not been possible to draw any firm conclusions (27-30). The question is: are NHL in elderly patients more aggressive or is the response to treatment worse owing to a decrease in delivered treatment with advanced age? The most important studies to have addressed this point have concluded that older patients fare worse than younger ones even if they have received full treatment. *Figure 1* shows the survival of patients treated with the LNH-84 regimen according to age. There is a statistically worse survival after 65 years. Most of the studies concluded that two thresholds exist: the first is at 55 and the second between 65 and 70 years.

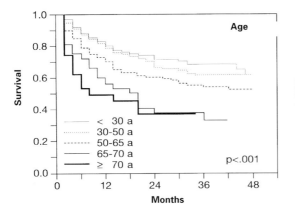

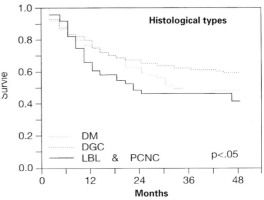

Fig. 1: Survival of 737 patients treated with the LNH-84 regimen (6) according to age. There was no difference between the administered doses as a function of age. Poor survival after 65 years is due to a higher death rate during treatment, a lower response rate and a higher relapse rate.

Fig. 2: Survival of 737 patients treated with the LNH-84 regimen (6) according to the histological subtypes (diffuse mixed NHL, large-cell NHL, and small non-cleaved and lymphoblastic NHL). Response rate was the same for each class but the relapse rate was statistically higher for lymphoblastic NHL patients.

Histology and immunology

Histology has long been the first prognostic factor used to choose between different therapeutic regimens whatever the classification used. Today the Working Formulation for Clinical Usage is used by most physicians to stratify patients into low-grade (SL, FSC, and FM NHL) and other "aggressive" types. The difference between all these aggressive types is not obvious. For most authors, lymphoblastic NHL should receive treatment more related to that used in acute lymphoblastic leukaemia than in other aggressive NHL, especially for patients with bone-marrow or CNS involvement (31). In childhood patients, small non-cleaved Burkitt-type NHL are treated with different regimens (*see pp. 157-160*). Do adult patients with small non-cleaved NHL need different therapeutic regimens from patients with large-cell NHL? No randomized trial gives the answer. In adult patients, the subject is complicated by the fact that this type comprises the Burkitt-type and the non-Burkitt-type NHL encountered in older patients (32). The two subtypes do not have the same presentation or the same response to treatment but they have the same aggressive course and are not easily distinguished by pathologists.

Survival by histological type in patients treated with the LNH-84 regimen was lower for patients with small non-cleaved and lymphoblastic NHL but not statistically different (6) *(fig. 2)*. As most of the American studies do not include small non-cleaved Burkitt-type NHL patients in the same regimen as large-cell NHL patients, and do not single out small non-cleaved, non-Burkitt-type patients, it is difficult to conclude whether these patients should receive the same regimen as other aggressive NHL patients or not. However, a recent study using a chemotherapy regimen as intensive as the LNH-84 regimen reported good results for patients with small non-cleaved NHL (33).

In contrast, diffuse small-cell NHL and follicular large-cell NHL certainly have a more aggressive course than low-grade NHL but probably do not respond to the same therapeutic regimens as well as large-cell NHL (10,34-37). As the number of patients with these histological types is low and as most of them are not included in the major therapeutic studies, it is difficult to determine whether these patients really fare worse or better than those with other aggressive NHL. Our current policy is to include them with the other aggressive NHL and to stratify them on the basis of the same prognostic factors.

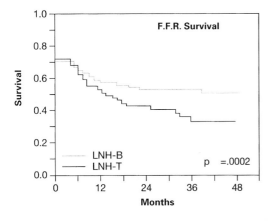

Fig. 3: FFR survival of 361 patients with diffuse mixed or large-cell NHL and a known phenotype included in the LNH-84 regimen according to the phenotype.

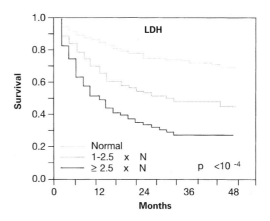

Fig. 5: Survival of 737 patients treated with the LNH-84 regimen (6) according to the LDH level: normal, increased but less than 2.5 times the normal value, and greater than 2.5 times the normal value.

There is no real difference in response to treatment or survival between diffuse mixed- and large-cell NHL if phenotype is the factor considered. Most of the peripheral T-cell NHL are included in the diffuse mixed and immunoblastic types (38). Patients with a peripheral T-cell NHL have a poorer survival rate than those with a B-cell NHL (39-41) *(fig.3)*. T phenotype is found to be a major prognostic factor for freedom-from-relapse (FFR) survival and overall survival in all the multivariate analyses that have included the phenotype in the analyzed variables (42,43).

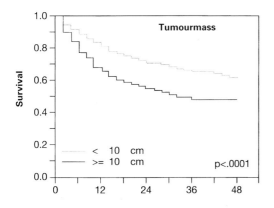

Fig. 4: Survival of 737 patients treated with the LNH-84 regimen (6) according to the largest diameter of the tumoral mass: < or ≥ 10 cm.

Tumoral mass

Tumoral mass has long been acknowledged as a major prognostic factor in NHL (15,17,23,28). Problems have come from the measurement of this tumoral mass. Numerous indexes have been described for measuring the tumoral mass (21,22,25,44). Stage as described in the Ann Arbor system for Hodgkin's disease is a reflection of the tumoral mass because it takes into account the number of involved sites (13,16,20). The number of nodal sites or extranodal sites has been used in most studies (17,23). The threshold between poor and good survival is between patients having zero or one site and those having more than one site of disease. The largest diametre of the nodal or extranodal sites is probably fairly closely related to the overall tumour mass but the threshold between low and high tumoral mass is a subject of debate: 7 or 10 cm. In our study, 10 cm was the best prognostic threshold *(fig. 4)* (26). More complex indexes have been described, such as the level of site-involvement, from the Memorial Sloan Kettering Cancer Center, (21) or the tumour burden, from the M.D. Anderson Cancer Center (22,25). These indexes have not increased the value of the preceding parameters (25).

LDH level is probably not only an indicator of tumoral mass but is also highly correlated with it (6,14,20-22,24-26). LDH level is the most important prognostic indicator of poor survival and poor FFR survival in virtually all the studies on prognostic parameters in aggressive NHL, except that of the Dana Farber Cancer Institute (23). Patients with above-normal serum LDH level have a less favourable prognosis and those with the highest levels have the least favourable prognosis (fig. 5).

β2-microglobulin level also reflects the tumour mass and is not related to LDH levels (24). However, very few prospective studies have included its measurement as a pretherapeutic stratification factor and its true relevance for choosing treatment is not defined. It is more valuable than LDH level for low-grade NHL, particularly follicular NHL. It seems a better marker than LDH level in the follow-up of treated patients for predicting relapse.

Performance status, weight loss and serum albumin level

A low performance status (2 or more on the ECOG/WHO scale) is highly correlated with a low response rate and poor survival in aggressive NHL as in other cancers (1,23,25,26,28). Weight loss greater than 10%, along with fever and night sweat, characterizes the B symptoms. It is the most important parameter of the three and has more statistical significance than the presence of B symptoms (26).

Serum albumin level lower than 30 g/l is highly correlated with a low CR rate, a high death rate during induction, and poor survival (20,26). Serum albumin level is highly correlated with performance status, weight loss and B symptoms and, in multivariate analyses, it has more statistical significance. However, the importance of hypoalbuminaemia is due first to starvation and to its association with acute phase syndrome and secretion of interleukins and TNF.

Karyotypic and kinetic abnormalities

The study of chromosomal rearrangements is a recent addition to the list of prognostic factors. Some chromosomal abnormalities are

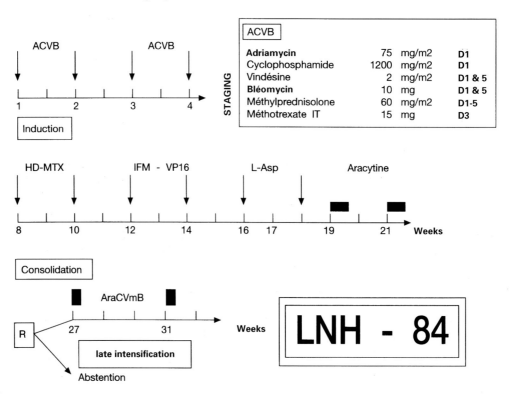

Fig. 6: LNH-84 regimen.

TABLE I

Description of the LNH-84 prognostic index

Index	Mass ≥ 10 cm	≥ 2 sites	Stage ≥ III	Increased LDH
1	-	-	-	-
2	1 or 2 adverse factors			-
2	-	-	-	+
3	+	+	+	-
3	1 to 3 adverse factors			+

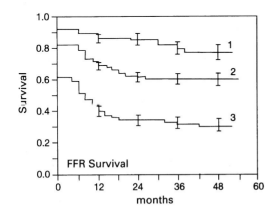 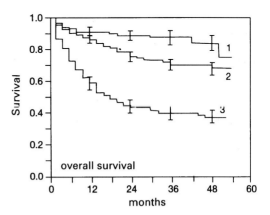

Fig. 7: Application of the LNH-84 index to the LNH-84 patients for FFR survival (A) and overall survival (B).

correlated with lymphoma characteristics, such as anomalies of chromosomes 5, 6, 7, 17 or 18 (45). Further studies on specific chromosomal abnormalities, gene alterations, and proto-oncogene modifications must be carried out before such parameters can be included in the determination of treatment.

Studies of the proliferative activity of lymphoma cells are highly correlated with survival (46). A higher percentage of cells in S phase of S+G2M phase has been associated with a poorer outcome but was not found to be statistically associated with survival in large trials analyzed with multiparametric methods. DNA aneuploidy and low proliferative activity predict a favourable outcome. High proliferative activity, defined by a high expression of Ki-67 antigen in lymphoma cells, was found to be a strong independent predictor of poor survival (47).

Specific involved sites

The involvement of certain sites in NHL, such as bone marrow (5,15,48), central nervous system (49-51), testis (52) skin, pleura or peritoneum, is associated with a poor prognosis in univariate analysis. However, these sites are correlated either with histological type or with tumour burden. The most statistically significant is bone-marrow involvement which is associated with a low response rate and a poor FFR survival and overall survival (48). None of these sites retain their statistical significance in multivariate analyses.

The gastrointestinal tract is the most frequent extranodal site involved: gastrointestinal NHL represent 30% of primary extranodal lymphomas and 15 to 20% of all

TABLE II

CHOP regimen

Drug	Dose	Days of therapy					
		1	2	3	4	5	22
Cyclophosphamide	600 mg/m^2	X					X
Adriamycin	50 mg/m^2	X					X
Oncovin	1 mg/m^2	X					X
Prednisone	40 mg/m^2	X	X	X	X	X	X

NHL cases. A better prognosis has often been associated with them but they comprise low-grade and high-grade NHL. Aggressive gastrointestinal NHL have the same prognosis as other nodal or extranodal lymphomas and should not be isolated amongst the lymphomas (6,53). The same prognostic parameters, such as tumoral mass, LDH level and age, carry the same poor prognosis.

Mediastinal tumour, for a long time synonymous with lymphoblastic NHL, has also been associated with an adverse prognosis. In the adult, mediastinal involvement is usually by large-cell B lymphomas with fibrosis or Ki-1-positive lymphomas (54-56). These subtypes are likely to present post-treatment fibronecrotic mass preventing patients from being considered in CR but they do not carry a worse prognosis.

Other prognostic factors

Anaemia is observed in 42% of patients with lymphoma. Anaemic patients have a shorter survival period (57) whether bone marrow is involved or not. This is probably a secondary prognostic factor but still an important one because it is related to host-tumour relationship. Factors associated with the response of host to lymphoma are B symptoms, performance status, serum albumin level and inflammatory manifestations. These abnormalities are mediated through interleukins and other related molecules such as TNF (58). In the near future, modulation of the host-tumour relationship could play an important therapeutic role.

Prognostic index and new staging systems

New staging systems have been described by large institutions (21-24). The staging systems described by the Dana Farber Institute, the Memorial Sloan Kettering Cancer Center, and the M.D. Anderson Cancer Center give good discrimination of patients into 3 or 4 subgroups but have rarely been tested on other sets of patients. Applied to our patients from the LNH-84 regimen, they give good results but not better than the LDH level alone (25). We have recently described another prognostic index based on stage, tumoral mass, number of extranodal sites and LDH level (26). This index is very simple to apply and was tested with success on patients from the Nebraska Lymphoma Study Group treated with another regimen. Such an index should be used to divide patients into subgroups of different prognosis with different treatments and to compare results from different regimens or different institutions. *Table I* gives the description of the LNH-84 index. Application of this index to patients from the LNH-84 regimen is shown in *Figure 7* for freedom-from-relapse survival and overall survival. An international study is currently being conducted under the auspices of the International Study Group on prognostic factors in large-cell lymphomas with more than 4300 patients from major institutions to describe and validate such a prognostic index. This index will permit a pre-therapy stratification of patients with lymphoma

TABLE III

M-BACOD and m-BACOD regimens

Drug	Dose	Days of therapy							
		1	**2**	**3**	**4**	**5**	**8**	**15**	**22**
Methotrexate	3000 mg/m^2							X+	
Bleomycin	10 mg/m^2	X							X
Adriamycin	45 mg/m^2	X							X
Cyclophosphamide	600 mg/m^2	X							X
Vincristine	1 mg/m^2	X							X
Dexamethasone	6 mg/m^2	X	X	X	X	X			X
+ 24 hours later, folinic acid rescue (25 mg x 4/d x 3)									
Methotrexate	200 mg/m^2						X+	X+	
Bleomycin	10 mg/m^2	X							X
Adriamycin	45 mg/m^2	X							X
Cyclophosphamide	600 mg/m^2	X							X
Vincristine	1 mg/m^2	X							X
Dexamethasone	6 mg/m^2	X	X	X	X	X			X
+ 24 hours later, folinic acid rescue (10 mg/m^2)									

into subgroups with the same outcome. It will permit the development of new strategies for patients with the poorest prognosis and comparisons of different types of chemotherapy regimens (59).

First-line treatment

Advanced disease

The first curative chemotherapy described in aggressive NHL was CHOP (cyclophosphamide, hydroxydaunorubicin [adriamycin], oncovin [vincristine] and prednisone) *(Table II)* (60). Numerous variations of CHOP were described under the term of CHOP-like regimens (C-MOPP, HOP/AC, BACOP, CHOP-B, COMLA) but none merited attention because they did not give better results and are no longer used. The CHOP regimen has been used in more than 500 patients in randomized studies and is the reference regimen. In the mid-1970s, investigators developed "second-generation" regimens. Such regimens were based on dose-intensification with flexible schedules, shorter duration of chemotherapy and addition of non-myelosuppressive drugs such as bleomycin. The intention was to increase the rate of response and thus of cure. Examples of such regimens are M-BACOD (methotrexate, bleomycin, adriamycin, cyclophosphamide, vincristine and dexamethasone) *(Table III)* (61,62) and ProMACE-MOPP *(Table IV)* (63) regimens. Third-generation regimens were created in an attempt to shorten the duration of therapy, and intensify the chemotherapy using non-cross-resistant agents. These relatively toxic and complex regimens are represented by LNH-84 *(Fig. 6)*, MACOP-B *(Table V)* (64), COPBLAM III *(Table VI)* (65) and CAP-BOP *(Table VII)* (29).

TABLE IV

ProMACE and ProMACE-CytaBOM regimens

Drug	Dose	Days of therapy			
		1	8	14	29
Etoposide	120 mg/m^2	X	X		X
Cyclophosphamide	650 mg/m^2	X	X		X
Adriamycin	25 mg/m^2	X	X		X
Methotrexate	1500 mg/m^2			X+	
Prednisone	60 mg/m^2	X ------------X ------------X			X
+ 24 hours later, folinic acid rescue (25 mg/m^2 x 6)					
Etoposide	120 mg/m^2	X			X
Cyclophosphamide	650 mg/m^2	X			X
Adriamycin	25 mg/m^2	X			X
Prednisone	60 mg/m^2	X ------------X ------------X			X
Cytarabine	300 mg/m^2		X		
Bleomycin	5 mg/m^2		X		
Vincristine	1,4 mg/m^2		X		
Methotrexate	120 mg/m^2		X+		
+ 24 hours later, folinic acid rescue (25 mg/m^2 x 6)					

TABLE V

MACOP-B regimen

Drug	Dose	Weeks of therapy											
		1	2	3	4	5	6	7	8	9	10	11	12
Methotrexate+	400 mg/m^2		X				X				X		
Adriamycin	50 mg/m^2	X		X		X		X		X		X	
Cyclophosphamide	350 mg/m^2	X		X		X		X		X		X	
Vincristine	1,4 mg/m^2		X		X		X		X		X		X
Bleomycin	10 mg/m^2				X				X				X
Prednisone	75 mg	X --X											
Co-trimoxazole	1000 mg	X --X											
Ketoconazole	200 mg	X --X											
+ 100 mg/m^2 IV bolus; then 300 mg/m^2 over 4 hours followed 24 hours later by folinic acid 15 mg x 6													

TABLE VI

COPBLAM III regimen

Regimen	Dose	Days of therapy										
		A:	1	2	5			B:	22		26	
Vincristine	1 mg/m^2		X+	X					X			
Bleomycin++	4 mg/m^2		X --------	--X								
Cyclophosphamide	350 mg/m^2		X						X			
Adriamycin	35 mg/m^2		X						X			
Prednisone	40 mg/m^2		X --------	--X					X --------	--X		
Procarbazine	100 mg/m^2		X --------	--X					X --------	--X		

+ 1 mg/m^2 infusion over 24 hours x 2 days
++ 4 mg/m^2 in bolus on day 1, followed by 4 mg/m^2 continuous infusion over 24 hours on days 1-5

	Week	1	4	7	10	13	16	19	22	25	28	31	34
	Cycle	A	B	A	B	A	B	A	B	A	B	A	B

No comparative study exists testing two or more of these regimens. Any advantages procured by the new regimens should be appreciated by comparison of response rate, relapse rate, and FFR or overall survival rates. However, in all the reports, the characteristics of patients are different, particularly the percentage of patients with adverse prognostic factors, and it is impossible to compare one study with others. Moreover, very few reports exist of the activity of one regimen when used by another institution and in some cases preliminary results are not confirmed (66). *Table VIII* presents some results obtained in aggressive NHL with the regimens described. In the absence of comparative data, no regimen should be recommended as the treatment of choice. Certain

TABLE VII

CAP-BOP regimen

Drug	Dose	Days of therapy			
		1	7	15	22
Cyclophosphamide	650 m/m^2	X			
Adriamycin	50 mg/m^2	X			
Procarbazine	100 mg/m^2	X ------	------X		
Bleomycin	10 mg/m^2			X	
Vincristine	1,4 mg/m^2			X	
Prednisone	100 mg			X ------	------X

TABLE VIII

**Results obtained in non-comparative studies for aggressive lymphomas
with the regimens described above**

Reference	Regimen	Number of patients	CR (%)	DFS	Survival
Coltman[60]	CHOP	418	53	50% (7 y)	30% (13.4 a)
Skarin[61]	M-BACOD	101	72	80% (5 y)	59% (5 a)
Shipp[62]	M-BACOD	81	61	71% (5 y)	55% (5 a)
Shipp[62]	m-BACOD	134	80	74% (5 y)	60% (5 a)
DeVita[85]	ProMACE-MOPP	52	84	NA	63% (2 a)
Klimo[64]	MACOP-B	61	84	88% (4 y)	75% (4 a)
Connors[67]	MACOP-B	125	84	76% (5 y)	69% (5 a)
Schneider[66]	MACOP-B	70	54	54% (2 y)	56% (3 a)
Coleman[65]	COPBLAM III	51	84	91% (2 y)	65% (2 a)
Vose[29]	CAP-BOP	157	65	NA	42% (3 a)
Coiffier[19]	LNH-80	100	84	NA	61% (5 a)
Coiffier[6]	LNH-84	737	75	67% (2 y)	62% (2 a)
CR: complete remission, DFS: disease-free survival, NA: not available					

regimens are known for their better results in some subtypes (i.e. MACOP-B in large-cell NHL) and others are associated with the same results whatever the subtype (i.e. LNH-84 regimen). *Table VIII* shows that results could be modified according to the time of publication and location of the study: a 5-year survival rate of 59% then 55% with the M-BACOD regimen (same patients) (62) or 75% then 69% with MACOP-B regimen (more patients) (67); a 69% 5-year survival rate in Canada with the MACOP-B regimen (67) and a 56% 3-year survival rate in New York with the same regimen (66). These discrepancies are due to the problems of heterogeneity of the lymphomas and the reproducibility and exportability of regimens.

One of the problems currently debated in relation to chemotherapy of aggressive lyphomas is the importance of dose intensi-ty (68-71). Most of the initial data on this problem have been obtained comparing intention-to-deliver dose intensity (70) and have concluded that regimens with higher doses seem to be associated with better results in terms of response and survival. But these studies have a lot of shortcomings, the principal one being that administered doses have not been taken into account. Moreover, it is extremely difficult to interpret retrospective results on this subject because of difficulty in analyzing the cases of patients dying during treatment from toxicity or disease. They have usually received one or two courses of chemotherapy with full doses and the inclusion or exclusion of such patients from the analysis is associated with bias. However, two studies have demonstrated a better outcome associated with either high-dose intensity of the initial cycles of therapy (71) or high-dose intensity of adriamycin (70). Only a prospective study comparing two schemes

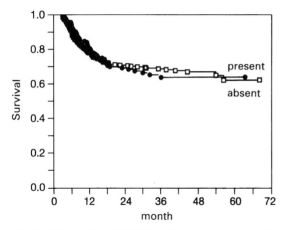

Fig. 8: FFR survival of LNH-84 patients according to the presence of a residual tumoral mass after induction.

with the same global dose of each drug but administered on a different schedule could draw conclusions on this point.

Localized disease

Localized stages of very aggressive NHL, i.e. Burkitt's and lymphoblastic lymphomas, should be treated as advanced stages by intensive chemotherapy regimens.

Patients with diffuse mixed- or large-cell NHL and a localized stage carry a different prognosis according to stage (I or II), presence of extranodal sites, or tumoral mass (17). In these patients, treatment should attain a > 95% CR rate and a > 80% 5-year overall survival. Extended radiotherapy has given good CR rates but is associated with a high relapse rate, even in patients with extensive staging procedure including exploratory laparotomy (17). Such an extensive staging procedure is not recommended today. If an examination shows a putative localization, the patient should be considered as a non-localized stage and treated by chemotherapy. Radiotherapy plus chemotherapy has always given better results than radiotherapy alone (72). Chemotherapy-only regimens have given better results than radiotherapy plus chemotherapy in some non-comparative trials (73,74). The problem, not yet resolved, is to assess the role of radiotherapy for stage I patients without adverse

prognostic factors. Our feeling is that four cycles of a non-intensive chemotherapy regimen (CHOP, m-BACOD) plus localized (involved field) radiotherapy will probably cure most of these patients and that more intensive chemotherapy should be reserved for relapsing patients or those with stage I and poor prognosis factors.

The problem of elderly patients

Patients older than 65 years have a worse prognosis than younger patients whatever the other prognostic factors (stage, tumoral mass, histological type, LDH level). Such patients require intensive therapy but their age, performance status and general condition do not permit these treatments (75). Depending upon the importance given to age as a prognostic factor, recommendations change for the treatment of elderly patients. However, most deaths of these patients occur during treatment for lymphoma as a very indirect consequence of these treatments in debilitated patients. The current randomized studies in these patients show, in the case of non-intensive chemotherapy, a low CR rate and a high death-rate from lymphoma and, in the case of adriamycin-based regimens, a high death-rate from neutropenia-related complications or from other disease not obviously related to the lymphoma but related to the fact that these patients have a lymphoma and are undergoing treatment. The use of mitoxantrone of growth factors could be a response to this dilemma (75).

Specific extranodal sites

In general, specific extranodal sites do not need a special therapeutic approach. The rules given for aggressive nodal lymphomas apply to extranodal lymphomas as well. Gastrointestinal sites, however, merit some comments on the role of debulking surgery. Patients with acute presentation (occlusion, gastric perforation) require exploratory laparotomy for diagnosis. When there is one gastrointestinal site among other nodal or extranodal sites (secondary gastrointestinal lymphomas), there is no need for special consideration of this site except in the case of a primary gastric site when diagnosis has been established by biopsies. Do these patients need a surgical resection of the stomach? If the biopsy specimen allows certain diagnosis of agressive lymphoma, durable CR may be obtained without gastrectomy (76-77). If there are some doubts regarding the diagnosis of lymphoma or its subtype, a partial gastrectomy should, if possible, be performed with staging of the lymphoma in the abdomen.

In cases of primary central nervous system lymphoma, curative radiotherapy (30 Gy) should be undertaken after chemotherapy. Radiotherapy alone has not permitted durable CR and should be abandoned (78,79).

Acute lysis syndrome can be seen in very proliferative lymphomas, particularly with high tumour burden: lymphoblastic, small non-cleaved and immunoblastic lymphomas. Acute lysis syndrome is suspected if LDH level is extremely elevated (greater than 3 times normal values), if creatinine level is increased, and if phosphoremia is increased (80). It should be treated with preventive measures before the installation of lactic acidosis or acute renal failure which are often followed by death. Prevention relies on high-volume diuresis and urate-oxidase before the start of chemotherapy.

HIV+ patients

Aggressive NHL is the most frequent tumour in HIV+ patients. The lymphoma can occur either in patients with a known positivity for HIV and severe opportunistic infections or as the first manifestation of AIDS. Histological subtypes are most often large-cell NHL or Burkitt's small non-cleaved type. The clinical presentation is usually aggressive with increased LDH level, impaired performance status, and several extranodal sites.

Results of treatment with moderately intensive regimens are poor (81) with a lot of patients dying from infectious complications or progressive lymphomas. A pilot study conducted in France shows that patients without opportunistic infections and without central nervous system involvement be can successfully treated by the LNH-84 regimen. Patients in CR should receive retrovir and prophylaxis of opportunistic infections. The adjunction of G-CSF or GM-CSF after chemotherapy should allow administration of the treatment without too much toxicity.

The problem of persisting residual masses

Patients with large initial tumoral mass, either thoracic, abdominal or peripheral, have a less favourable prognosis. Nevertheless, a considerable proportion of these patients achieve clinical CR. The discovery of a radiographically detectable residual mass at the time when all evidence of disease has disappeared is a common problem in this group of patients and represents a major dilemma for the physician. Biopsies of these residual masses have been performed and fibronecrotic tissue found in more than 80% of patients (82,83). Prognosis is not adversely associated with these masses as shown in *Figure 8* and as shown by others in mediastinal (82) or abdominal (83) masses. Persistent fibronecrotic masses are observed most often in large-cell lymphomas with high initial tumour mass, either mediastinal or abdominal, rarely peripheral. Diagnosis of persistent fibronecrotic masses is dynamic: patients should present an important decrease in tumour volume after the first chemotherapy course and then stabilization of this volume. Morphological examination, either by puncture or biopsy, is rarely necessary to diagnose a persistent fibronecrotic mass. This must to be done in the case of peripheral masses or persistent masses with high tumour volume, greater than 5 cm, or masses greater than 50% of the initial volume.

Rules for choosing a therapeutic regimen in aggressive lymphomas

Active therapeutic regimens have been described for aggressive NHL. Most of them probably have the same efficacy, CR rate, FFR survival and overall survival. It is not necessary to find the best of these regimens for all patients but rather to stratify patients according to prognostic indicators and to define the best therapeutic approach for each subgroup. No such study has yet been published but some are currently being performed and results will not be available for a few years.

Until such results are available, recommendations for treating patients with aggressive NHL should be those put forward by Armitage and Cheson (7):

- The intention of first-line therapy should be cure. With the exceptions already described for aged or debilitated persons, all new patients should be given a chance of cure.

- For a regimen to be curative, it must achieve a high rate of complete remission. The only exception is for patients who present bulky disease in the mediastinum or abdomen and who retain some residual tumour despite apparently successful chemotherapy. These patients should be considered in good clinical CR if no pathological examination has been re-performed.

- Cure must be obtained with front-line chemotherapy. Many drug combinations have been developed to attempt effective salvage treatment for relapsing or progressing patients but the response rate of the best of these regimens is only 40%. However, without intensive chemotherapy and bone-marrow transplantation, 10 to 15% of these patients are free from disease at 2 years and 10% at 3 years. In patients not adequately treated by current standards, the most intensive salvage therapy can only achieve a 30 to 35% survival rate at 2 years. All these studies show that prior chemotherapy or radiotherapy exposure jeopardizes response to subsequent treatment.

- Drugs must be delivered at curative doses. Patients treated with reduced doses because of age or poor-risk conditions have fared worse than those treated with full doses in all the studies where dose-intensity has been studied. Reduction of the dose of the first course of chemotherapy has been found to increase the risk of relapse in LNH-84 patients (6). In general, dose reduction based on arbitrary criteria should be discouraged and patients treated at full dose whenever possible.

Questions for the future

Aggressive lymphomas, and probably follicular lymphomas, should be stratified into two or three prognostic groups before deciding on treatment. However, the future indexing system is not yet recognized by all the major institutions. Preliminary studies must be confirmed before diffusion throughout the world.

Current intensive chemotherapy regimens have different activities and toxicities. Comparisons by randomized studies must be made after stratification into the different prognostic groups. New chemotherapy regimens will probably not be needed before thorough appraisal of the previous regimens.

Intensification was a major factor in the progress of treatment of aggressive lymphomas (84). Should intensification be continued, at what time of the treatment regimen, and for which groups of patients? These points have been settled and will be resolved in the near future. Randomized studies are in progress and will be completed in 2 to 3 years. Points being studied are: the place of intensification with growth factors (G-CSF or GM-CSF) to decrease the extent of neutropenia in front-line chemotherapies or in consolidation; the place of intensive therapy with autologous stem-cell rescue, early in the case of partial response, or in consolidation for poor-risk patients.

These growth-factor treatments will probably provide a response in the current dilemma concerning elderly patients. They will probably permit curative chemotherapy regimens to be undertaken without the haematological toxicity currently observed.

T-cell lymphoma patients do not have the same response to treatment and progression B-cell lymphoma patients. Are different therapeutic approaches required for B- or T-cell lymphomas?

The refractoriness to treatment of relapsing lymphoma is probably due to the appearance of drug-resistant clones of tumoral cells characterized by chromosomal abnormalities (85) and alteration/activation of oncogenes (86). Such clones have been described and therapeutic modulations have been proposed to circumvent this resistance (87,88).

References

1. ARMITAGE JO, WEISENBURGER DD, HUTCHINS M et al.

   Chemotherapy for diffuse large-cell lymphoma. Rapidly responding patients have more durable remissions.

   J Clin Oncol, 1986; 4: 160-164.

2. BOYD DB, COLEMAN M, PAPISH SW et al.

   COPBLAM III: infusional combination chemotherapy for diffuse large-cell lymphoma.

   J Clin Oncol, 1988; 6: 425-433.

3. CANELLOS GP, SKARIN AT, KLATT MM et al.

   The m-BACOD combination chemotherapy regimen in the treatment of diffuse large-cell lymphoma.

   Sem Hematol, 1987; 24 (suppl.1): 2-7.

4. COIFFIER B, BOSLY A, CALLIGARIS-CAPPIO F et al.

   European School of Oncology: management of non-Hodgkin's lymphomas.

   Conclusions of the European School of Oncology meeting, 1986. Europ J Cancer Clin Oncol, 1987; 23: 1691-1695.

5. COIFFIER B, BRYON PA, BERGER F et al.

   Intensive and sequential combination chemotherapy for aggressive malignant lymphomas (Protocol LNH-80).

   J Clin Oncol, 1986; 4: 147-153.

6. COIFFIER B, GISSELBRECHT C, HERBRECHT R, TILLY H, BOSLY A, BROUSSE N

   LNH-84 regimen. A multicenter study of intensive chemotherapy in 737 patients with aggressive malignant lymphoma.

   J Clin Oncol, 1989; 7: 1018-1026.

7. ARMITAGE JO, CHESON BD

   Interpretation of clinical trials in diffuse large-cell lymphoma.

   J Clin Oncol, 1988; 6: 1335-1337.

8. *The non-Hodgkin's lymphoma pathologic classification project: National Cancer Institute-sponsored study of classifications of non-Hodgkin's lymphomas. Summary and description of a Working Formulation for Clinical Usage.*

   Cancer, 1982; 49: 2112-2135.

9. SIMON R, DURRLEMAN S, HOPPE RT et al.

   The non-Hodgkin lymphoma pathologic classification project. Long-term follow-up of 1153 patients with non-Hodgkin's lymphomas.

   Ann Int Med, 1988; 109: 939-345.

10. BRITTINGER G, BARTELS H COMMON H et al.

    Clinical and prognostic relevance of the Kiel classification of non-Hodgkin's lymphomas. Results of a prospective multicenter study by the Kiel Lymphoma Study Group.

    Blut, 1984; 2: 269-306.

11. CARBONE PP, KAPLAN HD, MUSSHOFF K et al.

    Report of the Committee of Hodgkin's disease staging.

    Cancer Res, 1971; 31: 1860-1860.

12. ROSENBERG SA

    Validity of the Ann Arbor staging classification for non-Hodgkin's lymphomas.

    Centre Treat Rep, 1977; 61: 1023-1027.

13. ANDERSON T, DE VITA VT, SIMON RM et al.

    Malignant lymphoma. II. Prognostic factors and response to treatment of 473 patients at the National Cancer Institute.

    Cancer, 1982; 50: 2708-2721.

14. FERRARIS AM, GIUNTINI P, GAETANI GF

    Serum lactic dehydrogenase as a prognostic tool for non-Hodgkin's lymphomas.

    Blood, 1979; 54: 928-932.

15. FISHER RI, HUBBARD SM, DE VITA VT et al.

    Factors predicting long-term survival in diffuse mixed, histiocytic, or undifferentiated lymphoma.

    Blood, 1981; 58: 45-51.

16. JONES SE, MILLER TP, CONNORS JM

    Long-term follow-up and analysis for prognostic factors for patients with limited-stage diffuse large-cell lymphoma treated with initial chemotherapy, with or without adjuvant radiotherapy.

    J Clin Oncol, 1989; 7: 1186-1191.

17. KAMINSKI MS, COLEMAN CN, COLBY TV, COX RS, ROSENBERG SA

    Factors predicting survival in adults with stage I and II large-cell lymphoma treated with primary radiation therapy.

    Ann Int Med, 1986; 104: 747-756.

18. KOZINER B, LITTLE C, PASSE S et al.

    Treatment of advanced diffuse histiocytic lymphomas. An analysis of prognostic variables.

    Cancer, 1982; 49: 1571-1579.

19. COIFFIER B, BRYON PA, FFRENCH M et al.

    Intensive chemotherapy in aggressive lymphomas: updated results of LNH-80 protocol and prognostic factors affecting response and survival.

    Blood, 1987; 70: 1394-1399.

20. COWAN RA, JONES M, HARRIS M et al.
Prognostic factors in high and intermediate grade non-Hodgkin's lymphoma.
Brit J Cancer, 1989; 59: 276-282.

21. DANIEU L, WONG G, KOZINER B, CLARKSON B
Predictive model for prognosis in advanced diffuse histiocytic lymphomas.
Cancer Res, 1986; 46: 5372-5379.

22. JAGANNATH S, VELASQUEZ WS, TUCKER SL et al.
Tumor burden assessment and its implication for a prognostic model in advanced diffuse large-cell lymphoma.
J Clin Oncol, 1986; 4: 859-865.

23. SHIPP MA, HARRINGTON DP, KLATT MM et al.
Identification of major prognostic subgroups of patients with large-cell lymphoma treated with m-BACOD of M-BACOD.
Ann Inter Med, 1986; 104: 757-765

24. SWAN F, VELASQUEZ WS, TUCKER S et al.
A new serologic staging system for large-cell lymphomas based on initial beta-2-microglobulin and lactate dehydrogenase levels.
J Clin Oncol, 1989; 7: 1518-1527.

25. COIFFIER B, LEPAGE E
Prognosis of aggressive lymphomas. A study of five prognostic models with patients included in the LNH-84 regimen.
Blood, 1989; 74: 558-564.

26. COIFFIER B, GISSELBRECHT C, VOSE JM et al.
Prognostic factors in aggressive malignant lymphomas: description and validation of a prognostic index that could identify patients requiring a more intensive therapy.
J Clin Oncol, 1991; 9: 211-219.

27. DIXON DO, NEILAN B, JONES SE et al.
Effect of age on therapeutic outcome in advanced diffuse histiocytic lymphoma: the Southwest Oncology Group experience.
J Clin Oncol, 1986; 4: 295-305.

28. TIRELLI U, ZAGONEL V, SERRAINO D et al
Non-Hodgkin's lymphomas in 137 patients aged 70 years or older: a retrospective EORTC lymphoma study group.
J Clin Oncol, 1988; 6: 1708-1713.

29. VOSE JM, ARMITAGE JO, WEISENBURGER DD et al.
The importance of age in survival of patients treated with chemotherapy for aggressive non-Hodgkin's lymphoma.
J Clin Oncol, 1988; 6: 1838-1844.

30. SOLAL-CELIGNY Ph, CHASTANG C, HERRERA A et al.
Age as the main prognostic factor in adult aggressive non-Hodgkin's lymphoma.
Amer J Med, 1987; 83: 1075-1079.

31. SALLOUM E, HENRY-AMAR M, CAILLOU B et al.
Lymphoblastic lymphoma in adults: a clinicopathological study of 34 cases treated at the Institut Gustave-Roussy.
Europ J Cancer Clin Oncol, 1988; 24: 1609-1616.

32. PAVLOVA Z, PARKER JW, TAYLOR CR, LEVINE AM, FEINSTEIN DI, LUKES RJ
Small non-cleaved follicular center-cell lymphoma: Burkitt's and non-Burkitt's variants in the US. II. Pathologic and immunologic features.
Cancer, 1987; 59: 1892-1902.

33. Mc MASTER ML, GREER JP, WOLFF SN et al.
Results of treatment with high-intensity brief-duration chemotherapy in poor prognosis non-Hodgkin's lymphoma.
Cancer, 1991; 68: 233-241.

34. AL-KATIB A, KOZINER B, KURLAND E et al.
Treatment of diffuse poorly differentiated lymphocytic lymphoma. An analysis of prognostic variables.
Cancer, 1984; 53: 2404-2412.

35. ANDERSON KC, SKARIN AT, ROSENTHAL DS et al.
Combination chemotherapy for advanced non-Hodgkin's lymphoma of other than diffuse histiocytic or undifferentiated histologies.
Cancer Treat Rep, 1984; 68: 1343-1350.

36. GLICK JH, McFADDEN E, COSTELLO W, EZDINLI E, BERARD CW, BENNET JM
Nodular histiocytic lymphoma: factors influencing prognosis and implications for aggressive chemotherapy.
Cancer, 1982; 49: 840-845.

37. HORNING SJ, WEISS LM, NEVITT JB, WARNKE RA
Clinical and pathologic features of follicular large cell (nodular histiocytic) lymphoma.
Cancer, 1987; 59: 1470-1474.

38. NATHWANI BN, METTER GE, GAMS A et al.
Malignant lymphoma, mixed-cell type, diffuse.
Blood, 1983; 62: 200-208.

39. COIFFIER B, BERGER F, BRYON PA, MAGAUD JP
T-cell lymphomas: immunologic, histologic, clinical and therapeutic analysis of 63 cases.
J Clin Oncol, 1988; 6: 1584-1589.

40. CHENG AL, CHEN YC, WANG CH et al.

Direct comparisons of peripheral T-cell lymphoma with diffuse B-cell lymphoma of comparable histological grades. Should peripheral T-cell lymphoma be considered separately?

J Clin Oncol, 1989; 7: 725-731.

41. LIPPMAN SM, MILLER TP, SPIER CM, SLYMEN DJ, GROGAN TM

The prognostic significance of the immunotype in diffuse large-cell lymphoma: a comparative study of the T-cell and B-cell phenotype.

Blood, 1988; 72: 436-441.

42. COIFFIER B, BROUSSE N, PEUCHMAUR M et al.

Peripheral T-cell lymphomas have a worse prognosis than B-cell lymphomas: a prospective study of 361 immunophenotyped patients treated with the LNH-84 regimen.

Ann Oncol, 1991; 1: 45-50.

43. ARMITAGE JO, VOSE JM, LINOER J et al.

Clinical significance of immunophenotype in diffuse aggressive non-Hodgkin's lymphoma.

J Clin Oncol, 1989; 7: 1783-1790.

44. VELASQUEZ WS, JAGANNATH S, TUCKER SL et al.

Risk classification as the basis for clinical staging of diffuse large-cell lymphoma derived from 10-year survival data.

Blood, 1989; 74: 551-557.

45. SCHOUTEN HC, SANGER WG, WEISENBURGER DD et al.

Chromosomal abnormalities in untreated patients with non-Hodgkin's lymphoma: associations with histology, clinical characteristics, and treatment outcome.

Blood, 1990; 75: 1841-1847.

46. COWAN RA, HARRIS M, JONES M, CROWTHER D

DNA content in high and intermediate-grade non-Hodgkin's lymphoma. Prognosis significance and clinicopathology correlations.

Brit J Cancer, 1989; 60: 904-910.

47. GROGAN TM, LIPPMAN SM, SPIER C et al.

Independent prognostic significance of nuclear proliferation antigen in diffuse large-cell lymphoma as determined by the monoclonal antibody Ki-67.

Blood, 1988; 71: 1157-1160.

48. BENNETT JM, CAIN KC, GLICK JH, JOHNSON GJ, EZDINLI E, O'CONNELL MJ

The significance of bone-marrow involvement in non-Hodgkin's lymphoma: the Eastern Cooperative Oncology Group experience.

J Clin Oncol, 1986; 4: 1462-1469.

49. POLLACK IF, LUNSFORD LD, FLICKINGER JC, DAMESHEK HL

Prognostic factors in the diagnosis and treatement of primary central nervous system lymphoma.

Cancer, 1989; 63: 939-947.

50. FORMENTI SC, GILL PS, LEAN E et al.

Primary central nervous system lymphoma in AIDS. Results of radiation therapy.

Cancer, 1989; 63: 1101-1107.

51. RECHT L, STRAUSS DJ, CIRRINCIONE C, THALER HT, POSNER JB

Central nervous system metastases from non-Hodgkin's lymphomas: treatment and prophylaxis.

Amer J Med, 1988; 84: 425-435.

52. NONOMURA N, AOZASA K, UEDA T et al.

Malignant lymphoma of the testis. Histological and immunohistological study of 28 cases.

J Urol, 1989; 141: 1368-1371.

53. AZAB MB, HENRY-AMAR M, ROUGIER P et al.

Prognostic factors in primary gastrointestinal non-Hodgkin's lymphoma. A multivariate analysis, report of 106 cases, and review of the literature.

Cancer, 1989; 64: 1208-1217.

54. JACOBSON JO, AISENBERG AC, LAMARRE L et al.

Mediastinal large cell lymphoma. An uncommon subset of adult lymphoma curable with combined modality therapy.

Cancer, 1988; 62: 1893-1898.

55. PERRONE T, FRIZZERA G, ROSAI J

Mediastinal diffuse large-cell lymphoma with sclerosis. A clinicopathologic study of 60 cases.

Amer J Surg Pathol, 1986; 10: 176-191.

56. CHAN JKC, NG CS, HUI PK et al.

Anaplastic large-cell Ki-1 lymphoma. Delineation of two morphological types.

Histopathology, 1989; 15: 11-34.

57. CONLAN MG, ARMITAGE JO, BAST M, WEISENBURGER DD

Clinical significance of hematologic parameters in non-Hodgkin's lymphoma at diagnosis.

Cancer, 1991; 67: 1389-1395.

58. SAPPINO AP, SEELENTAG W, PELTE WF, ALBERTO P, VASSALLI P

Tumor necrosis factor/cachectin and lymphotoxin gene expression in lymph nodes from lymphoma patients.

Blood, 1990; 75: 958-962.

59. COIFFIER B, SHIPP MA, CABANILLAS F, CROWTHER D, ARMITAGE JO, CANELLOS GP

Report of the first workshop on prognostic factors in large-cell lymphomas.

Ann Oncol, 1991; 2 (suppl.2): 213-217.

60. COLTMAN CA, DAHLBERG S, JONES SE et al.

CHOP is curative in thirty percent of patients with large-cell lymphomas: a twelve-year Southwest Oncology Group follow-up.

Proc Amer Soc Clin Oncol, 1987; 5: 197 (abstr).

61. SKARIN AT, CANELLOS GP, ROSENTHAL DS et al.

Improved prognosis of diffuse histiocytic and undifferentiated lymphoma by use of high-dose methotrexate alternating with standard agents (M-BACOD).

J Clin Oncol, 1983; 1: 91-98.

62. SHIPP MA, YEAP BY, HARRINGTON DP et al.

The m-BACOD combination chemotherapy regimen in large-cell lymphoma: analysis of the completed trial and comparison with the M-BACOD regimen.

J Clin Oncol, 1991; 8: 84-93.

63. DE VITA VT, HUBBARD SM, YOUNG RC, LONGO DL

A randomized study of radiotherapy plus chemotherapy in stage I-II non-Hodgkin's lymphomas.

Sem Hematol, 1988; 25 (suppl.2): 2-10.

64. KLIMO O, CONNORS JM

MACOP-B chemotherapy for the treatment of diffuse large-cell lymphoma.

Ann Int Med, 1985; 102: 596-602.

65. COLEMAN M, GERSTEIN G, TOPILOW A et al.

Advances in chemotherapy for large-cell lymphoma.

Sem Hematol, 1987; 24 (suppl.1): 8-20.

66. SCHNEIDER AM, STRAUSS DJ, SCHLUGER AE et al.

Treatment results with an aggressive chemotherapeutic regimen (MACOP-B) for intermediate- and some high-grade non-Hodgkin's lymphomas.

J Clin Oncol, 1990; 8: 94-102.

67. CONNORS JM, KLIMO P

Updated clinical experience with MACOP-B.

Sem Hematol, 1987; 24 (suppl.1): 26-34.

68. EPELBAUM R, FARAGGI D, BEN-ARIE Y et al.

Survival of diffuse large-cell lymphoma A multivariate analysis including dose intensity variables.

Cancer, 1990; 66: 1124-1129.

69. KWAK LW, HALPERN J, OLSHEN RA, HORNING SJ

Prognostic significance of actual dose intensity in diffuse large-cell lymphoma : results of a tree-structured survival analysis.

J Clin Oncol, 1990; 8: 963-977.

70. ZUCKERMAN KS, LOBUGLIO AF, REEVES JA

Chemotherapy of intermediate-grade and high-grade non-Hodgkin's lymphomas with a high-dose doxorubicin-containing regimen.

J Clin Oncol, 1990; 8: 248-256.

71. MEYER RM, HRYNIUK WM, GOODYEAR MDE

The role of dose intensity in determining outcome in intermediate-grade non-Hodgkin's lymphoma.

J Clin Oncol, 1991; 9: 339-347.

72. NISSEN NI, ERSBOLL J, HANSEN HS et al.

A randomized study of radiotherapy versus radiotherapy plus chemotherapy in stage I-II non-Hodgkin's lymphomas.

Cancer, 1983; 52: 1-7.

73. JONES SE, MILLER TP, CONNORS JM

Long-term follow-up and analysis for prognostic factors for patients with limited-stage diffuse large-cell lymphoma treated with initial chemotherapy with or without adjuvant radiotherapy.

J Clin Oncol, 1989; 7: 1186-1191.

74. CABANILLAS F

Chemotherapy as definitive treatment of stage I-II large-cell and diffuse mixed lymphomas.

Hematol Oncol, 1985; 3: 25-31.

75. SONNEVELD P, MICHIELS JJ

Full-dose chemotherapy in elderly patients with non-Hodgkin's lymphoma: a feasibility study using a mitoxantrone-containing regimen.

Brit J Cancer, 1990; 62: 105-108.

76. MAOR MH, VELASQUEZ WS, FULLER LM, SILVERMINTZ KB

Stomach conservation in stages IE and IIE gastric non-Hodgkin's lymphoma.

J Clin Oncol, 1990; 8: 266-271.

77. SALLES G, HERBRECHT R, TILLY H et al.

Aggressive primary gastrointestinal lymphomas. Review of 91 patients treated with the LNH-84 regimen. A study of the Groupe d'Etude des Lymphomes Agressifs.

Amer J Med, 1991; 90: 77-84.

78. BAUMGARTNER JE, RACHLIN JR, BECKSTEAD JH et al.

Primary central nervous system lymphomas. Natural history and response to radiation therapy in 55 patients with acquired immunodeficiency syndrome.

J Neurosurg, 1990; 73: 206-211.

79. BRADA M, DEARNALEY D, HORWICH A, BLOOM HJG

Management of primary cerebral lymphoma with initial chemotherapy: preliminary results and comparison with patients treated with radiotherapy alone.

Intern J Radiat Oncol Biol Phys, 1990; 18: 787-792.

80. COHEN LF, BALOW JE, MACGRATH IT, POPLACK DG, ZIEGLER JL

A review of 37 patients with Burkitt's lymphoma.

Amer J Med, 1980; 68: 486-491.

81. BERMUDEZ MA, GRANT KM, RODVIEN R, MENDES F

Non-Hodgkin's lymphoma in a population with, or at risk for, acquired immunodeficiency syndrome. Indications for intensive chemotherapy.

Amer J Med, 1989; 86: 71-76.

82. SHIPP MA, KLATT MM, YEAP B et al.

Patterns of relapse in large-cell lymphoma patients with bulk disease. Implications for the use of adjuvant radiation therapy.

J Clin Oncol, 1989; 7: 613-618.

83. SUBORNE A, LONGO DL, DE VITA VT et al.

Residual abdominal masses in aggressive non-Hodgkin's lymphoma after combination chemotherapy: significance and management.

J Clin Oncol, 1988; 6: 1832-1837.

84. ARTIMAGE JO, WEISENBURGER DD, HUTCHINS M et al

Chemotherapy for diffuse large-cell lymphoma. Rapidly responding patients have more durable remissions.

J Clin Oncol, 1986; 4: 160-164.

85. CABANILLAS F, PATHAK S, GRANT G et al.

Refractoriness to chemotherapy and poor survival related to abnormalities of chromosome-17 and chromosome-7 in lymphoma.

Amer J Med, 1989; 87: 167-172.

86. YUNIS JJ, MAYER MG, ARNESEN MA, AEPPLI DP, OKEN MM, FRIZZERA G

Bcl-2 and other genomic alterations in the prognosis of large-cell lymphoma.

N Engl J Med, 1989; 320: 1047-1054.

87. DALTON WS, GROGAN TM, MELTZER PS et al.

Drug-resistance in multiple myeloma and non-Hodgkin's lymphoma. Detection of P-glycoprotein and potential circumvention by addition of verapamil to chemotherapy.

J Clin Oncol, 1989; 7: 415-424.

88. MILLER TP, GROGAN TM, DALTON WS, SPIER CM, SCHEPER PJ, SALMON SE

P-glycoprotein expression in malignant lymphoma and reversal of clinical drug resistance with chemotherapy plus high-dose verapamil.

J Clin Oncol, 1991; 9: 17-24.

Intensive chemoradiotherapy and bone-marrow transplantation in non-Hodgkin's lymphomas

A. BOSLY, M. SYMANN

The rationale for high-dose chemotherapy (HDC) and/or radiotherapy rests upon the steep dose/response curve observed for many cytotoxic agents. Experimental studies have shown the efficacy of increasing doses of cyclophosphamide against lymphoma cells transplanted in animals (1) and clinical studies have shown improvement of complete response rates in aggressive NHL with third-generation protocols [MACOP-B (2), LNH-80 (3), LNH-84 (4)] in comparison to the first-generation regimens [CHOP (5)]. In these protocols cyclophosphamide and adriamycin dosages are two to three times higher than in CHOP. Unfortunately, the same chemosensitivity is exhibited by the normal haemopoietic stem cells. Thus, increasing the dosage of chemotherapy eventually results in the killing of all the normal stem cells. Bone-marrow transplantation is thus used to rescue the patient from an otherwise lethal chemotherapy. This transplantation can be allogenic, syngenic or autologous (ABMT). At present, the widest experience with ABMT has been obtained in aggressive lymphomas and will be discussed first. ABMT in follicular lymphomas and allogenic BMT will then be summarized.

Autologous bone marrow transplantation (ABMT) in aggressive lymphomas

When can high-dose chemotherapy with ABMT be clinically useful? Three situations can be considered: as induction treatment, as salvage therapy and as a consolidation regimen in responding patients.

Few reports have been published about ABMT as initial therapy (6,7) but their results are not clearly superior to those achieved with standard induction chemotherapy regimens (2,4). Thus at present there is no reason to use HDC and ABMT as an induction regimen in NHL.

In relapsing patients, the rationale for using HDC + ABMT is the poor long-term prognosis with conventional salvage chemotherapy regimens (8) and the persistent sensitivity of NHL to cytotoxic agents and radiation even in relapse. The first use of ABMT in NHL in relapse was reported by Appelbaum et al., (9) who obtained long-term survival in

TABLE I

ABMT in adult non-Hodgkin's lymphomas in relapse
(recent studies)

Authors	Ref.	Regimen		Total	Toxic early deaths	Survivors NED	Duration (months)
PHILIP (1987) France, USA United Kingdom and Belgium	10	chemo. chemo. + TBI	61 39	100	21	19	21+-75+
PETERSEN (1990) Seattle	11	CY + TBI chemo. + TBI BU + CY	67 22 12	101 (20 HD)	21	28	12+-66+
PHILLIPS (1990) St-Louis	12	CY + TBI		68	14	15	37+-109+
BRAINE (1987) Baltimore	13	CY + TBI		10	1	5	12+-42+$
TAKVORIAN (1987) Boston	14	CY + TBI		49	2	34	2+-52+
GULATI (1988) New York	16	CY + TBI		17	2	4	35+-64+
VERDONCK (1987) Utrecht	17	CY + TBI		8	1	2	3+-14+
COLOMBAT (1990) Tours; Paris	18	chemo. chemo. + TBI	25 4	29	4	13	8+-36+
BOSLY (1990)	19	chemo.	21				
GELA, France and Belgium		chemo. + TBI	7	28	-	9	14+-38+
				410	66(16%)	129(31%)	3+-109+

Abbreviations: chemo. = chemotherapy (other than high-dose cyclophosphamide) ; TBI = total body irradiation; BU = Busulfan; NED = no evidence of disease ; CY = cyclophosphamide; HD = Hodgkin's disease

refractory and relapsing patients with BACT (BCNU-Cytarabine-Cyclophosphamide-Thioguanine) chemotherapy. In this study, Appelbaum showed that ABMT can reduce aplasia duration. *Table I* summarizes recent studies concerning the use of HDC in adults in relapse of NHL. Few patients were resistant to initial therapy. The most frequent conditioning regimen used was the association of cyclophosphamide (120 mg/kg) followed by TBI as usually performed before allo-

genic bone-marrow transplantation. Among 410 patients, early toxic deaths occured in 16%. Thirty-one percent were alive with no evidence of disease with quite a long follow-up, ranging from 3 to 109 months. The largest series has been reported by T. Philip (10). This study, which includes 100 patients, is heterogeneous: patients were treated in 10 different institutions in 4 countries with very different pre-transplantation anti-tumour regimens. For instance, less than half of the

TABLE II

ABMT in adult NHL in first partial remission

Authors	Ref.	Regimen	Total	Toxic deaths	Survivors NED	Duration (months)
PHILIP (1988) Lyon	24	chemo.	17	2	13	8+-82+
GULATI (1988) New York	16	CY + TBI	8	1	6	33+-64+
VERDONCK (1987) Utrecht	17	CY + TBI	5	1	2	18+-56+
BRAINE (1987) Baltimore	13	CY + TBI	4	-	2	6+-22+
COLOMBAT (1990) Tours; Paris	18	chemo. 4 CY + TBI 1	5	-	5	6+-82
			39	4(10%)	28(72%)	median 36+
Abbreviations: see *Table I*						

TABLE III

ABMT in adult NHL in first complete remission

Authors	Ref.	Regimen	Total	Toxic deaths	Survivors NED	Duration (months)
GULATI (1988) New York	16	CY + TBI	6	-	5	31+-59+
VERDONCK (1987) Utrecht	17	CY	7	-	5	3+-59+
COLOMBAT (1990) Tours; Paris	18	chemo. CY + TBI	7 5	12	2	8+-104+
			25	2	18(72%)	median 50+
Abbreviations: see *Table I*						

patients received total body irradiation. However, the main interest of this study is its success in pointing to 3 groups of patients with different outcomes following the high-dose treatment. The best prognosis group comprises patients whose relapse is still sensitive to rescue regimen before intensive therapy. For this group, the 3-year-disease-free survival rate was 36%. The group of relapsing patients whose disease continued to develop during rescue regimen had a poor prognosis: the 3 year-disease-free survival rate was 14%. The worst prognosis group is composed of patients who never achieved response with the induction regimen or with salvage therapy. For this group, the actuarial 3-year disease-free survival rate was zero. Out of 208 NHL patients initially treated with the third-generation protocol (LNH-84) and who failed after treatment (resistance or relapse), 28 were submitted to HDC + ABMT (19). The three-year survival rate after relapse was 30% but was not superior to that of patients who relapsed after LNH-84 and were treated with chemotherapy without ABMT (12%, p = 0.1). However, failure-free survival was longer for transplanted patients than for non-transplanted patients (p = 0.0044) and in Cox's multivariate analysis, bone-marrow transplantation was an independent good prognosis factor for survival and failure-free survival. Nevertheless, patients transplanted in second complete remission (CR) fared no better than ungrafted second-CR patients (p = 0.5). Thus, whether HDC + ABMT improves the prognosis of patients with aggressive NHL in relapse remains unresolved and randomized studies between ABMT and conventional salvage chemotherapy are required. Such a study is in progress in the International PARMA protocol. In this protocol, aggressive-NHL patients in first relapse are treated with salvage DHAP regimen (Dexamethasone, high-dose Cytarabine, Cisplatin) (20). After two courses, CR or partial remission (PR) patients are randomized between two arms; the first includes involved-field radiotherapy (IFR), high-dose chemotherapy BEAC (BCNU-Etoposide-Cytarabine-Cyclophosphamide), and unpurged ABMT, and the second includes continuation of DHAP regimen + IFR (21).

The next step was to use HDC + ABMT in the treatment of NHL patients in PR. In most studies, PR patients have a poor prognosis with a probability of survival of 21% for M-BACOD (22) of 19% for Pro-MACE-MOPP (23). Few reports of ABMT in PR patients have yet been published. *Table II* summarizes recent reports (13,15-17,24). For a total of 39 patients, 72% were alive with no evidence of disease after a median follow-up of 36 months. Obviously, these very impressive results are encouraging.

High-dose chemotherapy in CR patients must be discussed in the light of prognostic factors defined in several studies in NHL (25-26-27). In these studies, two different parameters are of importance. The first is related to the disease (LDH level, histology, bone-marrow involvement, tumoral mass or number of extranodal sites) and the second to the host (age or performance status). For poor-risk patients probability of long-term survival is only between 26 and 40%. In these cases, HDC + ABMT might be beneficial. *Table III* shows three series (15-17) with a total of 25 patients with bulky tumours and/or high LDH serum level treated with HDC + ABMT. Seventy-two percent were in continuous complete remission after a median follow-up of more than 50 months. Gulati's study (15) illustrated the value of HDC + ABMT as a consolidation for poor-prognosis patients responding to induction therapy. Patients submitted to ABMT at consolidation fared better than those who received ABMT at relapse. However, this study is not randomized. One such study is currently being conducted by the French group GELA with the LNH-87 protocol. In this study, patients aged from 15 to 55 years with at least one poor prognosis factor (namely, lymphoblastic or Burkitt-subtype, tumour mass greater than 10 cm, two or more sites of extranodal involvement, poor performance status, bone-marrow or CNS involvement) and in whom a response greater than 75% was achieved after induction treatment are randomized between either a conventional consolidation treatment or an intensive chemotherapy regimen (Cyclophosphamide-BCNU-VP 16) followed by ABMT. This study started in October 1987 and up to now, more than 800 patients have been included in it.

TABLE IV

Allogenic BMT in non-Hodgkin's lymphomas

Authors	Ref.	Regimen	Total	Survivors	Duration (months)
IN RELAPSE					
APPELBAUM (1987) Seattle	34	CY + TBI	49	12	12-36+
ERNST (1987) EB	35	CY + TBI	37	15	7+
			86	27 (31%)	
IN COMPLETE REMISSION					
ERNST (1987) EBMT	35	CY + TBI	31	23	7+
Abbreviations: see table I EBMT = European Bone-Marrow Transplantation Group					

ABMT in follicular lymphomas

Despite their indolent course over many years, follicular lymphomas (FL) have a worse prognosis at twenty years, with only 26% of patients surviving (28). Moreover, patients with initial adverse prognosis factors (large tumoral mass or B symptoms) or who respond poorly to therapy, or even in whom histological transformation occurs, have a poorer prognosis (28,29). Classical treatments (such as radiotherapy and/or chemotherapy at conventional dosages) do not influence natural disease history (30). In FL patients of young age, HDC + ABMT is therefore an attractive approach.

Few studies document the feasibility of this approach (31,32). In the Nebraska study (32) outcome in 18 FL patients depended on the presence or absence of histological transformation at the time of ABMT and thus the outcome of patients with FL was better for patients transplanted early in the course of their illness. In the Dana Farber study 69 patients with low-grade NHL have been reported. They were treated with cyclophosphamide + TBI and ABMT purged with one or several monoclonal anti-B antibodies. The 2-year disease-free survival is 53% for patients with untransformed low-grade NHL. Only PR versus CR at ABMT was significantly associated with adverse DFS (15).

If HDC + ABMT in FL is to be considered in young patients, the best time to give this treatment is still unknown (after CR, or relapse, or in cases of resistance or histological transformation).

Allogenic bone-marrow transplantation (BMT) in lymphomas

If the use of ABMT obviates the need for an HLA-matched donor and post-transplant immunosuppressive therapy as well as the risk of graft-versus-host disease, allogenic BMT eliminates the potential risk of reinfusion of tumour cells and also perhaps involves a graft-versus-tumour effect (33).

BMT in lymphomas have been reported by the Seattle group (34) and the European Bone-Marrow Transplantation group (35) (*Table IV*). Results of BMT after relapse are very similar (30% continous complete response) to those of ABMT. In the same centre (34), the source of marrow (syngenic, allogenic or autologous) was not found to significantly influence disease-free survival. However, in a series of BMT of 118 patients with NHL and Hodgkin's disease, the relapse rate after BMT for sensitive relapse was only 18% after allogenic BMT compared with 46% after autologous BMT.

Thus allogenic BMT induces a clinically significant graft-versus-lymphoma effect but beneficial anti-tumour effect was offset by higher transplant-related toxicity and survival was not improved (47).

Unresolved issues in marrow transplantation for NHL

To define the precise usefulness of ABMT in NHL, three major issues have to be resolved. The first is the role of purging of residual tumour cells in bone-marrow. If we assume that 10^{10} nucleated marrow cells are needed to achieve a full haematopoietic reconstitution and that this marrow is contaminated with one tumour cell out of 10^3 (a contamination that obviously does escape the best of pathologists), we ultimately reinfuse 10^6 tumour cells. Of course, the biological significance of this is not known, but recent reports (36) of leukaemia occurring after high-dose chemotherapy with autologous bone-marrow transplantation in Burkitt-type lymphomas illustrate the potential danger of bone-marrow contamination. The most extensive study of bone-marrow purging in malignant lymphoma has been reported by Takvorian et al. in 49 B1-positive NHL patients treated with chemoradiotherapy and ABMP purged with anti-B1 monoclonal antibody (14). Sixteen patients had bone-marrow involvement of up to 5% by lymphoma cells. Probability of relapse-free survival of these 16 patients is no different from that of the 33 patients with normal bone marrow. Thus, this important study suggested that purging bone mar-

row of tumour cells may indeed be of clinical relevance. Moreover, the same team reported results of immunological purging performed in 114 patients with B-cell non-Hodgkin's lymphoma. In 57 patients no lymphoma cells could be detected after purging. These patients had an increase in disease-free-survival in comparison with those whose marrow contained detectable residual lymphoma cells. These results provide evidence of the clinical usefulness of *ex vivo* purging of autologous bone-marrow (48).

The second unresolved problem is the optimal conditioning regimen. Even though the classical association of Cyclophosphamide + TBI has been the most widely used, there is no convincing evidence in favour of combining radiotherapy with chemotherapy versus chemotherapy alone. In the European survey conducted by Tony Goldstone, no difference was observed in the response rate or in survival between patients conditioned with chemotherapy alone or with chemotherapy + TBI (31). However, analysis of the progression site in transplanted patients (10) showed that 76% of relapses occurred in the initial tumour site. Local disease control is a major factor and involved-field radiotherapy with chemotherapy followed by BMT seems to be the best strategy.

Finally, the most recent question is about the role of haemopoietic growth factors such as GM-CSF or G-CSF after ABMT.

The use of CSFs in the acceleration of haemopoietic reconstitution after bone-marrow transplantation offers the prospect of substantially reduced mortality and morbidity, as well as lowering the expense of high-dose therapy. The straightforward work of Sheridan et al. (38) shows that administration of G-CSF shortens the period of neutropenia after high-dose busulphan and cyclophosphamide and ABMT. Points of particular interest are the significant reduction of days of parenteral antibiotic therapy, of isolation in reverse-barrier nursing and in the length of the hospital stay. Mucositis was also significantly reduced. Comparable to this study are the investigations of Brandt et al. (39) and Nemunaitis et al. (40), where patients received dose-intensive chemotherapy followed by ABMT and then GM-CSF. Only one of these two phase I/II dose-escalation studies reported significant shortening of time to > 500 neutrophils/µl in patients receiving > 60 µg/m^2/day GM-CSF compared to historical controls. Three interesting features distinguish the study by Sheridan et al. (38). First, an optimal dose of G-CSF (20 µg/kd) was administered to all patients as opposed to the phase I studies, where some patients received too little CSF and others presumably too high a dose. Second, the G-CSF was administered as a continuous subcutaneous infusion which may be better than short i.v. infusion. Third, once the granulocyte count exceeded 10^9/l, the dose of G-CSF was reduced using a carefully devised sliding scale allowing treatment on an out-patient basis. Taken together, these studies strongly suggest that CSF have a biological activity in marrow transplantation and shorten the duration of neutropenia. Whether this will translate into a decrease in early mortality has not yet been established. Larger prospective, placebo-controlled, randomized phase III trials are under way to define more precisely the therapeutic and economic advantages offered by CSF.

Results (41,49) of two randomized trials showed clinical and biological benefits of GM-CSF use after ABMT in lymphoid malignancies and no adverse long-term consequence of treatment with GM-CSF on disease evolution (41).

Other haemopoietic growth factors such as Interleukin-2 may play a role in immunoreconstitution and in immunotherapy against residual disease. In the first Rosenberg reports, the few lymphoma patients treated with IL-2 + LAK cells responded to the therapy (42). The use of IL-2 after ABMT in leukaemic or lymphoma patients (43,44) is feasible and may be of benefit in reducing relapse rate.

Many unanswered questions regarding BMT in patients with lymphoma are an incentive to design clinical trials in this area (45).

References

1. FREI E, CANNELLOS GP
   Dose: a critical factor in cancer chemotherapy.
   Am J Med, 1980; 69: 585-594.

2. KLIMO P, CONNORS JM
   MACOP-B chemotherapy for the treatment of diffuse large-cell lymphomas.
   Ann Intern Med, 1985; 102: 596-602.

3. COIFFIER B, BRYON P, BERGER F et al.
   Intensive and sequential combination chemotherapy for aggressive malignant lymphomas (Protocol LNH 80).
   J Clin Oncol, 1986; 4: 147-153.

4. COIFFIER B, GISSELBRECHT C, TILLY H, HERBRECHT R, BOSLY A, BROUSSE N
   LNH 84 intensive chemotherapy for aggressive lymphomas.
   J Clin Oncol, 1989; 7: 1018-1026.

5. ARMITAGE JO, DICK FR, CORDER MP, GARCEAU SC, PLATZ CE, SLYMAN DJ
   Predicting therapeutic outcome in patients with diffuse histiocytic lymphoma treated with cyclophosphamide, adriamycin, vincristine and prednisone (CHOP).
   Cancer, 1982; 50: 1695-1702.

6. GORIN NC, NAJMAN A, DOUAY L et al.
   Autologous bone-marrow transplantation in the treatment of poor-prognosis non-Hodgkin's lymphomas.
   Eur J Cancer, 1984; 20: 217-225.

7. TURA S, MAZZA P, GHARLIZONI F et al.
   High-dose therapy followed by autologous bone-marrow transplantation (ABMT) in previously untreated non-Hodgkin's lymphomas.
   Scan J Hematol, 1986; 37: 347-352.

8. CABANILLAS F, HAGEMEISTER FB, McLAUGHLIN P. et al.
   MIME combination chemotherapy for refractory or recurrent lymphomas.
   J Clin Oncol, 1987; 5: 407-415.

9. APPELBAUM FR, HERZIG GP, ZIEGLER JL, GRAN RG, LEVINE AS, DEISSEROTH AB
   Successful engraftment of cryopreserved autologous bone-marrow in patients with malignant lymphoma.
   Blood, 1978; 52: 85-95.

10. PHILIP T, ARMITAGE JO, SPITZER G et al.
    High-dose therapy and autologous bone-marrow transplantion after failure of conventional chemotherapy in adults with intermediate-grade or high-grade non-Hodgkin's lymphoma.
    N Engl J Med, 1987; 316: 1493-1498

11. PETERSEN FB, APPELBAUM FR, HILL R et al.
    Autologous bone-marrow transplantation for malignant lymphoma. A report of 101 cases from Seattle.
    J Clin Oncol, 1990; 8: 638-647.

12. PHILIPS GL, FAY JW, HERZIG RH et al.

   The treatment of progressive non-Hodgkin's lymphoma with intensive chemo-radiotherapy and autologous marrow transplantation.

   Blood, 1990; 75: 831-838.

13. BRAINE HG, SANTOS GW, KAIZER H et al.

   Treatment of poor prognosis non-Hodgkin's lymphoma using cyclophosphamide and total body irradiation regimens with autologous bone-marrow rescue.

   Bone Marrow Transplant, 1987; 2: 7-14.

14. TAKVORIAN T, CANELLOS GP, RITZ J et al.

   Prolonged disease-free survival after autologous bone-marrow transplantation in patients with non-Hodgkin's lymphoma with a poor prognosis.

   N Engl J Med, 1987; 316: 1499-1505.

15. FREEDMAN AS, RITZ J, NEUBERG D et al.

   Autologous bone-marrow transplantation in 69 patients with a history of low-grade B-cell non-Hodgkin's lymphoma.

   Blood 1991, 77, 2524-2529.

16. GULATI SC, SHANK B, BLACK P et al.

   Autologous bone-marrow transplantation for patients with poor-prognosis lymphoma.

   J Clin Oncol, 1988; 6: 1303-1313.

17. VERDONCK LF, DEKKER AW, VENDRIK PJ et al.

   Intensive cytoreductive therapy followed by autologous bone marrow transplantation for patients with hematologic malignancies or solid tumors.

   Cancer, 1987; 60: 289-294.

18. COLOMBAT P, GORIN NC, LEMONNIER MP et al.

   The role of autologous bone marrow transplantation in 46 adult patients with non-Hodgkin's lymphomas.

   J Clin Oncol, 1990; 8: 630-637.

19. BOSLY A, COIFFIER B, LEPAGE E et al.

   Aggressive non-Hodgkin's lymphomas (NHL) in failure after treatment with LNH 84 protocol. Evolution and prognosis factors in 208 patients (abst).

   4th International Conference on Malignant Lymphoma. Lugano, 1990.

20. VELASQUEZ WS, CABANILLAS F, SALVADOR P et al.

   Effective salvage therapy for lymphoma with cisplatin in combination with high-dose Ara-C and dexamethason (DHAP).

   Blood, 1988; 71: 117-122.

21. PHILIP T, CHAUVIN F, ARMITAGE J et al.

   Parma International protocol; pilot study of DHAP followed by involved-field radiotherapy and BEAC with autologous bone marrow transplantation.

   Blood 1991; 77: 1587-1592.

22. SKARIN AT, CANNELLOS GP, ROSENTHAL DS et al.

   Improved prognosis of diffuse histiocytic and undifferentiated lymphoma by use of high-dose methotrexate alternating with standard agents (M-BACOD).

   J Clin Oncol, 1983; 1: 191-198.

23. FISHER RI, DE VITA VT, HUBBARD SM et al.

   Diffuse aggressive lymphomas: increased survival after flexible sequences of Pro-MACE and MOPP chemotherapy.

   Ann Intern Med, 1988; 98: 304-309.

24. PHILIP T, HARTMAN O, BIRON P et al.

   High-dose therapy and autologous bone-marrow transplantation in partial remission after first line induction therapy for diffuse non-Hodgkin's lymphoma.

   J Clin Oncol, 1988; 6: 1118-1125.

25. SHIPP MA, HARRINGTON DP, KLATT MM et al.

   Identification of major prognostic subgroups of patients with large-cell lymphoma treated with m-BACOD or M-BACOD.

   Ann Intern Med, 1986; 104: 757-762.

26. COIFFIER B, BRYON PA, FFRENCH M et al.

   Intensive chemotherapy in aggressive lymphomas : updated results of LNH 80 protocol and prognostic factors affecting response and survival.

   Blood, 1987; 70: 1394-1399.

27. COIFFIER B, LEPAGE E

   Prognosis of aggressive lymphomas. A study of five prognostic models with patients included in the LNH 84 regimen.

   Blood, 1989; 74: 558-563.

28. GALLAGHER GJ, LISTER TA

   Follicular non-Hodgkin's lymphoma.

   Baillière's Clinical Haematology, 1987; 1: 141-155.

29. ROSENBERG SA

   The low-grade non-Hodgkin's lymphomas: challenges and opportunities.

   J Clin Oncol, 1985; 3: 299-310.

30. HORNING SJ, ROSENBERG SA

   The natural history of initially untreated low grade non-Hodgkin's lymphomas.

   N Engl J Med, 1984; 311: 1471-1475.

31. ROHATINER AZ, PRICE CG, ARNOTT S et al.

   Myeloablative therapy with autologous bone-marrow transplantation as consolidation of remission in patients with follicular lymphoma.

   Ann Oncol. 1991; 2 suppl 2: 147-150.

32. SCHOUTEN HC, BIERMAN PJ, VAUGHAN WP et al.

   Autologous bone-marrow transplantation in follicular non-Hodgkin's lymphoma before and after histologic transformation.

   Blood, 1989; 74: 2579-2584.

33. WILLIAMS SF, SCHILSKY RL, ULTMANN JE, SAMUELS BL

The role of high-dose therapy and autologous bone-marrow reinfusion in the treatment of malignant lymphomas.

Cancer Invest, 1988; 6: 427-437.

34. APPELBAUM FR, SULLIVAN KM, BUCKNER CD et al.

Treatment of malignant lymphoma in 100 patients with chemotherapy, total body irradiation, and marrow transplantation.

J Clin Oncol, 1987; 5: 1340-1347.

35. CANELLOS GP, ARMITAGE J, ERNST P et al.

Bone-marrow transplantation in malignant lymphoma.

Hematol Oncol, 1987; 5: 295-298.

36. VAUGHAN WP, WEISENBURGER DD, SANGER W, GALE RP, ARMITAGE JO

Early leukemic recurrence of non-Hodgkin lymphoma after high-dose anti-neoplastic therapy with autologous marrow rescue.

Bone Marrow Transplant, 1987; 1: 373.

37. GOLDSTONE AH

EBMT experience of autologous bone-marrow transplantation in non-Hodgkin's lymphoma and Hodgkin's disease.

Bone Marrow Transplant, 1986; 1: 289-292.

38. SHERIDAN WP, MORSTYN G, WOLF M et al.

Effects of granulocyte colony stimulating factor (G-CSF) following high dose chemotherapy and autologous bone-marrow transplantation.

Lancet, 1989; 2: 891-895.

39. BRANDT SJ, PETERS WP, ATWATER SK et al.

Effect of recombinant human granulocyte-macrophage colony-stimulating factor on hematopoietic reconstitution after high-dose chemotherapy and autologous bone-marrow transplantation.

N Engl J Med, 1988; 318: 869-876.

40. NEMUNAITIS J, SINGER JW, BUCKNER CD et al.

Use of recombinant human granulocyte-macrophage colony-stimulating factor in autologous marrow transplantation for lymphoid malignancies.

Blood, 1988; 72: 834-836.

41. NEMUNAITIS J, SINGER JW, BUCKNER CD et al.

Long-term follow-up of patients who received recombinant human granulocyte macrophage colony-stimulating factor after autologous bone-marrow transplantation for lymphoid malignancies.

Asco proc, 1990; 34.

42. ROSENBERG SA, LOTZE MT, MUU LM et al.

Observations on the systemic administration of autologous lymphokine-activated killer cells and recombinant Interleukin-2 to patients with cancer.

N Engl J Med, 1985; 313: 1485-1493.

43. HIGUCHI CM, THOMPSON JA, PETERSEN FB, BUCKNER CD and FEFER A.

Toxicity and immunomodulatory effects of Interleukin-2 after autologous bone-marrow transplantation for hematologic malignancies.

Blood, 1991; 77: 2561-2568.

44. BOSLY A, BRICE P, HUMBLET Y, DOYEN C et al.

Interleukin-2 after autologous bone-marrow transplantation as consolidative immunotherapy against minimal residual disease.

Nouv Rev Fr Hematol, 1990; 32: 13-16.

45. ARMITAGE JO

Bone-marrow transplantation in the treatment of patients with lymphoma.

Blood, 1989; 73: 1749-1758.

46. HAIOUN C, LEPAGE E, GISSELBRECHT C et al.

Autologous bone-marrow transplantation (ABMT) versus sequential chemotherapy in first complete remission aggressive non-Hodgkin's lymphoma (NHL). 1st interim analysis of the LNH 87 protocol (A bst)

ASCO proceedings 1992, in press.

47. JONES RJ, AMBINDER RF, PIANTADOSI S et al.

Evidence of a graft-versus-lymphoma effect associated with allogenic bone-marrow transplantation.

Blood 1991; 77: 649-653.

48. GRIBBEN JG, FREEDMAN AS, NEUBERG D et al.

Immunologic purging of marrow assessed by PCR before autologous bone-marrow transplantation for B-cell lymphoma.

N Enge J Med 1991; 325: 1525-1533.

49. GORIN NC, COIFFIER B, HAYAT M et al.

Rhu GMCSF shortens aplasia duration after ABMT in non-Hodgkin's lymphoma: a randomized placebo-controlled double-blind study.

Bone Marrow Transplant 1991; 7: suppl 2,82.

Salvage therapy in aggressive non-Hodgkin's lymphomas after failure

A. BOSLY

One of the major successes of cancer therapy during the last two decades has been the development of curative therapies for advanced-stage aggressive lymphomas.

Third-generation protocols can now achieve a cure rate of more than 50% (1,2). However, patients who were resistant to initial therapy (c. 10%) or who were in relapse after complete response (c. 25%) have an extremely poor prognosis and the probability of freedom-from-progression survival at 10 years is less than 10% (3).

It should be possible to achieve improvements on these poor results through either new agents or new therapeutic approaches.

A current, more appropriate approach to achieve a significant cure rate in failed patients is chemotherapy at very high dose (IC) associated or not with radiotherapy and followed by bone-marrow rescue (BMT) (4). This concept and clinical results are discussed *on pp. 361-369.*

However, long-term results of IC + BMT are better if an effective salvage therapy is given before IC (5). On the other hand, many patients are not eligible for IC because of age, general conditions, poor performance status or bone-marrow involvement. For these patients too, the best salvage treatment must be determined.

The most widely used combination regimen was based on the association of ifosfamide, VP16 and methotrexate, with or without AMSA or Methyl-GAG. In the MD Anderson Hospital experience, objective response rate with MIME (5) was 60% with a CR rate of 24%.

Recent reports from European Groups using the same combinations showed either the same results (6,7) or lower response rates (8).

Mitoxantrone is an anthracenedione which shows structural similarities to doxorubicin. In phase II trials, mitoxantrone showed a high response rate and low toxicity profile in heavily pre-treated patients. In 122 accessable patients, an overall response of 40% with 8% CR and 32% PR was observed with mitoxantrone alone (9). In combination with Ara-C, VP16-platinum or ifosfami-de-VP16, mitoxantrone exhibited a high complete response rate ranging from 26 to 67% (10).

A third type of salvage combination therapy was constructed on the combination of high-dose Ara C, platinum and steroids (DHAP) (11) or the same association plus etoposide (ESAP) (12). These regimens also used in the MD Anderson Hospital in 191 relapsing patients showed high overall (57%) and complete (30%) response rates.

A comparison between the three major types of salvage regimens (ifosfamide-VP16, mitoxantrone, AraC-platinum) is difficult because of the heterogeneity of induction regimens before failure.

We have reviewed (13) 244 patients initially treated with a 3rd-generation protocol

(LNH-84 regimen) and who were in failure, either in relapse after first CR (160 patients), or in first progression either after CR or after no initial response (84 patients) and were retreated. Prognosis of these patients after failure was poor. Median survival was 7 months, median freedom- from-progression (FFP) survival was 4 months and median freedom-from-relapse survival for second CR was 16 months.

The 4-year estimated survival rate was 16% for overall survival and 8% for FFP survival. A second CR was observed in 23% and a second PR in 35%. Probability of survival was no different if the salvage regimen was a combination with ifosfamide-VP16 (I), with mitoxantrone (M) or with Ara C (A) (24 to 28%), but was better than salvage regimen with doxorubicin (12%). In contrast with I, M or A, doxorubicin was given during the induction therapy.

In accordance with these results, patients ineligible for the LNH-87 regimen were treated with the combination of mitoxantrone, ifosfamide and VP16 (14). 52 patients are now assessable: 42% have achieved a CR and 18% a PR. Ten of the 22 complete responders relapsed within 2 to 15 months and 12 are still in CR after 2 to 20 months.

These data confirm a high response rate at relapse but also demonstrate that only a small fraction of patients with aggressive lymphoma can be cured by conventional salvage regimen after relapse. Improving these results remains a great challenge.

References

1. COIFFIER B, GISSELBRECHT C, HERBRECHT R, TILLY H, BOSLY A, BROUSSE N
   LNH 84 regimen: a multicenter study of intensive chemotherapy in 737 patients with aggressive malignant lymphoma.
   J Clin Oncol, 1989; 7: 1018-1026.

2. KLIMO P, CONNORS JM
   MACOP-B: chemotherapy for the treatment of diffuse large-cell lymphoma.
   Ann Intern Med, 1985; 102: 596-602.

3. SINGER CRJ, GOLDSTONE PH
   Clinical studies of ABMT in non-Hodgkin's lymphoma.
   Clinics in Haematology, 1986 ; 15 : 105-150.

4. PHILIP T, ARMITAGE JO, SPITZER G et al.
   High-dose therapy and autologous bone-marrow transplantation after failure of conventional chemotherapy in adults with intermediate-grade or high-grade non-Hodgkin's lymphoma.
   N Engl J Med, 1987; 316: 1493-1498.

5. CABANILLAS F, HAGEMEISTER FB, McLAUGHLIN P, SALVADOR P, VELASQUEZ WS, RIGGS S, FREIREICH EJ
   Results of MIME salvage regimen for recurrent or refractory lymphoma.
   J Clin Oncol, 1987; 5: 407-412.

6. HERBRECHT R, GARCIA JJ, BERGERAT JP, DUFOUR P, DUCLOS B, OBERLING F
   VP-16, Ifosfamide and Methotrexate combination chemotherapy for aggresive non-Hodgkin's lymphomas after failure of LNH 84 regimen.
   Cancer Chemother Pharmacol, 1989; 24: 338-339.

7. HUIJGENS PC, OSSENKOPPELE GJ, VAN DER LELIE J, THOMAS LLM, WIJNGAARDEN MJ, REIJNEKE RMR
   Ifosfamide and VP 16-213 combination chemotherapy combined with ablative chemotherapy and autologous marrow transplantation as salvage treat-ment for malignant lymphoma.
   Eur J Cancer Clin Oncol, 1988; 24: 483-486.

8. SANGSTER G, PATTON WN, HARRIS RI, GRIEVE RJ, LEYLAND ML
   Treatment of refractory and relapsed non-Hodgkin's lymphoma with Ifosfamide, Methotrexate and Etoposide.
   Cancer Chemother Pharmacol, 1989; 23: 263-265.

9. CASE DC, GAMS RA, JONES SE, STEIN RS, SILVER RA, STUART JJ, DUKART G
   Report of a multicenter phase III trial of Novantrone for non-Hodgkin's lymphoma. Update on treatment for diffuse large-cell lymphoma.
   In: Skarin ed. Wiley and Sons, 1986: 91-96.

10. Data on File Lederle Laboratories.

11. VELASQUEZ WS, CABANILLAS F, SALVADOR P
    Effective salvage therapy for lymphoma with Cisplatin in combination with high-dose Ara C and Dexamethasone (DHAP).
    Blood, 1988; 71: 117-122.

12. VELASQUEZ WS, SWANN F, REDMAN J, et al.
    Combination of Etoposide, high-dose Ara C and Solumedrol with or without platinol in relapsing or recurrent lymphoma (abst.).
    Proc. ASCO, 1989: 256.

13. BOSLY A, COIFFIER B, GISSELBRECHT C et al.
    Bone-marrow transplantation significantly prolongs survival after relapse in aggressive lymphoma patients treated with the LNH-84 regimen.
    1991, submitted.

14. HERBRECHT R, COIFFIER B, TILLY H et al.
    Mitoxantrone, Ifosfamide and Etoposide (MIV) in aggressive lymphomas failing after treatment with the LNH 87 regimen.
    ASCO proceedings, Abstract 968.

Treatment of non-Hodgkin's lymphomas in children

C. GISSELBRECHT, C. PATTE

Before 1975, the course of childhood NHL was often fatal, with less than 30% of children surviving 5 years after diagnosis. Most of these long-living patients had a localized stage and could be cured by surgery and radiotherapy. The other patients died from absence of local control, as well as bone-marrow or central nervous system relapse.

Major advances in the management of lymphomas have been the result of development of aggressive multi-agent chemotherapy so that more than 70% of children with this disease are now considered curable.

Surgery no longer has a therapeutic role. It may be useful for initial diagnosis or for histological study of a mass persisting after treatment (1,2). Radiotherapy of the tumour masses present at diagnosis is also no longer indicated, even in localized disease (3,4). Only CNS radiation treatment may be proposed in patients with meningeal involvement.

Systemic chemotherapy is indicated for all patients with childhood NHL, even in limited-stage diseases. In the seventies, the treatment was the same whatever the histological type and relied on systemic chemotherapy with meningeal prophylaxis by intrathecal methotrexate (MTX) and CNS irradiation. From the relevant studies (3-9), the following conclusions may be drawn:

(a) Complete remission (CR) rates ranged from 85 to 95%.

(b) Despite prophylaxis, CNS relapses occurred in 7 to 15% of patients.

(c) Cure rates were 70 to 85% in localized forms, but only 30 to 50% in disseminated disease.

(d) Furthermore, the results were different depending upon the immunohistological type.

(e) Intensive and discontinuous regimens such as COMP (7) or COPAD (3,5) gave the best results in B-cell NHL, whereas long and continuous regimens, similar to those used in acute leukaemias, such as LSA2-L2 (7,8) or BFM (6), yielded the best results in T-cell lymphoblastic lymphomas. For example, in a randomized study, 2-year survival in patients treated with COMP or LSA2-L2 showed (7) was:

- 76% for LSA2-L2 vs. 26% for COMP in lymphoblastic NHL;

- 57% for COMP vs. 28% for LSA2-L2 in non-lymphoblastic disseminated NHL.

(f) Relapses occurred early in children with B-cell NHL (before 1 year) but could occur later in lymphoblastic NHL (up to 4 years).

(g) High-dose MTX is active in patients with systemic and/or CNS disease (10).

(h) Relapsing patients may be cured by an intensive chemotherapy followed by autologous bone-marrow transplantation (11,12).

Current therapeutic modalities of childhood NHL are based on these conclusions.

Treatment of disseminated lymphoblastic NHL

The treatment begins with of intensive chemotherapy similar to the treatment of high-risk childhood acute lymphoblastic leukaemias.

Two regimens are most often used with similar results:

– The LSA2-L2 regimen, initially described by Wollner (8) and subsequently modified by adjunction of CNS irradiation (13) or high-dose methotrexate (14) to improve the efficacy of CNS prophylaxis with intrathecal MTX.

In a group of 33 stage III and 43 stage IV patients so-treated from the Institut Gustave - Roussy, the long-term survival was 79% and 72% (14) respectively.

– The BFM regimen (6) is used in several European centres. In the initial report (1979), the survival rate was 78% in 43 stage III or stage IV patients. Subsequent results (1981 and 1983) showed a 79% rate among 33 patients.

The results of other series are reported in *Table I*.

Treatment of disseminated Burkitt's lymphoma

Cyclophosphamide, vincristine, doxorubicin, prednisone and intermediate- or high-dose methotrexate are the most important drugs in regimens for non-lymphoblastic NHL. Cytarabine and teniposide are also active.

The Société Française d'Oncologie Pédiatrique (SFOP, French Society for Paediatric Oncology) has recently developed several regimens (termed LMB regimens) for B-cell lymphomas and leukaemias.

(a) Intensive chemotherapy is preceded by a low-dose COP chemotherapy cycle which allows metabolic complications to be cured before the occurrence of marrow aplasia.

(b) Intensive chemotherapy includes 2 cycles of COPAD-M (high-dose cyclophosphamide, vincristine, adriamycin, high-dose methotrexate, prednisone).

(c) Consolidation relies on continuously administered cytarabine.

(d) High-dose systemic and intrathecal methotrexate are used for CNS prophylaxis.

The first protocol (LMB 81) gave a 75% cure rate in stage III patients and 54% in stage IV among 114 patients (20). These good results did not worsen when the duration of chemotherapy was decreased to 4 months (protocol LMB 84) (21).

In these studies, initial bone-marrow involvement was were no longer associated with a bad prognosis (20). High-dose methotrexate helps prevent CNS involvement (risk less than 3%). Nevertheless, CNS involvement at diagnosis is still associated with a bad prognosis. Thus, patients with CNS involvement are treated at present with very high- dose methotrexate (8 g/m^2) and cytarabine administered continuously and by intermittent high-dose. The results of this study, called LMB 86, are encouraging, with actuarial survival of 75% in 24 patients (23).

The degree of remission at the end of induction may be difficult to assess when there is a persisting mass. In approximately 2/3 of cases, surgical removal shows a non-tumoral fibronecrotic mass (2) and complete remission may be obtained. If the response is only partial, a cure may nevertheless be obtained by intensification of chemotherapy and autologous bone-marrow transplantation (24).

Studies in Germany using the BFM protocol - either as initially developed or with its subsequent modifications - gave similar results. Studies performed in the years 1981-1983 showed a 73% survival rate in 75 stage III patients, a 57% rate in 15 stage IV patients, and 45% in 46 patients with a leukaemic form (more than 25 % of blast cells in the bone marrow) (6).

These studies are reported in *Table II* together with others including lower numbers of patients.

TABLE I

Chemotherapy regimens in childhood lymphoblastic NHL

Authors (ref.)	Regimen	Patient numbers	Stage	CR (%)	Event-free survival %
Wollner (8)	LSA2-L2	9	III	88	88 (DFS)
Sullivan (9)	LSA2-L2 modified	24	III	96	55 (FFS)
Anderson (7)	LSA2-L2 modified	31	III-IV	-	76 (FFS)
Patte (14)	LSA2-L2 + HD MTX	33 43	III IV	94 98	79 (FFS) 72 (FFS)
Muller (6)	BFM	42	III-IV	-	78 (FFS)
Dahl (16)	X-H	22	III-IV	96	73 (DFS)
Weinstein (17)	APO	21	III-IV	95	58 (DFS)
Anderson (7)	COMP	24	III-IV	-	26 (FFS)
Magrath (18)	77-04	10	III	100	70 (FFS)
Hvizdala (19)	A-COP	33	III	-	54 (DFS)
Abbreviations : DFS: Disease-free-survival FFS: Failure-free-survival					

TABLE II

Chemotherapy regimens in disseminated B-cell lymphomas of childhood

Authors	Regimen	Stage	Patient numbers	Event-free survival (%)
Anderson (7)	COMP	III-IV	38	57
Magrath (18)	NCI7704	III IV	30 9	57 13
Murphy (15)	Total B	III IV + LAL-B	38 12	81 17
Muller (6)	BFM81/83	III IV	73 15	75 57
Patte (21,22)	LMB0281 LMB84	III IV + LAL-B III IV + LAL-B	72 42 167 34	73 48 80 68
Sullivan (23)	HD-CPM HD-MTX	III	12	66

Treatment of non-Burkitt B-cell NHL

These histological subtypes - most often diffuse large-cell NHL - are not usually distinguished from Burkitt's lymphoma. When these patients are treated with regimens proposed for non-lymphoblastic NHL, their prognosis is similarly good. The results in these patients of regimens for adult aggressive NHL are not known.

Localized disease

The prognosis of localized forms is excellent, with cure rates higher than 85%. Therefore, there is at present a tendency to decrease the intensity of treatment, especially of CNS prophylaxis.

Conclusion

Progress in the treatment of childhood NHL has been impressive, allowing 70 to 80% of patients to be cured. Several problems have still to be resolved, namely how to:

- find other prognostic parameters (cytogenetics, markers, etc.) which should allow the intensity of treatment to be decreased for the nost favourable forms and increased early for the most aggressive forms;

- prevent some complications, especially sterility in boys (26); and

- decrease the infection rate in patients treated with the most intensive regimens using haemopoietic growth factors.

These improvements will be achieved more quickly if children are treated in specialized centres with multicentre cooperative protocols.

References

1. WAKIM A, HELARDOT PG, SAPIN E
The surgeon facing malignant non-Hodgkin's lymphoma of the abdomen in children.
Chir Pediatr, 1989; 30 (5): 197-200.

2. HELARDOT PG, WAKIM A, KALIFA C, LECLERE J, LACOMBE MJ, PATTE C
The place of surgery in the remission assessment of childhood abdominal malignant non-Hodgkin's lymphoma (NHL).
Med Ped Oncol, 1989; 17: 322 A.

3. PATTE C, RODARY C, SARRAZIN D, BERNARD A, LEMERLE J
Résultats du traitement de 178 lymphomes malins non hodgkiniens de l'enfant de 1973 à 1978.
Arch Fr Ped, 1981; 38: 321-327.

4. LINK MP, DONALDSON SS, BERARD CW, SHUSTER JJ, MURPHY SB
Results of treatment of childhood localized non-Hodgkin's lymphoma with combination chemotherapy with or without radiotherapy.
N Engl J Med, 1990; 322: 1769-1774.

5. LEMERLE J, BERNARD A, PATTE C, PLO JK
Malignant B-cell lymphoma of childhood.
In: Cancer in children, Clinical Management published by Barrett A, Bloom HJG, Lemerle J et al. Eds. UICC Handbook, Springer, 1986: pp. 137-151.

6. MULLER-WEIHRICH SE, HENZE G, ODENWALD E, RIEHM H
BFM trials for childhood non-Hodgkin's lymphoma.
In: Malignant lymphomas and Hodgkin's disease, Cavalli F, Bonadonna G, Rosencweig G Eds. Experimental and therapeutic advances. Boston, Martinus Nijhoff, 1985: pp. 633-642.

7. ANDERSON JR, WILSON JF, JENKIN DT, MEADOWS AT, KERSEY J, CHILCOTE RR, COCCIA P, EXELBY P, KUSHNER J, SIEGAL S, HAMMOND D
Childhood non-Hodgkin's lymphomas: results of a randomised therapeutic trial comparing a 4-drug regimen (COMP) to a 10-drug regimen (LSA2-L2).
N Engl J Med, 1983; 308: 559-565.

8. WOLLNER N, EXELBY PR, LIEBERMAN PH
Non-Hodgkin's lymphoma in children. A progress report on the original patients treated with the LSA2-L2 protocol.
Cancer, 1979; 44: 1990-1999.

9. SULLIVAN M, BOYETT J, PULLEN J, CRIST W, DOERNING EJ, TRUEWORTHY R, HVIZDALA E, RUYMANN F, STEUBER CP
Pediatric oncology group experience with modified LSA2L2 therapy in 107 children with non Hodgkin's lymphoma (Burkitt's lymphoma excluded).
Cancer, 1985; 55: 323-336

10. PATTE C, BERNARD A, HARMANN O, KALIFA C, FLAMANT F, LEMERLE J
High-dose methotrexate and continous infusion Ara-C in children's non-Hodgkin's lymphoma.
Pediatr Hematol Oncol, 1986; 3: 11-18.

11. PHILIP T, BIRON P, HERVE P
Massive BACT therapy with autologous bone-marrow transplantation in 17 cases of non-Hodgkin's lymphomas with a very bad prognosis.
Eur J Cancer, 1983; 19: 1379-1383.

12. HARTMANN O, PEIN F, BEAUJEAN F et al.
High-dose polychemotherapy with autologous bone-marrow transplantation in children with relapsed lymphomas.
J Clin Oncol, 1984; 2: 979-985.

13. VECCI V, PESSION A, SERRA L, ROSITO P, MANCINI AF, PAOLUCCI G
Non-Hodgkin's lymphoma in children: results of treatment with the modified LSA2-L2 protocol.
Med Ped Oncol, 1981; 9: 483-491.

14. PATTE C, KALIFA C, FLAMANT F et al.
Results of the LMT 81 protocol, a modified LSA2-L2 protocol with HD-methotrexate on 84 children with non B-cell (lymphoblastic) lymphoma.
Med Ped Oncol, 1992: in press.

15. MURPHY S, BOWMAN W, ABRAMOVITCH M et al.
Results of treatment of advanced stage Burkitt's lymphoma and B-cell (S-Ig+) acute lymphoblastic leukemia with high-dose fractionated cyclophosphamide and coordinated high-dose methotrexate and cytarabine.
J Clin Oncol, 1986; 4: 1732-1739.

16. DAHL GV, RIVERA G, PUI CH et al.
A novel treatment of childhood lymphoblastic non-Hodgkin's lymphoma: early and intermittent use of tenoposide plus cytarabine.
Blood, 1985; 66: 1110-1114.

17. WEINSTEIN HJ, CASSADY JR, LEVEY R
Long-term results of the APO protocol (Vincristine, Doxorubicin (Adriamycin), and Prednisone) for treatment of mediastinal lymphoblastic lymphoma.
J Clin Oncol, 1983; 1: 537-541.

18. MAGRATH IT, JANUS C, EDWARDS BK et al
An effective therapy for both undifferentiated (including Burkitt's) lymphomas and lymphoblastic lymphomas in children and young adults.
Blood, 1984; 63: 1102-1111.

19. HVIZDALA EV, BERARD C, CALLIHAN G et al
Lymphoblastic lymphoma in children: a randomized trial comparing LSA2 L2 with the A-COP + therapeutic regimen:p a pediatric oncology group study.
J Clin Oncol, 1988; 6: 26-33.

20. PATTE C, PHILIP T, RODARY C et al
Improved survival rate in children with stage III and IV B-cell non-Hodgkin's lymphoma and leukemia using multi-agent chemotherapy: results of a study of 114 children from the French Pediatric Oncology Society.
J Clin Oncol, 1986; 4: 1219-1226.

21. GENTET JC, PATTE C, QUINTANA E et al.
Phase II study of cytarabine and etoposide in children with refractory or relapsed non-Hodgkin's lymphoma: a study of the French Society of Pediatric Oncology.
J Clin Oncol, 1990; 3: 661-665.

22. PATTE C, PHILIP T, RODARY C et al.
High survival rate in advanced-stage B-cell lymphomas and leukemias without CNS involvement with a short intensive polychemotherapy. Results of a randomized trial from the French Pediatric Oncology Society (SFOP) on 216 children.
J Clin Oncol, 1991; 9: 123-132.

23. PATTE C, LEVERGER G, PEREL Y et al.
Updated results of the LMB 86 protocol of the French Pediatric Oncology Society (SFOP) for B-cell non-Hodgkin's lymphoma with CNS involvement and B ALL.
Med Ped Oncol, 1990; 18: 397.

24. PHILIP T, HARTMANN O, BIRON P et al.
High-dose therapy and autologous bone-marrow transplantation in partial remission after first-line therapy for diffuse non-Hodgkin's lymphoma.
J Clin Oncol, 1988; 6: 1118-1124.

25. SULLIVAN H, RAMIREZ I
Curability of Burkitt's lymphoma with high-dose cyclophosphamide - high-dose methotrexate therapy and intrathecal chemoprophylaxis.
J Clin Oncol, 1985; 3: 627-636.

26. AUBIER F, FLAMANT F, BRAUNER R, CAILLAUD JM, CHAUSSAIN JM, LEMERLE J
Male gonadal function after chemotherapy for solid tumors in children.
J Clin Oncol, 1989; 7: 304-309.

Index

Achevé d'imprimer par Corlet, Imprimeur, S.A.
14110 Condé-sur-Noireau (France)
N° d'Imprimeur : 4464 - Dépôt légal : juillet 1993

Imprimé en C.E.E.